Two Monographs On Malaria and the Parasites of Malarial Fevers

Amico Bignami

TWO MONOGRAPHS

ON

MALARIA

AND THE

PARASITES OF MALARIAL FEVERS.

I.—MARCHIAFAVA AND BIGNAMI.

II.—MANNABERG.

LONDON:
THE NEW SYDENHAM SOCIETY.

1894.

ON

SUMMER-AUTUMN MALARIAL FEVERS.

BY

E. MARCHIAFAVA, M.D.,

PROFESSOR OF PATHOLOGICAL ANATOMY IN THE UNIVERSITY OF ROME;

AND

A. BIGNAMI, M.D.,

FIRST ASSISTANT IN THE ANATOMICO-PATHOLOGICAL INSTITUTE.

TRANSLATED FROM THE FIRST ITALIAN EDITION

BY

J. HARRY THOMPSON, A.M., M.D.,

LATE PROFESSOR OF PHYSIOLOGY AND OPERATIVE SURGERY,
GEORGETOWN UNIVERSITY;
SURGEON-IN-CHIEF, COLUMBIAN HOSPITAL, WASHINGTON, U.S.A.

WITH NOTES AND APPENDICES BY THE AUTHORS.

EDITOR'S PREFACE.

WHEN invited by the Council of the Sydenham Society to make myself responsible for Dr. Thompson's translation of Marchiafava and Bignami's work on the malarial fevers occurring during summer and autumn round Rome, and to introduce the volume to English readers in a preface, after due consideration I consented to do so. I soon found, however, that to accept the responsibility of another man's translation in its wider sense, practically involved re-writing the work with the aid of the previous translation—an undertaking I was quite unprepared for. In the narrower sense of carefully reading over the proofs, and correcting obvious slips in any hurried translation, substituting a more exact word or phrase, transposing a word or a clause to make the English run more smoothly, I have attempted somewhat that might justify me in saying I have accepted the responsibility. In this, as in all translations, passages occur that might be considerably improved by being re-written, laying aside entirely the Authors' forms of expression, not translating the words so much as recasting the ideas; this, too, I do not pretend to have undertaken. Even in the discharge of such limited functions as I have laid down for myself numerous difficulties cropped up, which to those interested will become evident on a comparison of the English with the Italian work. As specifying them will not, as a rule, assist in arriving at a correct appreciation of the Authors' meaning, I pass them all by except two. I wish to call attention to the fact that I have perhaps a little strained the meaning of the two terms *relapse* and *recurrence* in adopting them for the Italian *ricaduta* and *recidiva*. In Italian even, the distinction involved is perhaps more conventional than classical. The first time the two words are met with I have appended an editorial note, which I trust will prevent any difficulty in grasping the necessary shade of meaning.

Torti's use of the words *solitaria* and *comitata* applied to malarial fevers constitutes also a difficulty. Our Authors use them so often, that in the translation these words appeared to me to disfigure the text, for anyone who had not mastered the distinction involved. To translate the Latin literally would not have conveyed Torti's meaning; so for better, for worse, I adopted *simple malignant fever* and *complicated malignant fever* as the nearest equivalents I could suggest. This, however, is only a compromise with the difficulty, and practically leaves every one still to master it for himself, though by the use of italics and quotation marks, I have tried to do what I could to assist the reader. No one will recognise more than I do how imperfectly my aim has been attained. The solitaria is in most cases not a *simple* fever, though it never has the single well-marked complication which gives to Torti's comitata its name. It must be noted that the distinction lies not between a case, strictly speaking, without a complication, and another with one, but between a case with a single complication, so well marked as to make it possible to mistake a malarial fever for cholera, apoplexy, &c., and another in which one or more complications may exist, to such a minor extent as not to make any similar mistake possible. Even here, however, it must be borne in mind that the morbid process causing the coma, profuse diarrhœa, &c., is one intimately connected with the disease, a part of it, and not a superadded complication, as a broken leg in a case of phthisis, a malarial fever attacking a surgical patient, or delirium tremens occurring in a case of pneumonia. This question of classification will not interest the general reader in England, while to anyone in India, or wherever questions relating to malarial fevers require minute examination, the distinction dwelt on by Torti will be easily arrived at by careful study of the text.

Several technical expressions occur which are not yet current in general medical literature. Those which, though new to myself, seemed to be probably familiar to younger men, I have generally passed by without notice. I have ventured, however, in a few instances to append an explanatory foot-note, to save others the trouble I have had in arriving at the meaning. I am aware that in a few years such aids will seem superfluous, as the younger generation will have grown up, using words that to many of us are new ones; I shall be content, however, if such foot-notes serve a useful though temporary purpose. The elaborate temperature charts, with synchronous annotations of the parasitic finds met with in the blood, appended to this volume, are worthy of the closest study. It may help in this if I point out that the headings M. and E. refer to day and night observations. Under each of these headings the four columns indicate three-hour periods which begin at 12 o'clock. Thus, when he desires to do so, the reader can arrive at a very close approximation of the hour when any of the recorded observations were made, or when a dose of quinine was administered.

While introducing the present treatise to English readers, it may perhaps assist them to arrive at a correct appreciation of the great work that the Italians have done in advancing and explaining Laveran's discovery, if I briefly recapitulate some of the points in which progress has been made in Italy. The subject is a vast one, and anything like a comprehensive critical examination of it cannot be attempted within the narrow limits of a preface.

After the discovery by Laveran of certain forms assumed by the parasite of malaria in 1880, many workers in Italy have undertaken serious researches on the subject. Among others Marchiafava, Celli, Golgi, Bignami, Bastianelli, Antolisei, Angelini, Grassi and Feletti, Canalis, &c. The young Roman school have been very successful in the prosecution of this work, and among them all I point out Marchiafava as having been not only first in the field, but at all times as having deserved well of us, by inciting others to work at the subject of malaria, as well as by making advances himself, and accepting and confirming all trustworthy advances made by others. To us his views may serve as the embodiment of all that it is safe to accept on the questions with which he deals. He has naturally followed carefully American, German, and Indian work.

As bearing closely on the present translation, reference may here be made to the previous researches made by Marchiafava into the question of the connection of melanæmia with malaria. Indeed, these investigations may in a sense be said to be a part of his present undertaking, as they certainly led up to it, and, in fact, are inseparable from it. The gradual and precise way in which he has been able to advance our knowledge is most instructive, as the routes he followed were different from those taken by Laveran. On the 6th of November, 1880, Laveran saw a flagellate organism free in the blood of a patient suffering from malaria, and at a single bound arrived at the conclusion that it was the parasite of malaria. Marchiafava travelled by no such royal road. By a slow and laborious process along with Celli—

(1) He established the fact that a manufactory existed in the red blood-corpuscle in which the hæmoglobulin was changed into melanin; 1879.

(2) On subjecting the red blood-corpuscle to the influence of methylene blue he found spots stained blue, which he remarked had a great analogy to micrococci; 1883.

(3) By attempting to grow these spots on cultivating media he differentiated them from micrococci; 1883.

(4) He therefore attributed them to degenerative changes in the discoplasma; 1883. Before 1883 he used lenses belonging to the dry system; after that date these observations were all made on dried blood and with an oil immersion lens, $\frac{1}{12}$ Zeiss. Now he changed, still using a Zeiss $\frac{1}{12}$ oil immersion lens, and began to examine freshly drawn living blood; and—

(5) He recognised amœboid movements even in the most minute, spot-like, hyaline, unpigmented protoplasm enclosed in the red blood-corpuscle, and knew for the first time he had a parasite to deal with; 1884.

From this time onwards his career year after year has been one of progress, and it is hardly too much to say, that all the advances which have been made, are due either to Marchiafava or his pupils. An obvious limitation to such a broad assertion has to be made in the case of Golgi's early work; also as regards the investigations undertaken by zoologists who have discovered similar organisms to the malaria parasite in the blood of healthy birds, as well as in that of other animals lower in the scale; and of good work into minute morphology and attempted classification of the parasite. Not less must we gratefully acknowledge laborious researches made by observers in every country confirmatory of the advances made by Golgi and the young Roman school.

Before he entered on this field of research, Laveran had described the parasites as being pigmented, at times adherent to the red blood-corpuscles, and giving rise to mobile filaments, the perfect form of the parasite being still held by him to be the mobile filament after it has become separated and has assumed an independent existence in the blood-plasma. In 1883–4 Marchiafava and Celli arrived at the conclusion, while studying the genesis of melanæmia, that the pigment was formed within the red blood-corpuscles after their invasion by minute bodies *probably of a parasitic nature.* At this time they did not confirm Laveran's discovery. Since then, however, they have arrived at the conclusion that the parasite of malaria consists of a minute particle of protoplasm, which, resembling a small amœba, enters into the red blood-corpuscle, and there converts the hæmoglobin into melanin. It is often endowed with amœboid movements, which may be very active and produce rapid changes in its shape. It lives in the interior of the red blood-corpuscle, and gathers the pigment it forms into its centre. It then divides into separate fragments, this segmentation taking place within the body of its host, the red blood-corpuscle. As regards the mobile filaments, the above-named authors demonstrated that they were flagella of a certain phase of the development of the parasite. On this Golgi came into the field with his very successful researches, 1885–6. He was able to differentiate the variety of the parasite which is connected with the tertian type from that which is found in quartan fevers. The distinctions between the two are morphological as well as biological, and were most clearly pointed out by him. To him, too, we owe the knowledge of the fact that the commencement of the paroxysm of the fever is synchronous with the stage of sporulation of the parasite. Passing over many points of minor importance that have been studied in Italy, I will now only refer to the later researches of Marchiafava and Celli, 1889–90, on the dangerous forms of fevers to be seen in Rome during the summer and autumn, where patients are brought for treatment from the surrounding districts —*the Roman Campagna*. A careful investigation into this group of fevers was rewarded by very important results. They were able to distinguish between the mild spring fevers, tertian and quartan, and the group they were engaged on, by clinical and epidemiological characters, as well as by distinctive appearances in the parasite, both in the circulating blood during life, and the living spleen, as well as in the blood-vessels of certain of the organs after death. They were thus able to separate the comparatively harmless forms of fever from those which might suddenly develop dangerous symptoms, though at any given moment they might not show by a single symptom, that they had such potential mischief in reserve. The cycle of the life of this parasitic variety is not completed in the circulating blood, so it had to be studied by procuring blood from the living spleen, and their observations had to be followed up in the deadhouse and in the pathological laboratory. It resulted from this prolonged and complicated research, that by a microscopic examination alone of the parasite it can be determined with certainty whether malignant or pernicious symptoms have to be guarded against. The high practical as well as scientific worth of this discovery requires no comment.

As connected with these researches we may refer to the work done by Bignami in 1890. He made afresh an anatomico-pathological inquiry into the morbid appearances met with after death in pernicious fevers. In this he studied the parasites found in the blood-vessels of the various organs, and the secondary alterations met with in the tissues. He connected what he saw with symptoms before death, and arrived at the pathological significance and causation of several symptoms met with during life, in the course of some forms of pernicious fever, especially of the comatose variety.

A very obscure question is that of the significance and clinical importance of the semilunar bodies first described by Laveran, which are only met with in the blood of the summer-autumn infections, and from which alone, originate the flagellate forms met with in this class of fevers. Golgi, Canalis, Grassi and Feletti, Antolisei, Angelini, and others had expressed various views on the subject when, in 1890, Bignami and Bastianelli undertook to study the whole question, especially from the point of view of the time at which these crescents could be first found in the circulating blood, and in the spleen, after the commencement of malarial fever. Their special attention was also directed to the genesis of this form of the parasite, and to its clinical significance. References to the exact data they were successful in accumulating are often made in the body of the present work.

The fact that the parasitic forms found in connection with dangerous fevers could be distinguished from those of other malarial fevers having been arrived at, it still remained to study more fully, both biologically and morphologically, at the bedside, their relations with the production of the fever; for many Italian observers, as well as those of other countries, looked on irregular atypic fevers as being dependent on the summer-autumn forms of parasite. From this investigation, undertaken by Marchiafava and Bignami in 1891, we have arrived at the knowledge of the fact, that although the dangerous types of fever often appear to be irregular at their commencement, nevertheless it can be established that there are two fundamental types only, the quotidian and the tertian, to which these dangerous fevers can be traced. Both of these types are quite distinct from those of the mild spring fevers.

In the present work Marchiafava and Bignami describe the summer-autumn fevers, the febrile types which they present, the parasitic varieties in connection with each type, and the peculiarities of malignant infection. To those engaged in practice in India, or in the British colonies where malarial fever prevails, this translation will afford assistance to be found nowhere else. In America also, from the same points of view, the work will prove extremely helpful. In England as well, where malarial fevers have become comparatively rare, the following pages are worthy of being studied, not merely on account of their intrinsic scientific interest, but on account also of the bearing of the various questions discussed on other pathological problems. They are most suggestive, and will doubtless supply the germs for new thoughts and fresh investigations on diseases other than malarial. Of many points on which my interest has been aroused I will mention only one, that came upon me as a surprise when I first knew it. A specimen of malarial blood being sent for examination to the laboratory, a microscopist can not only furnish full details as to the questions of malaria, but, should he find an excess of white blood-corpuscles, can reply to the clinical observer,—if your patient is not already in the act of dying, or does not suffer from diarrhœa, and has no other condition with which the leucocytosis is associated, he has an acute inflammatory affection beginning; and if you examine the lungs you will probably find a commencing pneumonia which you possibly have not detected. I do not look forward to a time when we shall have to depend on our microscopes for diagnosing our pneumonias for us, but still regard the thought as a pregnant one.

Perhaps it may not be considered out of place for me to mention here, that I have enjoyed the great privilege of being allowed to renew my acquaintance with malaria in the wards of the Santo Spirito Hospital, and in the laboratory which is under the direction of Dr. Bastianelli; also in the post-mortem theatre, to study the appearances found after death by Professor Marchiafava and Dr. Bignami. Under such favorable circumstances, while following cases in the wards of the summer-autumn fevers, I was able to recognise with my own eyes what the Authors describe in the book that has just been translated. I have been able to convince myself of the general correctness of the descriptions, and feel certain of the practical utility of their methods of studying the subject. On this account I commend the views expressed in this work with confidence for the acceptance of English readers, in preference to those of other investigators. It will take some time before the subject has been fully worked out, and amid conflicting statements, it is of some advantage to be able to choose reliable guides.

The Authors do not fail to note that there are many lacunæ in our knowledge of the biology of the parasite of these dangerous fevers. The contradictory opinions that have been dwelt on relative to certain of the questions, both in the original Italian work, and in the various notes and appendices prepared for the present translation, may serve as so many starting-points for fresh investigations. These may help to fill up such lacunæ, and to advance our knowledge in this most important field of study.

From the above remarks it will be seen how thoroughly abreast the Authors are with the most modern clinical and pathological methods, and that the volume is a model of conscientious research.

The inquiry undertaken by our Authors into the question of the curative action of quinine, and the influence exerted by the drug on the parasites of malaria, will be followed with great interest. According to them, very little change can be observed in the structure of the parasite. The remedy seems to inhibit the nutritive processes which enable the hæmatozoon to develop and grow, up to the time that it has become ready to undergo segmentation. On the changes involved by the process of multiplication, quinine seemed to have no visible effect. When once the spores have become free in the blood-plasma, the specific appears to exert a deleterious action on them, and to render them incapable of penetrating within the red blood-corpuscle, where alone they seem able to accomplish their life-cycle. At all events, a generation of spores, on becoming free in the blood-plasma sufficiently charged with quinine, disappears, and proves for the time harmless. Mannaberg's researches on this point represent some of his very best work, and according to him, the fortress having been stormed at the citadel by the drug has left the garrison impotent for evil. Though the bulk of the garrison has not been touched, yet the fortress, having been taken at a vital point, is incapable of offering resistance. To drop metaphor, Mannaberg found that when careful staining processes were resorted to, though the parasites as a whole seemed to retain much of their usual appearances, the nuclei (chromatin substance) had been fatally damaged, and were found in a necrotic condition. This apparent discrepancy between the Roman researches and those of the Austrian observer seemed to depend on fresh specimens of the parasites only having been studied in Rome, while it was owing to staining, that the changes otherwise invisible had been brought out. This seemed to have advanced the subject much, simplifying the question, and rendering it intelligible. Later researches by our Authors, in which they had recourse to staining, have not, on all points, in the case of summer-autumn fevers borne out Mannaberg's careful work. Perhaps it may be found that the observations made by Mannaberg, being chiefly in the spring tertians and quartans, as is shown by his illustrations, while those made in Rome were on the summer-autumn parasites, the differences in the results arrived at depend on the spores of the parasite of the tertian type of fever being more susceptible to the influence of quinine, while those of the parasites of the dangerous forms of fever possess greater powers of resistance to the influence of the drug.

If some such simple explanation is arrived at by careful microscopic research, the apparent differences will be reconciled. But for the present we must be content to wait.

Our Authors have not dealt with the structure of the malarial parasite in this work, but I may just refer the reader to an important communication on the subject made by Drs. Bignami and Bastianelli to the Royal Academy of Medicine in Rome, which has an important bearing on the question under consideration. The results they arrive at are somewhat different from those of other investigators. They distinguish between two substances in the youngest forms of amœbæ: the one situated on the exterior, a cytoplasm which can be stained with hæmatoxylin; the other incapable of taking this stain, and occupying a deeper position. In the first they found one or more granules of chromatin. They describe the changes they observed in the subsequent development of these structures thus differentiated, and in the process of spore-formation, dwelling on details of description which cannot be condensed into the form of a *résumé*. They conclude that in the summer-autumn variety of the malarial parasite it is not possible to recognise any formation provided with the anatomical elements which constitute a true nucleus. According to them the chromophil granule, which constitutes part of the ectoplasm, and which is diffused in the cytoplasm when it prepares for multiplication, represents that part of the parasite which fulfils the functions of a nucleus; therefore it would appear that the parasites of the summer-autumn fevers are not provided with a true nucleus, but with a nucleiform structure, as Hertwig styles it. Their communication has not yet been published, but is expected to appear in the 'Transactions of the Roman Royal Academy of Medicine' in April or May, 1894.

With the view of assisting the reader in accepting the advanced teaching of the Authors, I may be permitted to allude here, shortly, to Laveran's views. With regard to the differences between the parasite of the quartan and that of the tertian, Laveran left us for long in doubt whether he accepted Golgi's advances or not. In his latest work, 'Paludisme,' published more than a year ago, it seems as if he had definitely decided, on not admitting the distinctions existing between the parasite of one type of fever and that of another (page 42). Again, he seems to think that polymorphism serves to explain the differences in the evolution of the hæmatozoa, and that these differences are not sufficient to authorise us in admitting distinct varieties (page 43). From his previous writings it was easy to understand the position that this great French observer took up, in combating any attempt to establish as species what were merely varieties of a single parasite. But it is not easy to find an explanation of the position which he has more lately assumed. The most trustworthy observers in all countries have confirmed the Italian work, and, as far as I know, the representative of the French school stands alone. As bearing on the question of his not being able to admit these differences, it must not be lost sight of that Laveran, even in his latest published work, holds to the view that the parasites are not endoglobular, while every other observer has confirmed Marchiafava's observation that they are endoglobular. Another point of a similar nature, which shows that Laveran differs from all other observers, consists in his constantly seeing free parasites and spores circulating in the blood. This is a most difficult observation to make, and all are agreed that they are not familiar with appearances that would justify such an interpretation. We may, of course, assume that Laveran is a better observer or is possessed of better appliances for observation than men of all other nationalities, in which case he may be right. But it is also open to us to assume that the microscope he uses has less perfect arrangements for illumination, and prevents him from seeing the shell or shadow of the red blood-corpuscle that has been fully occupied by the parasite, and has had its contents removed to furnish the hæmatozoon with nourishment. All must be most unwilling to explain the position by assuming any want of skill on the part of Laveran, as we marvel at his acuteness in having with imperfect means arrived at the discoveries he announced in 1880. Whatever the explanation adopted, the fact of his having assumed isolated, if not untenable, positions in regard to many of the questions discussed in this work, must not be overlooked.

As the preface has already outgrown the limits within which I had hoped to be able to compress what I thought it necessary to say, I have thrown into a tabular form some of the differences between the views of our Authors and those of Laveran. Besides avoiding a lengthened disquisition, as the points that might have been dwelt upon are numerous, I hope this bird's-eye view will serve to show at a glance in what these differences consist, and how much modern medicine owes to Italy in the subjects taken up in this treatise.

TABLE SHOWING SOME OF THE DIFFERENCES BETWEEN THE VIEWS HELD BY LAVERAN AND THOSE OF THE ITALIAN SCHOOL.

	VIEWS HELD BY LAVERAN.	ORIGINAL OR ADOPTED VIEWS OF OUR AUTHORS.
1. *The mature form of the parasite.*	A mobile filament.	A spherical form which has undergone segmentation and is forming spores.
2. *Its cystic nature.*	Lays great stress on the parasite being contained in a cyst.	Deny that any cyst is under any circumstances connected with the parasite.
3. *The* causa causans *of the fever.*	Vague and uncertain. Possibly accumulation in the blood of a secretion from, or rapid multiplication of, the parasites.	The liberation of the spores from the red corpuscle, and their becoming free in the blood-plasma; probably some toxine secreted during segmentation being the pyrogenic agent. This is a point on which much turns.
4. *The cause of the intermittence.*	In part phagocytosis, in part substances elaborated by the parasite inhibiting the production of other parasites.	Completion of the protrusion of spores into the blood-plasma in any generation of parasites. No other stage of growth in the parasite being capable of producing fever; the intermittence being thus dependent on the life cycle of the parasite.
5. *The cause of the periodicity.*	Intermittence far from constituting a constant character of paludism; other diseases also being intermittent. Precise explanation not attempted.	Each variety of parasite has its own cycle of development of a definite length, and this regulates the length of time between the paroxysms.
6. *The cause of recurring fevers.*	Vague and indefinite, although recurrence is the rule.	Undestroyed spores being preserved in the system, possibly in the spleen and bone marrow.
7. *The different stages of the parasite's growth.*	Recognises the early stage of the parasite as being unpigmented, also later stages as being connected with the formation of pigment; but beyond this, his views are vague and ill-defined.	Dwell on the unpigmented stage of the parasite; trace the gradual formation of pigment, beginning at the periphery, and later tending toward the centre. The formation of the pigment into a central block, marking a pre-segmental stage, and being followed by the formation and extrusion of spores.

	Views held by Laveran.	Original or Adopted Views of our Authors.
8. *Still forms with central pigment.*	Regards as cadaveric forms of the parasite.	Look on them as of the utmost importance in the life of the parasite, showing it is about to form spores.
9. *Significance of the flagellated forms.*	An all-important stage of the parasite's growth, leading up to the mobile filaments.	Not in necessary connection with the fever. Probably represents an artificial degenerative phase.
10. *Significance of the crescents.*	An important form connected with chronic fevers and cachexiæ.	Forms not met with in spring tertians and quartans. In summer-autumn fevers only met with after about the seventh day. Are perhaps sterile forms, and never represent the fever-producing agency. Much yet remains to be worked out regarding them.
11. *The position that the parasite holds in relation to the red blood-corpuscle.*	That it is extra-globular, often attaches itself to the corpuscle, but is very frequently to be seen quite free.	It is essentially endoglobular; when it is free, except in the stage of a spore, it is often seen undergoing degenerative processes.
12. *Varieties in the pigmentation, size, and action on the blood-corpuscles of the parasite.*	Accidental, and unconnected with the type of fever in any individual case.	Each variety recognisable as the parasite which causes a special type of fever. Tertian, quartan, &c., each variety only giving rise to a progeny with the power of causing the same type of fever.
13. *Recognition of these varieties.*	Unimportant.	Pointing out with undeviating precision whether any case of fever is devoid of danger. Directing attention not only to existing malignancy, but to the possible advent of a pernicious paroxysm. The malignity of the summer-autumn fever being connected with the special varieties of the parasite.

14. *The causes of the type, tertian, quartan, &c.*	Vague conditions in the individual attacked; his having been acclimatised or not; having had previous attacks of fever; condition of his nervous system, especially its irritability, &c. The types of fever are often transformed one into another.	Invariably and uniformly solely dependent on the variety of parasite that can alone cause the special type of any malarial fever; the conditions of the parasite and not of the individual being involved. Apparent transformations depend on double tertians and triple quartans counterfeiting the quotidian type.
15. *Quotidians may be double tertians or triple quartans.*	Does not at all see the grounds for such an important distinction.	Dwell on its importance. The recognition of two generations of parasites in the blood of double spring tertians being a matter of daily observation, quartana triplex being also capable of verification. The only true quotidian is a summer-autumn form.
16. *Explanation of a prolonged paroxysm.*	External heat; vigorous reaction in strong full-blooded individuals; a first attack of fever; intensity of palustral infection.	Maturation of one generation of parasites in successive groups instead of all about the same time.
17. *Polymorphism.*	Insists on the different forms presented being evidence of its being a polymorphic hæmatozoon. In many difficulties alludes to polymorphism as being a sufficient explanation.	Believe in the unpigmented amœboid organism growing and developing, through successive stages, till spores have been formed; the flagellated and crescent forms being only sterile individuals. The different parasitic varieties have not been proved capable of being transformed one into the other. There are no facts that authorise an assumption that there is only a solitary polymorphic parasite.
18. *Action of quinine on the hæmatozoa.*	Prevents the mobile filaments escaping from the cysts, and makes the hæmatozoa assume their cadaveric form.	The young generation of parasites is prevented from entering the red blood-corpuscles and disappears. When given too late to act thus the drug inhibits the nutrition of the parasites, the more advanced forms only going on to segmentation; has little influence on their segmentation phase. Many of the spores even after full doses of quinine present no visible alteration.
19. *Confirmation by outsiders.*	On most of the above points, Germans, Austrians, Russians, Americans, &c., do not follow Laveran.	There is a very great consensus of opinion, among observers of different nationalities, that the Italian school is right in most of the above points.

During the year and a half since the Italian edition of this work was published a considerable amount of additional material has been accumulated by the Authors, new controversies have sprung up, and a considerable amount of recent work requiring notice has been published. This virtually necessitated a second edition being prepared. Unfortunately the work had been translated, and was partly in type, before the necessity for a second edition became very clear. The Authors would have preferred making the called-for additions in the form of notes appended to each page, but, perhaps fortunately, the work was too far advanced to permit of such a compromise, and the additional material has been thrown into various chapters at the end of the volume. The first consists of "Notes" referring to the text by means of cross-references. A second chapter, described as the "First Appendix," refers to the principal classifications of the parasites of malaria, and the Authors explain the various reasons for which they consider that they are unable to adopt any of the schemes for classification as yet published. The "Second Appendix" treats of those parasitic finds that are more seldom met with in the pernicious fevers, and the Authors return again to the localisation of the parasites in the various viscera in dangerous cases. The "Third Appendix" discusses the various points at which the results of our author's researches differ from those published by Golgi in November and December, 1893.

After this preface was in print the valuable postscript to Appendix III was sent to me. The quotation from Celsus is probably unique in its exactness; but others also among ancient writers describe the same thing with great clearness. In fact, the intimate knowledge they show of all the varieties of malarial fever known to us is very surprising. Hippocrates speaks of true tertians (spring) and of semi-tertians (summer-autumn), the one not fatal, and the other a very formidable fever. Pernicious paroxysms he ascribes to the supervention of other acute diseases. One year specially he observed that the (συνεχεῖς) continued malarial fevers (summer-autumn) were distinguished by an exacerbation every alternate day, after the manner of (spring) tertians.

Galen distinguished between continued fever, synochus (typhoid, typhus), and subcontinued malarial (συνεχής): some (summer-autumn) subcontinued fevers having a daily remission like the quotidian (tertiana duplex and quartana triplex), others assuming the type of (spring) tertians, or, very rarely, of (spring) quartans.

Rhases dwells on the distinctions between the *febris continens* (typhoid, typhus) and the *febris continua* (malarial subcontinued), and clearly points out the close relation of the latter to intermittents.

Avicenna calls the quotidian intermittent (spring, tertiana duplex, and triple quartan) *febris phlegmatica periodica;* and the subcontinued quotidian (summer-autumn) *febris phlegmatica inseparabilis* or *latica.* The (spring) tertian is his *tertiana periodica,* and the (summer-autumn) subcontinued tertian his *tertiana continua.* The two quartans he distinguished likewise as *periodica* and *continua.*

Paul of Ægina says, "The subcontinued fevers (summer-autumn) are allied to each of the (spring) intermittents;" thus to the true tertian (spring) is allied the *causus* or ardent fever (summer-autumn); to the quotidian (double tertian, triple quartan) that fever which has a paroxysm every day, but does not terminate in a complete freedom from fever (summer-autumn); and in like manner to the (spring) quartan, is related that which has an exacerbation every fourth day (a malignant quartan not known in Rome). Those who wish to pursue this subject further will find abundant materials for doing so in the learned prefaces, and notes full of erudition, which Francis Adams wrote for his translations of the Greek, Roman, and Arabian authors, published by the Sydenham Society.

In the appendices, as well as in the notes, our authors accentuate those portions of their researches that are subsequent to the Italian text,—researches in part confirmatory of previous work, in part entering on new ground. With these notes and appendices in our hands we may safely feel that up to the beginning of the year 1894 we are abreast of our times. These notes and appendices were made over to me in English by the Authors.

The question of the reproduction of the various types of malarial fever by injecting blood containing the parasites has up till now remained in an unsatisfactory state. The experiments have seemed to be more or less contradictory of one another, and some seemed to be wanting in precision. In the autumn of 1893 Drs. Bignami and Bastianelli carried out experiments on the inoculation of the parasites of the summer-autumn fevers, which have given important results, by contributing to our knowledge of the incubation period of malarial fever thus induced. They hold that the time that elapses between the injection of blood containing parasites and the first paroxysm of fever depends chiefly on two factors: 1st, on the number of parasites introduced; 2nd, upon the rapidity of the cycle of their development. They have brought to light a fact not hitherto demonstrated, that the incubation period for these summer-autumn parasites may be extremely short, extending over only two days or even less. Comparing such a result with those noted regarding the incubation in the case of quartan fevers, they have shown that the minimum period in the one case is much shorter than the minimum in the other.

The inoculation of the blood containing young parasites has always given positive results. The inoculation of blood, on the other hand, containing only semilunar bodies did not, in the single case observed, give rise to fever. This affords very strong confirmation of the view held by our authors that the semilunar bodies represent sterile forms. The results of this inquiry were lately communicated to the Royal Academy of Medicine in Rome, and are expected to appear in the Transactions of that body in April or May, 1894.

In concluding these prefatory remarks I have the pleasing duty to perform of expressing my deep sense of the obligation due by me to the Authors for having revised the translation. In several cases they have pointed out that their meaning was not conveyed by the translation; they have suggested important corrections; and throughout the work have so carefully scanned each line as to detect printer's errors that the sharp eyes of a London proof reader had failed to discover, and my less practised eyes had not noticed. Such a critical acquaintance with a foreign language, as it should be written, may serve as an example most of us would like to follow; and with such help I think I have fair grounds for hoping that the translation will be found free from, at least, grave mistakes.

T. Edmondston Charles, M.D.,
Honorary Physician to H.M. the Queen.

72, Via di San Nicolo da Tolentino,
Rome.

CONTENTS.

CHAPTER IV.

THE QUOTIDIAN FEVER.

CHAPTER V.

THE SUMMER-AUTUMN TERTIAN.

CHAPTER VI.

DIFFERENTIAL DIAGNOSIS OF THE PARASITIC VARIETIES AND THE MIXED INFECTIONS.

CHAPTER VII.

MALIGNANT FEVERS.

CHAPTER VIII.

ACTION OF THE SALTS OF QUININE ON THE PARASITES OF MALARIA.

ON THE

SUMMER AND AUTUMN MALARIAL FEVERS.

INTRODUCTION.

The work which we now publish has two special objects. We propose in the first place to set forth the results of the researches carried out by us on the fevers which prevail in Rome during the summer and autumn[1]—researches which have in part recently been described in a preliminary paper.[2] It is the exact statement of facts, supplemented by proofs, that forms the only means by which a useful criticism of the conclusions advanced by us can be rendered possible.

The study of the clinical forms, no less than the nomenclature of these fevers, has been hitherto the object of many discussions. We find the classification varying according to different authors, the delineation of this group of fevers uncertain; while the errors in diagnosis, which have been the means of multiplying beyond measure the number, already very great, of the clinical forms which malaria produces in man, are not infrequent. The knowledge, then, of a sure means of diagnosis, *the examination of the blood,* sufficiently justified new and patient researches into the various febrile types of this group. In addition to this, it is necessary to study the biological cycle of the parasite in relation to the alternations of the fever. We could not, of course, flatter ourselves that such a study—in the nature of things—could prove

[1] Marchiafava e Celli, 'Riforma Medica,' 13 Settembre, 1889; e 'Atti dell' Accad. Med. di Roma,' 1890–91.

[2] Marchiafava e Bignami, "La quotidiana e la terzana estivo autumnale," 'Rif. Med.,' Settembre, 1891.

complete; indeed, it is established that although the morphology of the malarial parasite, as far as it is known at present, is the same wherever it has been studied, whether in tropical or temperate climates, nevertheless the clinical forms of malaria, to judge from the descriptions of various writers, can run their course under very diverse appearances. Consequently our descriptions, estimates, and conclusions must refer solely and exclusively to the observations made during the last few years by us and by others on the summer and autumn endemic malaria of the Roman Campagna. Since the parasite of malaria became known, we and others have not had an opportunity of observing several clinical forms which have been described as malarial, and naturally it is as regards these that the question remains open.

In the second place, we have a practical aim in view. We wish to place within reach of all medical men those most important facts brought to light by modern research which are a sure guide in diagnosis, and which can also afford useful criteria in determining the prognosis and directing the treatment. The results, in fact, which are obtained from the study of the parasite of malaria possess not merely a scientific interest; it is an opinion by this time shared by all, that the examination of the blood is in some cases necessary for diagnosis. For the same reason we have thought it useful to consider also the action of quinine on the malarial parasite, as well as other questions which are of practical interest.

With this view, moreover, we have recapitulated in shorter form all we now know about the tertian and quartan fevers, chiefly for the purpose of determining the difference between the summer tertian described by us and the mild tertian which prevails in the Roman Campagna during the spring. We have also supplemented our work with illustrative plates and thermometric charts, by which can be seen at a glance the difference between the parasitic variety of each type and of each group of fevers.

CHAPTER I.

CLASSIFICATION OF THE MALARIAL FEVERS.

The fevers of the winter and spring, and the summer-autumn fevers—The malignant infections form part of this latter group.

The knowledge recently acquired with respect to the biology of the parasites of malaria harmonises perfectly with all that is known through clinical and epidemiological research. Supported by the facts demonstrated by epidemiology, clinical study and parasitology divide the malarial fevers into two great groups.

The first group comprises the quartan and the tertian. These two types of fever are usually found together in districts affected by mild malaria throughout the whole of the malarial season. They are only prevalent from the close of winter to the end of spring in the regions where malaria is severe, but they may also be found in the summer and autumn, along with the so-called summer and autumn fevers, but much less frequently than these latter; they are frequently observed in persons coming from parts of the district relatively less unhealthy. Clinically speaking, they are alike in the great regularity of their development in the majority of cases—a regularity which is much greater, however, in the quartan than in the tertian.

In fine, they have this in common, that, excepting the tendency to recur, which is frequently very obstinate, as is the case with the majority of malarial fevers, in most cases they do not tend to become aggravated, and recovery sometimes follows spontaneously.

Complex fevers may ensue,—for example, double tertian, double and triple quartan, subintrant ("intra ire") fevers, and very rarely true subcontinued; *but malignant fevers never.*

This assertion rests on Marchiafava's experience of nearly ten years' duration, since the parasite of malaria has become known; we may say that almost all the cases of malignant fever in the hospital of S. Spirito have been studied from the point of view of the biology of the parasite, *and not once have the forms of the parasite which belong to the tertian or quartan group of fevers been found.*[1]

These two types of fever are produced by two varieties of parasite (the amœba of the tertian and the amœba of the quartan fever), morphologically and biologically differing from each other; but their difference is much less than that which differentiates them from the parasites of the following group.

The second group of fevers, which is the subject of the present work, includes those fevers which constitute the summer and autumn endemic in the districts of severe malaria, fevers which all those practising in these regions at once distinguish from the common fever (tertian and quartan) which they place in contradistinction to them. They are observed only exceptionally in the regions of mild malaria. These fevers present a combination of clinical characteristics by which they form a natural group which cannot be split up. Two fundamental clinical types belong to this group: a quotidian type (*true quotidian*), which must be distinguished from the quotidian caused by the doubling of the tertian of the first group, and from the rare form of quotidians of quartan origin (*triple quartans*); and a tertian type, the summer and autumn, or malignant tertian (we call it malignant that it may not be forgotten that even forms relatively mild have a tendency to become aggravated progressively, and not seldom till malignant symptoms set in).

But the regular course of fevers of this group is often complex and obscured to such an extent that it becomes difficult or almost impossible to discern the fundamental type. Whether the attacks are prolonged or become approximated, or whether the subsequent attacks vary in length, or in the time of onset, or in the gravity of the symptoms, &c., it will be seen how all this produces such a complex of facts that the study of this group of fevers is rendered arduous enough.

To the two types—summer-autumn quotidian and tertian—belong the greater part of the subcontinued fevers, *and all the cases of malignant fever which have as yet been studied.*

In the second place, these fevers ought to be comprised in a

[1] This agrees also with what Bignami observed in the twenty dissections of cases of Perniciosa, of which he has availed himself for the work "Sull' Anatomia Patologica delle Perniciose" ('Atti dell' Accad. Med. di Roma,' 1890), as well as with all that has been noticed in the districts of mild malaria; so also Golgi, who for many years has been engaged in the study of malarial infection, admits that he has not seen one case of malignant fever.

single group because they present a characteristic parasitic variety. In correspondence with the two fundamental clinical types, we distinguish the amœba of the quotidian and the amœba of the summer or malignant tertian. These two parasitic varieties (we shall discuss later on the question whether this name is really a suitable one for them) differ from each other chiefly in certain biological characteristics, as well as in a different rapidity in development, but they approach and resemble each other in numerous other characteristics; while morphologically and biologically they are sharply separated from the parasitic varieties which belong to the mild tertian and quartan fevers. From the facts which we shall set forth on this point it results that from the clinical, as well as from the parasitic point of view, the group of summer and autumn fevers is sharply defined.

All this leads us to believe that the following division and classification of malarial fevers answers to the body of facts known to epidemiology, to clinical medicine, and to parasitology.

1. Mild malarial fevers prevailing in the winter and spring. This group comprises—

(*a*) The quartan, the double quartan, and some quotidians of quartan origin (triple quartans), fevers due to the life cycle of a parasite, which is completed in three days (Golgi).

(*b*) The tertian, the double tertian, some quotidians of tertian origin, very rarely subcontinued, fevers due to the development of a parasite which takes two days to mature (Golgi).

2. Severe malarial fevers of the summer and autumn, comprising—

(*a*) The quotidian, caused by the life cycle of an amœba which is developed within twenty-four hours.

(*b*) The malignant tertian due to the life cycle of an amœba which is matured within forty-eight hours. (We call it malignant that it may not be forgotten that even forms relatively mild have a tendency to become aggravated progressively, and sometimes till malignant symptoms set in.) To this group belong the malignant intermittent fevers, and the greater number of the subcontinued.[1]

[1] In connection with this division of fevers into winter-spring and summer-autumn groups, we cannot but remember the classification of Sydenham (T. Sydenham, 'Opera omnia medica,' Patavii, 1700). He divides the intermittent fevers into two classes, those of the winter and those of the autumn. "It is true that some fevers occur at intermediate times; but since these are less frequent, and may, moreover, be referred to the others above mentioned (that is to say, to those which they most resemble), I shall include all fevers in these two classes, the spring and the autumn. February

and August are the months when, as a rule, they specially predominate, although sometimes their onset is sooner, sometimes later than this" (p. 87).

This distinction of the fevers, according to Sydenham, is so necessary, that without taking it into account it is impossible to rightly determine the prognosis or direct the cure. As to the type, winter fevers are almost all quotidian or tertian, while those of autumn are tertian and quartan. The winter fevers are not dangerous; by the frequent repetition of the paroxysms, and by the long duration of the disease, the patient may be badly reduced, but recovery is the constant result; if treated in the wrong way, *e.g.* by bloodletting and purgatives, they may be much prolonged, but are not fatal, so much so that the winter tertians may even be left to themselves without danger.

The autumn fevers proceed in an entirely different manner; in respect to these it is well known that in the first days of the attack the type is difficult to recognise; that, as regards the cure, they stubbornly resist treatment; that, as regards gravity, the epidemic tertian of the autumn is not devoid of danger; that, as regards after results, while but few symptoms follow the intermittent fevers of the winter, the autumn fevers are succeeded by more numerous and more serious ones, as dropsy, induratio ventris, &c. This division of the fevers is, according to Sydenham, fundamental and essential. There are tertians in winter and spring, just as in autumn; nevertheless "I have no doubt," writes Sydenham, "that these fevers are different essentially and in their entire nature."

CHAPTER II.

QUARTAN AND TERTIAN.[1]

Cycle of evolution, Biological and morphological characteristics of the Amœba febris quartanæ—*Biological and morphological characteristics of the* Amœba febris tertianæ—*In the quartan as in the tertian the beginning of an attack coincides with the coming to maturity of a parasitic generation—Difference in the cycle of evolution and in the morphological and biological characteristics between the* Amœba febris quartanæ *and the* Amœba febris tertianæ.

§ 1. The fundamental facts known about the amœba of the quartan and the amœba of the tertian are due for the most part to the investigations of Golgi.[2]

As we shall have frequently to refer to these two parasitic varieties, in order to determine their points of difference and resemblance to other malarial parasites, and to facilitate the following description we give here a short account of these facts.

§ 2. Quartan fever is caused by an amœba (*Amœba febris quartanæ*, Golgi) which completes its life cycle in three days. If the blood of a patient with quartan fever be examined on the morning of the first day of apyrexia we shall find within the red corpuscles amœbæ varying in size from a sixth to a fifth part of the corpuscle itself, with granular pigment at the periphery, of a hyaline appearance, endowed with sluggish movements, as is shown by the slow transformations of their contour. The red globules which contain them remain of normal size and

[1] For clearness' sake we ought to note that when we write "tertian" without further qualification we always intend reference to the common or mild tertian, as it is called, the parasitic cycle of which has been described by Golgi, a tertian which we distinguish from the summer or summer-autumn or malignant tertian.

[2] C. Golgi, "Sull' infezione malarica," 'Arch. delle Scienze Mediche,' vol. x, 1886.

C. Golgi, "Sullo sviluppo dei parassiti malarici della febbre terzana," 'Arch. per le Scienze Mediche,' vol. xiii, 1889.

appearance. During the whole period of apyrexia the dimensions of the amœbæ slowly increase, and they preserve the same aspect; the pigmentation becomes more abundant, and the development goes on in this manner until at last nothing is left of the red globules but a very fine margin. About six, eight, or ten hours before the fresh paroxysm those changes in the amœba, which lead to segmentation (spore formation), begin to appear.

At this point in its development the parasite has become so large that it fills up entirely or almost entirely the red blood-corpuscle, the periphery of which appears like a membrane round the amœba. Some of these bodies are apparently free, and the pigment is no longer distributed on the periphery but irregularly. Then, while the process of segmentation is beginning, the pigment is usually disposed in radial striæ, which have a tendency to form a central cluster. This concentration of the pigment continues to take place until a collection of black granules or a single mass has been formed at the centre, and at the same time the divisional striæ in the substance of the parasite become gradually more clear. The result of this process is the formation of from nine to twelve ovoid or round spores, which are arranged like the petals of a daisy round the central mass of pigment.

This segmentation (*sporulation*) *is completed a little before or coincidently with the commencement of the paroxysm of fever.* When the fever has developed the segmented forms disappear, and within the red globules the young amœbæ can be seen without pigment, and endowed with amœboid movement. These slowly develop, forming pigment meanwhile, and so the life cycle is repeated as described.

The process of segmentation may happen in a less regular way. Instead of the pigment being concentrated in a single central mass it may form into smaller masses, or it may remain distributed among the spores, &c. Moreover the spore formation may take place even before the amœba has attained the dimensions of the red globule, with at the most six to eight spores (*Antolisei*[1]). But this is found only exceptionally. It is possible to meet with forms of segmentation even from seven to eight hours before the paroxysm; and the young forms of the parasite may appear even two hours before the commencement of the fever, and go on increasing as the fever progresses. These facts, however, do not shake the law, which is that *the beginning of each paroxysm coincides with the maturation of a generation of parasites.*

[1] E. Antolisei, "Sull' ematozoo della quartana," 'Rif. Med.,' 1890.

The life cycle of a quartan amœba is completed entirely in the blood as it circulates, in such a way that all its phases are very easily open to observation. On an examination of blood extracted from the spleen *Bastianelli* and *Bignami*[1] found no notable differences in the distribution of the parasite forms when they compared what they found with what was seen at the same time in the blood of the finger (while the differences are very remarkable, as we shall see, in the summer forms); they found in the spleen a much larger number of leucocytes containing pigment, or containing parasites and spores.

Every paroxysm of fever is concomitant with the inclusion of a certain number of spores in the white blood-corpuscles (Golgi). *Bastianelli* and *Bignami* have also established the fact that all the adult forms do not arrive at sporulation, but that a part, after becoming free in the plasma, die (although this happens to a much less extent than what is observed in the tertian); this fact, taken in conjunction with the foregoing, explains how it is that the red blood-corpuscles, invaded by the young amœbæ during the paroxysm of fever, *are never as numerous as we should expect to see them, taking into consideration the pre-existing adult forms, and forms of segmentation.*[2]

§ 3. The tertian is caused by a parasite (*Amœba febris tertianæ*, Golgi) which completes its life cycle in two days.[3] The development of this amœba takes place in the following way:—Some hours after the paroxysm the plasmodia described by *Marchiafava* and *Celli* are seen in the red blood-corpuscles; they are of small size (one quarter to one fifth of the red blood-corpuscle in diameter) and endowed with amœboid movements, which are more lively than in the similar forms of the quartan fever; the pseudopodia are fine and very long, so that they extrude themselves almost to the circumference of the red blood-corpuscle; sometimes they are so fine that their connection with the body of the parasite would escape detection were it not that as one follows them they are seen to retract, while other pseudopodia go ploughing up the substance of the red blood-corpuscle in other directions.

At a somewhat more advanced stage of development fine granules of black pigment are noticed; these have a tendency to

[1] Bastianelli e Bignami, "Sull' infezione malarica primaverile," 'Rif. Med.,' 1890,

[2] See Plate I *a*, figs. 1—14.

[3] See Plate I *a*, figs. 14—33.

accumulate towards the extremities of the pseudopodia, which are usually slightly thickened.

Already at this stage the tendency in the red blood-corpuscles to shrivel is less pronounced than in the normal ones, and they appear somewhat larger than the others (the healthy red blood-corpuscles).

On the day of apyrexia the amœboid bodies have become considerably larger, so that they now fill half to two thirds of the red blood-corpuscle, and contain a great deal of pigment; at the same time the amœboid movements are much less lively. The red blood-corpuscles which contain them are very pale, and much larger than the others.

This phase of life is followed by those internal changes which precede segmentation, as well as by the segmentation itself. The segmentation is effected, according to Golgi, in various ways; the pigment collects together at the centre of the amœba in a mass, while the body of the parasite divides itself in such a way that a cluster of ovoid or round spores is formed. This is Golgi's second mode of segmentation.

The third method of segmentation which *Golgi* points out—but with reserve—is, according to what the latest investigations would lead us to believe, a process of disintegration and death.

Golgi's first mode of segmentation has not been remarked by other observers (Antolisei); it is as follows:—After the pigment has been collected at the centre, the circumference of the parasite's body separates itself, and becomes like a ring; the substance of this ring divides itself into from fifteen to twenty spores, at first oval, then globular, which arrange themselves like a crown round the pigmented disc in the centre.

Not all the adult pigmented bodies of the tertian reach sporulation. Many become provided with flagella, to the frequency of which, as forming part of the life cycle of the tertian amœba, *Antolisei*[1] especially has called attention. Others form vacuoles and disintegrate into a hyaline spherule; this has been described by *Celli* and *Antolisei,* and regarded as a process of degeneration and death.

The sporulation does not always happen in the manner described; in the anticipating tertians and irregular quotidians of tertian origin, *Bastianelli* and *Bignami*[2] have described small sporulations formed of from five to ten spores collected round little granules, or on a single granule of pigment; they extend

[1] Antolisei, "Sull' ematozoo della terzana," 'Rif. Medica,' 1890.

[2] Loc. cit.

hardly halfway (or perhaps a little more) into the red blood-corpuscle.

Moreover the degeneration of the red blood-corpuscle which has been invaded does not always take place in the way described. Sometimes one notices a complete discoloration of the red blood-corpuscle before the parasite has invaded more than a small part of it. Much more rarely the colouring substance of the red corpuscle becomes like old gold, while the globule itself shrivels up, in a way analogous to what is seen in the summer fever.[1]

Unlike what we see in the quartan, the adult forms of the parasite *have a tendency in the tertian to accumulate in the internal organs.* Thus in the spleen the forms of segmentation are found in considerable quantities, and the pigmented hyaline spheres, which arise from the necrotic disintegration of the adult bodies, can be seen collected in large numbers within the macrophagi.

§ 4. In the tertian as in the quartan *the beginning of the paroxysm coincides with the maturation of a generation of parasites.* The double tertian is caused by two parasitic generations, in the same way as the double and triple quartan (quotidian of quartan origin) are due to the presence and development in the blood of two and three generations respectively (*Golgi*). Subcontinued fevers caused by quartan and tertian parasites are met with only exceptionally. In two cases of subcontinued fever with quartan parasites Antolisei found parasites in all the stages of development in one and the same preparation, and forms of sporulation smaller than usual (premature sporulation).

§ 5. The quartan parasites are distinguished morphologically and biologically from those of the tertian (*Golgi*). We may notice the following:

(*a*) *Differences in the cycle of evolution.*—The tertian parasite completes its life cycle in two days, the quartan in three.

(*b*) *Differences in the character of the amœboid movements.*—In the tertian the amœboid bodies within the red blood-corpuscles have much more lively movements than those in the quartan.

(*c*) *Differences in the mode of action of the parasite as regards the substance of the red blood-corpuscle.*—The tertian parasite discolours the red blood-corpuscle much more energetically and rapidly than does the quartan. And further, while the red blood-corpuscles which have been invaded by the quartan parasite tend to shrivel up, those invaded by the tertian parasite, on the contrary, are seen to be expanded, and they tend to become larger than the normal red blood-corpuscles.

[1] Loc. cit.

(*d*) *Differences in morphological characteristics.*—The quartan amœbæ have more sharply defined contours than the tertian. The granules of pigment in the tertian amœba are of extreme fineness; in the quartan amœbæ they are coarser.

The following differences are seen in the forms of sporulation:—(1) The number of spores arising from the division is from fifteen to twenty in the tertian, from six to twelve in the quartan; (2) the size of the single segments is larger in the quartan; and further (3), in the interior of each segment, which is the result of the division of the quartan amœba, we find a central shining sphere (probably the nucleus), while in the tertian spore no such bright spot is seen (*Golgi*).

The resemblances between the two varieties are so marked that there is no need of their being dwelt on; we shall now discuss much greater differences by which they are distinguished from the parasites of the summer-autumn fevers.

CHAPTER III.

SUMMER-AUTUMN FEVERS—HISTORICAL SKETCH.

Classification of Torti's *fevers, and especially of the malignant infections; complicated* (comitata) *and subcontinued* (subcontinua) *malignant fever; distinction between a* benign continuity *and a* malignant continuity; *origin of the subcontinued fevers through* the overlapping of paroxysms; *instance of subcontinued infection produced by the prolongation of the febrile paroxysms*—Guéguen; *researches on the course of temperature in the intermittent and ephemeral fevers*—Baccelli; *differential diagnosis between subcontinued* (subcontinua), *proportioned* (proportionata), *and subintrant* (subintrans) *fever; origin and conception of the subcontinued infection—Condition and quantity of the parasites in the different types of fever*—Colin; *clinical characteristics of the* remittent *or* simple continued fevers; *symptoms of the two forms of subcontinued infection, "the summer subcontinued and the autumn subcontinued"—Transformations of the types of fever*—Laveran; *clinical characteristics of the* marsh continued fevers; *condition of the parasites in the continued fevers and in quotidians of first invasion*—Sternberg; *different forms of* remittent *malarial fever*—Kelsch *and* Kiener; *classification of all the malignant malarial fevers in two groups,* simple malignant (solitaria) *and* complicated malignant (comitata); *various clinical forms of the "solitaria" fever*—Schellong; *observations on the malarial fevers of New Guinea; recent researches on the parasite of the summer-autumn fevers* (Marchiafava *and* Celli, Golgi, Canalis, Antolisei *and* Angelini, Sakharoff, *&c.*).

§ 6. It is not our object to give a complete history of the dangerous malarial fevers—the fevers, that is to say, which *Marchiafava* and *Celli* have collected under the group of summer-autumn fevers. This task would carry us too far, and would draw us away from the aim we have set before us. Still we cannot refrain from stating the opinions which have been expressed with regard to these fevers by some of the principal writers on malaria, and we shall consider especially the fevers called by various authors subcontinued, continued, or remittent.

Of the subject of these fevers, even recent authors, *e. g. Sternberg*, say with *Dutroulau*, "It is all chaos."

The contradictory descriptions, the inexact data which we possess on this subject, depend to a large extent on the fact that the majority of the writers who have engaged in the study of these fevers, through not having a sure means of diagnosis, such as we now have in the examination of the blood, have frequently confounded fevers of a different nature with malarial fevers—a mistake by no means difficult to make unless one has as guide that salient characteristic of malarial fevers, the intermittence and periodicity. Now these are exactly the characteristics which very often are wanting, or at least are not detected, in the fevers with which we are dealing.

Another cause of obscurity in this matter lies in the different use of terms and in the different significations given not infrequently by different observers to the same word.

Although the biology of the hæmatozoon which is the cause of these fevers in relation to the course of the disease must be our chief subject of consideration, still we could not, without becoming obscure, quite omit to notice these fevers from the clinical point of view, and this especially when we remember how much light is thrown on the disease in its course by the knowledge of the parasite's biology, and how this knowledge explains in a satisfactory way why the intermittence in these types of fever disappears either wholly or in part, and how the complex types of malarial fever are generated, and how, finally, it elucidates the genesis of many malignant symptoms.

§ 7. The best part of our clinical knowledge with regard to these fevers is derived from the classical book by *Torti* on the treatment of the periodic malignant fevers; his classification of the fevers has been followed by the majority of subsequent writers.

Torti[1] divides fevers into *simple* and *putrid*, and the latter into *continued* and *intermittent*. The intermittent he divides into *discrete* and *subintrant*, calling them (the intermittent) *discrete* or *legitimate* when the paroxysms are well distinguished, *subintrant* or *masked* ("*notæ*") when before one paroxysm is finished another succeeds it; and these latter he divides into *communicating* when the fresh paroxysm comes on just as the

[1] Torti, 'Therapeutice specialis ad febres periodicas perniciosas,' Venetiis, 1743. lib. v, cap. I.

preceding one approaches its termination, and *subintrant properly so called* when the end of the paroxysm is still distant. The discrete fevers are divided according to their type into *quartan, tertian*, and *quotidian*.

Malignancy belongs, for the most part, to tertian fever, which is subdivided into *benign* and *malignant*. Malignant fevers are divided into simple (*solitaria*) and complicated (*comitata*). "That is to say, they comprise the fever which, of its own evil nature passes into an acute, malignant, and pernicious malady, as well as the kind which suddenly becomes serious owing to the addition of some peculiar and dangerous symptom, worse than the disease itself which it counterfeits, and the fever which it accompanies." The complicated are divided into *colliquative* (choleraic, hæmorrhagic, cardiac, diaphoretic) and *coagulative* (syncopal, algid, lethargic).

In Book III, chap. i, p. 123, *Torti* defines the two forms of the malignant fevers as follows :—"Now, as a general rule, there are two varieties of this periodic malignant infection : in the one the intermissions continue, and the severe nature of the disease is only shown by the circumstance that the paroxysm is attended by some severe and peculiar symptom, the deadliness of which is but little affected beneficially by the intermediate apyrexia which in other cases, according to Hippocrates, gives assurance of safety ; in the other variety the period of intermission becomes lost little by little, and the fever tends to assume a continued and acute form, usually gradually, but sometimes abruptly, while various severe symptoms continue up to the actual time of the intermission, which is itself not complete."[1]

[1] Puccinotti keenly criticises Torti's conception of the "solitaria" fever, and apropos of this sets forth facts and conclusions which, in part, are certainly in conformity with truth.

In the same group of Torti's "comitatæ" fevers (he says) some present the subcontinued type; "just as, on the other hand, if I were to properly examine his 'solitaria' subcontinued fevers, I should constantly find in every case a predominating symptom, by virtue of which they would have to be admitted again into the family of the 'comitatæ.' In the first I should find the paroxysms accompanied by a comatose condition, in the second by mental aberration, in the third by serious delirium, in the fourth by clonic convulsions, &c. . . . . Now, however much these forms may occasionally be interchangeable, nevertheless the rule is that these symptoms present a more considerable constancy than the type of the fever." And he goes on to notice that many malignant "comitatæ" fevers can be, as far as regards the type, subcontinued, "just as the subcontinued are capable of developing any primary symptom of the malignant fever." ('Opere mediche di Francesco Puccinotti,' Milano, 1856, vol. i, p. 162, *et seq.*)

The malignant fevers in which the state of fever is continued and accompanied by serious symptoms of different sorts constitute Torti's eighth species of the malignant fevers, called by him "febris subcontinua perniciosa" or "malignans." With regard to the continuity of the fever which is by nature intermittent, Torti distinguishes a "benign" and a "malignant" continuity. Thus, in speaking of the subcontinued fever, he says, "I am not, therefore, here speaking of that mild and benign form of accidental continuity which an intermittent fever sometimes acquires when, from being originally simple, it becomes double or triple, and then finally subintrant,—in a word, exactly so far continued as it can be made from a certain slight prolongation of paroxysms which, in their own nature, perfectly admit of coming to an end; in this case, of course, one attack is often anticipating, and supervenes on another before this latter has completely passed away, &c. I am not now discussing fevers of this sort, which assume a purely accidental and, at the same time, benign continuity," &c.

Nevertheless he maintains that such fevers as have acquired the benign continuity can "proceed to an essential and dangerous continuity, nay, even to the highest degree of virulence and malignancy" (p. 130); and a little further on, speaking of the intermittent fever, "which, when it becomes continued, becomes also acute and serious, for it is only with the advent of continuity that the disease takes a severe form," he adds, "whether this takes place by means of subintrant paroxysms, or in any other way, if indeed any other way be possible (which I should hardly believe)."

As results from this position, Torti maintained that the more usual way in which an intermittent fever would become a malignant subcontinued one would be "per viam paroxysmorum subingredientium." This fact is also recognised in the cases which he mentions.[1]

The transition from an intermittent fever to a subcontinued one takes place at different periods and in various ways. Sometimes the intermittent fever becomes subcontinued suddenly, at the very beginning of the illness, sometimes during its course.

In this case the transition happens either rapidly, or else gradually after many paroxysms.

In his statement of the symptomatology of the subcontinued fevers, illustrated by some cases, it is clearly seen how some of these belonged to other infections, chiefly of a typhoid nature.

[1] Torti, lib. v, chap. ii, p. 199.

In discussing the subcontinued fever which is malignant "ab initio morbi," he gives an example of a fever which had become so through the paroxysms being prolonged.[1] "That students may better understand the state of the question, which may be studied in an analytical way, we will give an example. Let us suppose the case of a duplex tertian fever; on the first day, its commencement in the morning is marked by a moderate amount of shivering and some vomiting, together with the other usual symptoms. This is succeeded by a heat which is strongly pungent to the touch, by thirst, and by a dryness of the tongue which cannot be easily moistened. The paroxysm is prolonged over the usual time; and at length a considerable, but not complete remission is ushered in by a sweating which is neither abundant nor general. On the afternoon of the following day, before the first attack has entirely passed away, a fresh access appears, accompanied by a very slight, short, and scarcely perceptible rigor; soon after this the heat and other symptoms of fever return in more than average intensity. At night the patient feels ill, and only secures sleep a little before daybreak; the sleep induces a general moisture on the body, which in the region of the forehead develops into perspiration; and so at last a sort of intermission occurs; but it can hardly be called such, strictly speaking. In the mean time, before the sweating has finished, another and very short fit of shivering takes place, and simultaneously there is a transitory lowering of the pulse. This leads on the third day to a paroxysm more serious and of greater length than the preceding, attended with the same symptoms, only more pronounced, and, it may be, with others also. We will suppose that this access of fever persists very decidedly until the following morning,—that is to say, the commencement of the fourth day." And then follows the discussion of the treatment of this form of fever.

These textual quotations from Torti determine, then, the fact that in the group of dangerous fevers he distinguished a series of cases in which one symptom exclusively determined the whole clinical physiognomy, and which he called "complicated" (*comitatæ*) malignant fevers; and a series of cases in which one predominating symptom did not exist, or at least was not very pronounced, but in which serious symptoms of different sorts existed, and the intermittence was not well marked; these he called "simple" malignant subcontinued fevers (*solitariæ*). In the group of fevers where the intermittence was obscured he drew a distinction between the subintrant, as benign fevers,

[1] Lib. ix, p. 239.

and the malignant subcontinued ones; he made no sharp division, however, between these two forms, as if they were essentially distinct, seeing that he admitted that the subintrant fevers could become malignant. This is shown also by the idea which Torti had of the way in which an intermittent fever becomes subcontinued,—that is, by the overlapping of the paroxysms. We find, then, in Torti's conception of the subcontinued fever no idea of its differing from the subintrant also in the way in which it is developed from a common intermittent. It was in the symptoms, in the gravity, in the clinical course of the disease, &c., that he found his reasons for differentiating these two clinical forms. In fact, the instance of subcontinued fever which he adduces as a type is nothing but a double tertian with prolonged and subintrant paroxysms.

We shall see in the sequel how far Torti's classification can be reconciled with the researches on the biology of the parasite, and on the thermometry of the dangerous fevers.

§ 8. All observers have noticed the importance of studying Torti, not only on account of his nosography—for it is difficult to be happier than he is in describing the various morbid forms,—but also because of the view, which he so strenuously maintained, that these fevers should be treated by cinchona bark. Almost all writers have adopted his classification and fundamental criteria for the division of these fevers, without adding facts or remarks of much importance; so much so that to find investigations worthy of attention we must come to the last few decades.

§ 9. Wunderlich had to admit that from the point of view of thermometry only the intermittent form of marsh infection is sufficiently exactly known.[1] This blank in our knowledge Guéguen set himself to fill up, and published an abundance of charts wherein certainly figure many fevers of non-malarial nature.

In his work 'Sur la marche de la température dans les fièvres intermittentes et les fièvres éphémères,'[2] completed at Guadaloupe, the author we have quoted endeavours to determine by exact thermometrical observations, the thermal curve of the intermittent fevers in hot countries, and especially of the remittent fevers. Although among his various types of the latter there may be some, as we have already said, which cannot be considered malarial in nature, still we shall briefly give Guéguen's classification of the remittent fevers, noticing that some examples of his

[1] Wunderlich, 'De la température dans les maladies,' trad. par le Dr. Labadie-Lagrave, 1872.

[2] Paris, Baillière et fils, 1878.

remittent tertian recall our summer or malignant tertian. The author does not devote much time to the nature of the febrile state, but studies only the charts of remittent fever. He makes the following divisions :

GROUP OF THE REMITTENT FEVERS.

A. *Remittent quotidian* (p. 34).—The temperature varies between 100·4° and 104° F., and it may also reach 98·6° F. or thereabout during the period of remission, but this defervescence is in all cases transitory, and the fever soon reappears with all its train of symptoms.

B. *Remittent tertian* (p. 35).—Here we find regular remissions every forty-eight hours. This regularity is not always exact, as one paroxysm sometimes comes before, and another after its time. If the intervals which separate the remissions are sometimes irregular, those which separate the apex of the curve are almost always regular.

C. *Subcontinued fever* (p. 36).—This is a fever which is continued for eight or ten days, the temperature varying between 102·2° and 104°; towards the twelfth day a more marked remission takes place, and the fever becomes an intermittent quotidian (Ex. 20). It does not follow from the description that this subcontinued fever of Guéguen is a malarial fever; on the contrary, it is only reasonable to suppose that it is not. According to the author it would be a seasonal fever for the acclimatised, because the Creoles and the natives are generally taken by it at the beginning of the winter or at the commencement of the cool season; the new-comers, on the contrary, may fall victims to it at any time.

D. *Remittent-intermittent fever* (p. 38).—Only two cases of this observed. Guéguen says the treatment (salts of quinine) has no effect on the order of the paroxysms.

E. *Intermittent fever with relapses.*—Of this fever there were only two cases seen. The symptoms are those of a typhoid fever. The author puts down this fever as bordering on the "*relapsing fever.*"

F. *Remittent typhoid fever* (Tracings 23, 24, 25).—Guéguen believes this to be a typhoid fever with a special curve of temperature. All the symptoms considered together, this fever resembles the typhoid of Europe.

To these forms he adds—

G. *The inflammatory fever.*

H. *The bilious remittent fever.* But the object we have in view does not oblige us to discuss these.

§ 10. Prof. Baccelli's Roman clinical studies on these fevers, and especially on the subcontinued group, extend back to the year 1866. The fundamental principles upheld by him as regards malarial infection, and recapitulated in the Report read before the Italian Medical Congress of 1889, are that "malaria as an infective agent produces in the human organism a morbid condition of blood and a neuro-paralysis through direct injury of the blood-corpuscle and of the ganglionic system, and that the process which results therefrom produces fever but never inflammation, as is taught by clinical science and pathological anatomy." In the first lecture[1] published by him on the subject, after determining the fundamental facts of which it is necessary to take account in diagnosing the subcontinued fevers, he considers the differential diagnosis between the subcontinued and the so-called "proportionata," and gives the following conception of the proportionata.

"By this last term is meant the union of two morbid processes, the one continued, the other intermittent, in such a way that to the continued course of the fever caused by the one process there is added the clearly defined onsets and remissions caused by the appearance and disappearance of the paroxysm produced by the other process" (p. 6).

On the other hand—

"The subcontinued is a simple process, and subordinates completely to itself every "crotopathia,"[2] and when the symptoms and the groups of symptoms are strictly examined it reveals its special nature as one of congestive dyscrasia. The preparations of quinine form the sole remedy" (p. 8).

After this he confines his observations to the pneumonic subcontinued fever, *i. e.* the subcontinued accompanied by the phenomena of pulmonary congestion. The temperature varies in these fevers between 98·6° and 104° F.

With regard to these forms of subcontinued fever the author[3] remarks that when the patients were subjected to large doses of quinine "to paralyse in a few hours the causal influence," "the congestive dyscrasic pneumonia passed into exudative pneumonia."

[1] 'Delle febbri subcontinue,' Lezione del Prof. Guido Baccelli, Roma, 1866.

[2] Dominant symptom.—ED.

[3] 'La perniciosità,' 1884, p. 44.

Later on, in another monograph[1] concerning the morbid forms of malaria, he considers specially the subcontinued and the subintrant fever.

"The subintrant (*subintrans*) is marked by the prolongation of the paroxysms, so that another begins before the first is ended. In this way the initial cold stage of the coming fever occurs in presence of, and almost in contact with, the sweating stage of the attack which is *passing away*. *This fever presents nothing serious*; the paroxysms become constantly longer and milder until they cease altogether, and for the most part the fever disappears with a last prolonged paroxysm" (p. 31).

"In the subcontinued fever (*subcontinua*) there is also the overlapping of paroxysms, and this is the reason why many people have confounded it with the subintrant. . . . Sometimes it begins as intermittent, sometimes it appears at once as subcontinued. In the first case it is clearly seen how the paroxysms, at first definite, and, so to say, autonomous, become afterwards more frequent; at last, as these attacks hurry more and more upon each other, their alternation is concealed under the appearance of continuity. In the second case the onset of the paroxysms is no longer shown, except by the rise and fall of the temperature *at short, very short, intervals*" (p. 31).

Further on the author unfolds his theory, and says "the subintrant owes its appearance of continued fever to the *prolonging of the paroxysms*, the subcontinued to the *numerical increase of the paroxysms in a fixed time*." The subintrant is a very mild form, "which may be treated up to its close by the mildest measures;" the other one is dangerous, "indeed, the only one which deserves the name *of malignancy by reason of the type*."

In his various later works on the same subject the author returns to the same idea of subcontinued fever, insists on the notion that the subcontinued is produced by the numerical increase of the paroxysms in a fixed time, and criticises the word "remittent" applied by the French and Germans to these malarial fevers. In his lecture on malignancy he expresses himself as follows:—"The malignancy of the type lies in its being subcontinued" (p. 35).[2] The way in which the intermittent fever becomes subcontinued is by "the numerical increase of the paroxysms in a fixed time." On the other hand, a continued fever which has become so from a prolongation of the paroxysms (as, for instance, the subintrant) is not malignant (p. 36). The

[1] 'La malaria di Roma,' Prof. G. Baccelli, 1878.

[2] "La Perniciosità," 'Lezione Clinica,' Roma, 1884.

malignant fevers which Torti called "*comitatæ*" the author believes to be due to the feeble resistance of the organ or organs, through which the culminating symptoms show themselves. "The masked fevers form an extreme which admits the maximum of malignancy" from the individual point of view, "then comes as a middle term, Torti's *comitatæ*, and lastly as the other extreme, the malignant fever (the *subcontinua*), which is devoid of culminating symptoms" (p. 40).

As far as concerns the clinical form, the difference between the *comitata* and *subcontinua* lies in this, that while "the malignant intermittent has a predominant qualifying symptom —lethargy, delirium, hiccough, syncope, hæmorrhage, and the like, . . . every subcontinued fever has no single symptom to qualify it, but a general morbid condition, *e. g.* pneumonic, bilious, rheumatic, typhoid, &c."[1]

The character of the thermoscopic curve of this fever consists in this, that "in a given cycle of time—twenty-four hours—it presents several breaks which correspond to the number of the paroxysms noted in the day's course" (l. c., p. 18). As regards its length and clinical course, Professor Baccelli writes that "the typhoid subcontinued fever has no necessary cycle" (p. 45).

Moreover, the most recent researches of this illustrious physician on the same subject—researches in which due account is also taken of the results of the discovery of the parasite—arrive at the same fundamental conclusions that we have deduced from the preceding works. We may notice this last study more fully for the special reason that it has to do also with that which more directly concerns the subject of our researches—we mean the examination of the blood.[2]

The subcontinued fever (*subcontinua*) (p. 142) may arise from every sort of febrile type; only a clear change must take place in the paroxysmal form of the type.

The first thing to be observed is the increased number of the paroxysms. A tertian becomes a double tertian, then a double redoubled tertian; in this way the type of a real subcontinued is reached at last. It is the summer forms, as a rule, that are more inclined to this change in the type.

In the form of subcontinued fever which is derived directly from intermittent paroxysms (tertian and quartan), the author has succeeded in determining by the microscope the co-existence of

[1] G. Baccelli, 'La subcontinua tifoide,' Roma, 1876.

[2] 'Verhandlungen des X Internationalen Medicinischen Congressen,' Berlin, 4—9 August, 1890, Bd. ii, Abtheilung v, 1891.

several generations of parasites in different degrees of development, the cycles of evolution of which "se pressent les uns sur les autres." The same was noticed in the summer fevers, which are remarkably liable to become subcontinued.

The thermoscopic charts of the tertian show, 1st, that the paroxysms tend to come nearer together; 2nd, that they tend to keep remote from the complete apyrexia; and 3rd, that they tend to increase in number.

Now raise these symptoms (says Prof. Baccelli) another degree higher, and you get the subcontinued; the subcontinued is nothing but the confused mass of these attacks of fever. But after the action of quinine the type may become more easy to recognise (p. 143).

As regards the search for the parasite, with reference to the so-called summer fevers and the tertian and quartan, Prof. Baccelli remarks as follows:

"In some circumstances, and this, too, only rarely in the first days of the original infection, *especially in the case of those fevers which are observed in the summer months*, the microscopic examination of blood taken from the finger has yielded a negative result. In the same way it has been negative in the first attacks of fever induced by way of experiment through intra-venous injections of malarial blood. In these cases the result was always positive when the blood of the spleen was examined."

Then, with regard to the connection between the number of the altered red corpuscles and the degree of the morbid process, our author determines the following laws:—In the primary quartan, tertian, and quotidian fevers, or in those of recurring infection, the more serious paroxysms correspond to a larger, the weaker paroxysms to a smaller number of parasites. In the primary quartan and tertian with a high temperature, the number of the parasites is limited in comparison with that found in the recurring forms (pp. 140 and 141). In the summer fevers the number of the parasites is so limited during the first days of the disease that sometimes they are not found at all in the blood of the finger; but they increase progressively in the following days in proportion to the aggravation of the fever.

We shall afterwards speak of the important observations which Prof. Baccelli has made as regards the effect of quinine on the malarial parasites.

§ 11. Colin,[1] who made his observations in Rome, draws a clear distinction between the group of summer fevers and the other

[1] L. Colin, 'Traité des fièvres intermittentes,' Paris, Baillière, 1870.

malarial fevers. However (and it is certainly for want of exact thermometrical observations), he does not at all recognise the intermittent course of these fevers in the majority of cases; indeed, he calls them *remittent* or *simple continued fevers*, convinced that their essential character is that of continuity. Anyone who goes by the account given by the patients themselves, and takes their temperature only at long intervals during the twenty-four hours, is very liable to fall into this mistake.

The following is Colin's description of this group of fevers:

They begin, as determined by Mayer, about the 5th or 6th of July, reach their maximum as regards their number of victims towards the 20th of July, and then decline rapidly; in September there are only isolated cases, while the intermittent fevers become extremely numerous.

As a rule the symptoms are very uniform. Our author distinguishes two forms—the gastric and the bilious.

The clinical characteristics of these fevers are—

1st. The inflammatory nature of their course.

2nd. The intensity of pains in the loins, epigastrium, and head,—pains which, when taken together with the vomiting, the laboured respiration, the flushed countenance, the injected conjunctivæ, form a sum-total of symptoms analogous to those of the first period of yellow fever, and to an attack of severe smallpox.

3rd. The frequent absence of initial shivering.

4th. The intensity of the paroxysms does not surpass the limits of the evening exacerbations of the other fevers.

This remittent fever is almost always initial, the fevers which are distinctly periodic follow on it.

This remittent fever of Colin is in all probability our primary summer tertian; it is just the difficulty which so often occurs of recognising the type of this fever that leads the author to assert that the malarial fevers are not necessarily periodic. At the beginning of summer—indeed, after the first days of July—almost all the primary malarial infections belong to this sort of fever.

As regards the malignant fevers Colin criticises Maillot's classification, which divides the malignant fevers according as their characteristic phenomena are related to one of the three great splanchnic cavities; certain malignant fevers—as, for example, the algid fever, the sweating fever, &c.—it would, indeed, be difficult to put under this head. The author retains Torti's division of the malignant fevers into *comitatæ* and *solitariæ*, and names these last the subcontinued or malignant remittent fevers. He mentions, however, that the same Torti, in giving to these fevers the name of *solitariæ*, did not mean to say that they presented none of the accidents which mark the *comitatæ*, but simply meant to point out that the *solitariæ* fevers offered no "cachet esclusif de perniciosité;" that they had not, like the *comitatæ* fevers, a more marked tendency to become "*coagulative*" or "*colliquative*," but that, on the contrary, they were liable to take indifferently, and with an almost equal tendency, the accidents peculiar to both the classes ("coagulatives et colliquatives") of the *comitatæ* fevers. He mentions also the observation of Puccinotti that the *solitariæ* fevers are attended *very frequently* by the symptoms of the *comitatæ;* the name of *solitariæ* is therefore less happy than that of continued, subcontinued, and remittent—names which indicate the tendency as to the duration without excluding the contingency of malignant accidents. The malignant fevers which Colin observed are the comatose (apoplectic, soporose, lethargic), the delirious, the convulsive, the algid, the choleraic, the icteric (hæmorrhagic), the diaphoretic, the cardialgic, the syncopal, the summer *solitariæ* or subcontinued, and the autumn *solitariæ* or subcontinued.

The existence of the dysenteric malignant fever, which Torti accepted, is denied by Colin, who maintains that it is a question of two diseases. Moreover, in the so-called pneumonic malignant fevers, it is a question, according to Colin, of pneumonia real and proper, which takes an exceptionally severe course in those suffering from malaria.

We will pass over Colin's observations on the *comitatæ* malignant fevers, and give our attention to the clinical picture which he draws of the subcontinued fevers, of which he distinguishes two forms.

1. Summer subcontinued (ataxic, typhoid, typhoid remittent). This fever is developed at the time of the greatest heat; it may follow on attacks of intermittent fever, but it specially falls on those who are suffering from *simple remittent* fever. The length of the remittent fever is prolonged, the symptoms become aggravated, and the patient falls into a typhoid condition. In some of these cases the lesions are found at the autopsy to be those most characteristic of typhoid fever; while in others the post-mortem examination shows nothing but the changes of the malignant fevers. There follow some examples in which, from the autopsy, the typhoid infection is clear, while there is no proof of the existence of malaria (*e.g.* see 'Case xxiii, p. 274). In those cases in which lesions similar to those of typhoid are found in the intestines, the author denies that it

is a question of mixed infection; he takes it to be a change from malarial to typhoid infection. We give this opinion simply in order to justify our statement that we can neither use Colin's clinical description, nor the observations which he collected on this subject, in order to obtain the clinical representation of the malarial subcontinued fever. Out of four cases reported by him three certainly belong to typhoid, as the autopsy demonstrated.

2. Autumnal subcontinued fever. This is the subcontinued of the cachectic; it comes on in individuals who have had, or are having, fevers clearly intermittent. It is a very long illness, and may last for five or six weeks. As the fever becomes continued the serious symptoms appear,—hæmorrhage from the nose, nocturnal delirium, spasmodic motions of the tendons, hypostatic pneumonia, decubitus, and parotitis. At the autopsy the small intestine is found intact. Colin adduces one example alone of this sort of subcontinued fever.

After this description it is doubtful whether it is a question of simple malarial infection in cases of this sort; and it is more than probable that the *continued fever* is kept up by other affections (such as hypostatic pneumonia, parotitis, infection from bed-sores), which easily arise in cachectic persons.

Colin's observations on the influence of the febrile type in producing the malignant fevers are also worth while mentioning. He notes the stress which the old writers laid on the tertian type; even the subcontinued fevers were in Torti's eyes transformed double tertians, "tertiana duplex per subintrantes accessiones continua" (v. Mercurialis, Morton, Mercatus, Torti). Colin, on the other hand, saw the malignant symptoms set in for the most part in patients suffering from quotidian or remittent fever. He explains the contradiction by taking account of the place and the subjects on whom his observations were made (foreigners, who for the most part displayed the primary types of fever —the quotidian and remittent) (?). According to Colin, the idea that the malignant fevers arose all of them from the tertian type was accepted by the authors of old time rather through scholastic tradition than through actual observation.

In Algeria, also, the malignant fevers are most numerous in patients suffering from remittent or *pseudo*-continued fever; they are less frequent among quotidian patients, and still less in the cases of tertian fever. The malignant fever, according to our author, is almost always continued. When a simple intermittent undergoes the transformation into a dangerous fever it loses, as a rule, its intermittent type (p. 220).

We mention this opinion, which is shared by many authors, because our own observations, which we shall set forth, demonstrate, on the contrary, the great importance of the tertian type; we believe we are not mistaken when we affirm that the greater part of the malignant fevers have their origin in the type known as "the summer or malignant tertian;" a type of fever which Colin and others, through want of exact observation, confounded with the remittent or continued fevers.

§ 12. Now that many maintain the multiplicity of parasitic species or variety corresponding with the different types of fever, the transformation of these types becomes a question of interest. This is how Colin expresses himself on the matter.

The transformations of the intermittent fevers are exceptional. As a rule, the patients who remain a long time in hospital present a series of paroxysms marked by a single and invariable rhythm; it is only later, after they have left, that these paroxysms may be replaced by another series with different rhythm, whence another type of fever.

In the cases where the change takes place under our eyes, this generally happens abruptly: thus a tertian turns usually into a quotidian, or *vice versâ*. Colin never observed that progressive change, spoken of by Griesinger, according to which the transformation from one type to another would be nothing but the consequence of a series of anticipating or postponing paroxysms. The remittent which follows an intermittent—this fever also always becomes confirmed suddenly, and without giving any sign of a progressive transformation; the paroxysms are not anticipating, and consequently they do not become confused together, as might be the case in an intermittent fever.

As a rule, the anticipating or postponing paroxysms are a sign of an approaching convalescence, and not of a change in the type.

These observations are clearly in perfect agreement with the idea of the multiplicity of the malarial parasites. As regards the tertian being followed by the quotidian, it is now known that many so-called quotidians (even when the paroxysms come on at the same time, and the degree of fever, &c., is the same, and which, as far as can be seen from purely clinical observation, are in truth quotidians) are nothing but double tertians; but they cannot be accurately recognised as such unless the blood be examined, and there be found in it the two generations of tertian parasites maturing at one day's interval.

§ 13. The observations of Laveran,[1] the discoverer of the para-

[1] Laveran, 'Traité des fièvres palustres,' 1884.

site of malaria, controlled as they are by the examination of the blood, have more interest for us than the preceding ones of Colin. He divides the malarial fevers into intermittent and continued. As regards the frequency of the various types of fever, and the season of the year in which they are most frequently met with, he remarks as follows:

The quotidian fever is the most usual clinical manifestation of malaria in Algeria; the intermittent fevers—tertian and quartan—are according to his experience essentially fevers that have recurred (p. 216). The continued marsh fevers are seen only in the hot season: at this time the quotidian fevers are of the intermittents the most common; on the other hand, during the cold season the continued fevers disappear while the tertians increase (p. 217).

With respect to the fevers he calls continued marsh fevers, the principal facts determined by Laveran are the following:

The majority of the continued fevers are seen in the months of July, August, September, and October (at Constantine).

The causes of the continuity are probably—the external heat,[1] which has a marked effect on all fever patients—the sharp reaction which a first attack of marsh fever produces, especially in strong and full-blooded individuals. The continued fever hardly ever attacks the natives and the old fever patients, but usually the people who have lately come to a swampy place (Annesly, Griesinger, Colin)—The intensity itself of the marsh infection.

The quotidian fever is the most common intermittent in hot countries, and it is seen to be almost exclusively the first form of fever that attacks people. The same causes which make the quotidian fever so frequent in hot countries may, it appears, produce the continued marsh fevers. To these causes we must add fatigue, alcoholic excesses, exposure to the sun, and neglect of treatment. With regard to the origin of these fevers, Laveran thinks with Dutroulau and Griesinger that the continued marsh fever is derived in a direct line from the intermittent quotidian; if we suppose prolonged and subintrant paroxysms of fever, without the initial shivering, we get the continued fever. There are no natural boundaries between the intermittent fevers and the continued marsh fevers: the intermittent fevers with prolonged or subintrant paroxysms form a sort of neutral territory between the two, in such a way that it is necessary to draw an

[1] And how about the subcontinued fevers in the advanced autumn?

artificial line, and say, for example, that the fever is continued when it lasts longer than forty-eight hours, and when the continuity does not manifestly arise from the overlapping of quotidian paroxysms.

The symptoms of the continued fevers are—Commencement for the most part without shivering; constant headache, usually frontal, sometimes pains in the loins; pungent heat; tongue white and furred, or red and dry at the point; burning thirst, complete anorexia, sometimes diarrhœa, more often constipation, frequent pains, either spontaneous or on pressure, in the spleen, which is slightly enlarged, but rarely to be felt on palpation; frequent hæmorrhage from the nose; nervous symptoms like those in typhoid fever; prostration and apathy, or else agitation, anxiety; delirium at night. In some cases there are signs of congestion of the lungs or of bronchitis, in other cases bilious vomiting with a jaundiced or subjaundiced complexion.

Left to themselves, these fevers may cause death; or the fever may subside, and this usually from the eighth to the tenth day; the continued fever may also be followed by an intermittent. If treated with quinine (24—32 grains as a dose) they seldom last longer than four or five days.

As regards the febrile type, the continued fevers must be put among those that are atypical. The author has never observed the period of onset. During the course of the fever there are varieties in the temperature more or less great; the evening temperatures are, as a rule, higher than those of the morning, but there are many exceptions. The subsidence is completed by crisis in twelve, twenty-four, or forty-eight hours.

The parasites found in continued fevers, as in the primary quotidians, consist of bodies No. 2,[1] which are the forms found most frequently in the blood; and sometimes only bodies No. 2 of small size are those almost exclusively met with.

Hence it results that in this clinical description of the continued fevers which Laveran gave, and which we have recapitulated, we do not find those varieties of type which are met with in other writers, *e.g.* Colin; those fevers of long continuance, which resist quinine, &c., which other authors tell us of, are no longer classed among the malarial fevers. The examination of the blood serves as a guide, and prevents mistakes in diagnosis which are otherwise easy.

With reference to the intermittent fevers, we will only mention what Laveran says about the parasites.

[1] Small, hyaline, mobile, frequently pigmented.—Ed.

According to this author, it is at the *beginning* of the paroxysms, and in the hours which precede their appearance, that the probability is the greatest of meeting the parasitic elements in their most characteristic form. The existence of *bodies* No. 2, and of *mobile filaments* in sufficiently large numbers in a patient who has been without fever for a certain time, allows one to be sure that the sufferer will soon have an attack. The examination of the blood of patients seized by intermittent fever for the first time often shows nothing but *bodies* No. 2 of medium or small size, either free or adhering to the blood-corpuscles. This author has several times in cases of this sort only met with *bodies No.* 2 of very minute size, not containing more than one or two granules of pigment. This author has not determined the differences between the parasitic elements of the blood in persons suffering from quotidian, tertian, and quartan fevers.

As regards the length of the febrile attacks, Laveran distinguishes short attacks, from four to eight hours; attacks of medium length, from eight to twelve hours; prolonged attacks, from twelve to twenty-four, and even thirty-six and forty hours. These prolonged attacks explain the mechanism of the subintrant paroxysms, each paroxysm necessarily beginning before the end of the one preceding it.

The author gives three charts of intermittent quotidian, in which two paroxysms are joined together in such a way that there is no apyrexia between them. (This looks like the paroxysms of our summer tertian.)

Laveran suggests no classification of the malignant fevers. He does not consider them malignant fevers properly so called, forming, so to say, a clinical species in themselves, but simply accidents, complications of the ordinary marsh fevers.

§ 14. Sternberg[1] brings together all the malarial fevers, which are not clearly intermittent, in his chapter on the *remittent fevers*, which in the United States attain their maximum frequency in August. He distinguishes various forms.

1. A simple remittent malarial fever. This is a fever with paroxysms of malarial origin, differing from the intermittent because the attack is more prolonged, is not followed by complete apyrexia, and the cold stage is for the most part badly defined or entirely absent. In severe cases there are frequently symptoms of gastric irritability and bilious vomiting. He gives cases of remittent quotidian, double tertian, and irregular tertian (pp. 211, 233, *et seq.*).

[1] G. M. Sternberg, 'Malaria and Malarial Diseases,' 1884.

2. "Ardent malarial fever" (p. 237). This is a fever more continued than remittent in type; it prevails in the tropics, but also in subtropical climates, and in the southern temperate zone during the hottest time of year; it attacks, by preference, strangers not yet acclimatised. It is Colin's "fièvre inflammatoire."

3. Adynamic remittent fever (p. 250). This is not a distinct form of malarial remittent fever, but for convenience of description the author classes under this name a series of cases which, *instead of yielding to the treatment in the usual time or ending in a simple intermittent fever*, linger on with adynamic symptoms accompanied by more or less fever of an irregular character. Synonyms are "typhoid remittent fever," "summer subcontinued fever."

Under this head are included Colin's summer and autumn subcontinued fevers, with regard to the malarial nature of which we have reasons for raising doubts.

4. Malignant remittent fever (p. 264). Under this name the author groups a large number of malignant fevers where the fever is remittent and the symptoms like those in Torti's "comitatæ" fevers.

5. Complicated remittent fever (p. 280); this may have cerebral, gastric, or enteric complications.

§ 15. Kelsch and Kiener[1] keep Torti's division of the malignant fevers into "solitariæ" and "comitatæ," and make use of the same division also for the non-malignant fevers—putting, for example, the "simple fever" among the "solitariæ." Kelsch and Kiener's classification is as follows:

"Solitariæ" fevers	Simple fever.
	Gastro-bilious fever.
	Adynamic typhoid fever.
"Comitatæ" fevers	1st group, characterised by cerebral symptoms.
	2nd " " gastro-intestinal symptoms.
	3rd " " dissolution of the blood.

"Solitariæ" fevers.—1st. Simple marsh fevers.

These are intermittent or remittent fevers which are not accompanied, at any rate in a noteworthy degree, *by any of the other morbid symptoms characteristic of malaria* (p. 346). These fevers correspond to a milder degree of poisonous infection.

The *remittent fever* consists of periods of fever more or less long, and of intermissions more or less incomplete, which are not in their succession subordinate to a regular and sustained type. These periods of fever, which may last for five or six days, are

[1] 'Traité des maladies des pays chauds,' I. B. Baillière, 1884.

composed either of a *single prolonged attack* or else of *several subintrant attacks* (p. 439).

In the *prolonged attack* the fever may keep above 104° F. for thirty-six hours and more, but if the paroxysm lasts longer than forty-eight hours the fever usually shows a slight remission in the morning, and a return in the evening, as in the continued fevers.

The fever is remittent through *subintrant paroxysms*, when one paroxysm begins before the close of the preceding, and this may happen either *by approximation of the paroxysms* or *by their prolongation*. This last cause is more usual (p. 440).

The *approximation of the paroxysms*, which Torti looked upon as the ordinary condition of continuity in the periodic fevers, and which Baccelli regards as pre-eminently the type of malignancy, is, according to these writers, in reality exceptional (p. 441).

2nd. Bilious and gastric fevers.

These are the fevers which prevail in the epidemic outburst which occurs every year at the return of the hot season. The predominating symptoms are due to functional disorder of the liver and gastro-intestinal derangement (pp. 449, 450). They may take the tertian, quotidian, or remittent type; this last is the most common.

The symptoms are pain in the epigastrium, bilious vomiting, diarrhœa; the region of the liver probably painful on pressure; complexion jaundiced or subjaundiced; the urine highly coloured, especially with urobilin; albuminuria frequent, but scanty and transitory; hæmorrhage from the nose; headache, &c.

Our authors insist on the excess of bile existing in these fevers, and explain by it the jaundice (hæmo-hepatogenic jaundice). But by this excess of bile they cannot explain the gastro-intestinal disturbances which may be co-existent with but a trifling degree of excess of bile. In cases of malignant fever accompanied by serious gastro-intestinal symptoms (vomiting, diarrhœa) they have found a subinflammatory condition of the omentum and the intestinal mucous membrane: these membranes were infiltrated by leucocytes and granules of pigment (p. 466).

3rd. Dangerous "solitariæ" fevers—typhoid and adynamic (p. 467). These fevers differ from the "comitatæ;" they give us, so to speak, the general outline of the clinical picture, the various details of which are presented by the "comitatæ" fevers. All the poisonous effects of malaria meet together here, but no single effect is represented in its full strength. (See Torti, Malignant subcontinued fever.)

(*a*) *Typhoid remittent fever.*—In the majority of cases the typhoid symptoms become pronounced from the third to the sixth day. Stupor, delirium, cardiac weakness, meteorism of the abdomen, dry mucous membranes, and signs of pulmonary hypostasis. When death is imminent, the stupor passes into coma, the adynamic condition is intensified, &c., or else there suddenly supervenes (so our authors say) a malignant paroxysm, algid, convulsive, &c. (A temperature chart which they give resembles that of our malignant tertian, p. 471.)

(*b*) *Adynamic remittent fever.*—This is the most serious of the "solitariæ" fevers. It corresponds to Colin's autumnal subcontinued fever (pp. 472–6). Instead of having a comatose malignant paroxysm, its development is gradual; "it lasts a long time, the suspension of the cerebral functions is incomplete, and there is the co-existence of other symptoms, such as profound anæmia, jaundice, collapsed temperatures, cardiac weakness, &c."

The anæmia is always pronounced, and there is frequently hæmoglobinuria (as also in the typhoid remittent fever), biliousness, jaundice, &c.

The temperature of the axilla is usually not very high, and, as a rule, it varies between 99·6° and 101·2° F. In the intermissions, which may become prolonged, it has a tendency to drop below the normal height, and varies between 96° and 98·6° F. The tendency to depressed temperatures is characteristic of this species of fever.

The typohid condition and the adynamic condition correspond to the two degrees of gravity which the infection shows.

The typhoid condition, according to our authors, should not be regarded as due to a specific property of the marsh poison. It is found in the same way in other acute infections. Perhaps it is caused by the retention in the system of the poisonous products formed by the retrograde metamorphosis of the tissues (as Robin tried to establish for typhoid fever); perhaps by a secondary infection through intestinal products (see Bouchard, p. 483).

In the adynamic state two factors must be taken into consideration: first, the depressing action of the marsh poison on the nervous centres: second, the anæmia, which acts in the same way, and, moreover, produces collapse temperatures and impending syncope.

Complicated fevers, "comitatæ" (pp. 485—514).—The cerebral complicated are the most frequent; in point of frequency they come immediately after the dangerous "simple malignant" fevers, *with which in other respects they are connected very frequently indeed.*

Our authors bring together under the heading of algid forms—

The cardialgic paroxysm.

The choleraic paroxysm.

The dysenteric paroxysm.

The diaphoretic and syncopal paroxysm.

The algid condition, one of the manifestations of marsh infection, is only a secondary phenomenon which may depend on manifold conditions, especially on a morbid determination to the gastro-intestinal canal, on the weakening of the cardiac function, or on depressed temperatures following on dangerous fevers.

§ 16. Schellong[1] divides the diseases of malarial infection, as observed by him in Kaiser-Wilhelm's Land (New Guinea, East Indian Archipelago), in the following way:

1. Malarial infection with fever. (*a*) Intermittent fevers; (*b*) continued or remittent fevers without type; (*c*) bilious hæmaturic fever; (*d*) malarial coma.

2. Malarial infection without fever. (Malarial anæmia, malarial cachexia, malarial neuroses.)

In the region where Schellong practised, as is general in the tropics (Hirsch), the quotidian type of the intermittent fevers prevails.

The paroxysms last, as a rule, for six or eight hours, and tend to become anticipating: badly marked intermissions, and disparity between the length of the paroxysms and that of the intervals are often found: and the shivering, which generally indicates the typical course of the fever, is frequently wanting.

Such atypic fevers, continued or remittent, or of mixed character, are distinguished by this, that the febrile rise or the decline of the fever, or both these, occur so leisurely that there are no intervals, but simple remittences; or else the fever has at the beginning or end, or during its whole course, a continued character, while the symptomatology corresponds to that of the ordinary intermittent fevers. These fevers, as a rule, last a week. They are found more frequently when the malarial epidemic is at its height. The symptomatology is in some cases mild, in others severe, and in others so severe that death ensues: in these the gastro-enteric affections are frequent, as well as states of stupor, &c. In these fevers the shivering is often wanting, and there is

[1] 'Die Malaria Krankheiten in Kaiser-Wilhelm's Land' (New Guinea), Berlin, 1890.

no distinct enlargement of the spleen. It is the Europeans who are more frequently attacked by them. *Quinine has no great effect on their course.*

The hæmorrhagic bilious malarial form is marked by acute jaundice and hæmoglobinuria; it is a very dangerous form, and denotes serious infection. The patients had previously been attacked by fever, and had not made a sufficient use of quinine.

Schellong rejects the distinction between the jaundiced form and the hæmoglobinuric form; he describes at length the chemical and microscopic changes in the urine, and sets forth the following data on which to base the diagnosis:—(*a*) after various attacks of intermittent fever have been passed through, the disease commences with severe shivering; (*b*) decided enlargement of the spleen and liver; (*c*) acute universal jaundice; (*d*) want of correspondence between the pulse and the temperature, so that the latter is even normal while the former is increased in frequency; (*e*) violent gastro-intestinal disturbance; (*f*) nervous agitation of the sufferers and sense of oppression on the chest. Death may be accompanied by uræmic phenomena.

The *malarial coma* is the most serious malignant form. Of the nine cases observed by Schellong seven had a fatal issue. This is a state of "collapse" not dependent on the fever or on the failure of the vital forces, or on complications, but it is the expression *of the predominating influence of the malarial poison over the nervous centres.* The author classes under this head other forms of malignant fever (eclamptic, tetanic, delirious, sweating, &c.). The disease may run its course without fever, or with fever in different degrees,—sometimes intermittent, sometimes atypic. The unconsciousness is sometimes complete, sometimes not. Of the reflex actions, that of the cornea is usually preserved. The coma supervenes at one time at the beginning, at another time during the course of the disease. Quinine given in repeated doses of 24 grains has but little influence, either on the cerebral phenomena or on the course of the temperature, according to Schellong.

§ 17. The principal object of the researches which have been published during the last few years with reference to this group of fevers is the study of the biology of the parasite in relation to the development of the type of fever, but the opinions and observations of the various writers are to a large extent contradictory. Above all, these fevers have been named in different ways, either from the point of view of their clinical course, or from that of the parasitic variety which produces them; hence they have been called *"fevers caused by the falciform hæmatozoon, irregular fevers, intermittent fevers of inconstant type*" (Golgi).

These names contain all of them, in our opinion, a false conception, as much with reference to the clinical course of these fevers as with regard to the biology of the parasite which produces them. We will now give the clinical characteristics of these fevers as they should be according to the different investigators. According to Golgi[1] there belong to this class many intermittent fevers of inconstant type, and not only the fevers which are intermittent at long intervals, but also many fevers with short intervals, as well as some quotidians, and even some subcontinued fevers and subintrant quotidians. Canalis[2] follows Golgi's view; the fevers of this group (he says) are for the most part irregular, quotidian, subcontinued, subintrant, and fevers with long intervals. Also Antolisei and Angelini admit that they have been unable to trace in these fevers a noticeable rhythm. "This variety of parasite" (they say) "gives rise to a course of fever so varied that it is impossible to tell from any of our thermographic charts how long the parasite requires to pass from the initial amœba phase to the final phase of sporulation; one cannot trace any rhythmic course in the fever." Sakharoff[3] has lately described a parasite "*of the irregular malarial fevers,*" thinking that he was depicting a new variety of the malarial parasite; but it is clearly a question of the same parasite which has already been studied in Rome, as is manifest from the description and from the photographs which illustrate it. And these fevers which he calls irregular are the same fevers which have already been described here, and marked off in a group, under the name of the summer-autumn fevers.

In all these researches there prevails, then, the idea of the irregularity of these fevers, and consequently of the uncertainty with which the parasite which causes them must complete its cycle of development. On the other hand, Marchiafava and Celli, as well in their preliminary monograph as in their extended work on this group of fevers, which they have been the first to clearly define, do not arrive at this conception; but, recognising indeed that these fevers are not clearly periodic, they trace in them the quotidian type, which is distinct through the tendency of the paroxysms to become prolonged and to approximate to

[1] 'Arch. per le scienze mediche,' 1890.

[2] Ibid.

[3] "Recherches sur le parasite des fièvres irregulières," 'Annales de l'Institut Pasteur,' No. 7, 1891.

each other, whence sometimes the fever becomes really continued, and they trace the parasite's biological cycle in correspondence with the paroxysm.

Such ideas having been expressed with regard to the clinical type of these fevers, it is natural that the way of considering and of constructing the biological cycle of the parasite should vary with the different investigators, for the one thing cannot be separated from the other; it is natural that he who believes the fevers to be irregular or taking place at long intervals should take a different view of the parasite's biology from the man who has quite another conception. But we shall return to this later on.

The existence of such contradictory opinions has convinced us of the need of a new series of observations with a view to determining the type, or the fundamental clinical types, of these fevers, and starting from these, the origin of the complex fevers, the subcontinued, the subintrant, &c., and at the same time to investigate the life cycle of the parasite side by side with the clinical course, for these two kinds of research cannot possibly be separated, but must necessarily proceed *pari passu*. We were, in fact, persuaded that the irregularity in this group of fevers was only apparent, lay simply on the surface, and concealed a regularity which it was difficult to detect.

To the above quotations from authors we might add what has been published by many others, did it not appear to us useless to mention the results of observations which, to a large extent, are not original, nor different from those we have already noticed, except in the way of grouping the facts, or in the classification of the fevers, &c.

The result of this long disquisition is that, in our opinion, the most recent analytical researches represent above all a work of delimitation and of elimination. We are especially led to adopt this view when we study what has been written by even recent authors concerning the dangerous malarial fevers, and above all the subcontinued (*subcontinua*), whether remittent or continued, without having their guide in the examination of the blood. When we compare their statements with what has been observed by men who have studied not only the clinical course of the fevers, but, in addition, the search for, and the biology of the parasite, up to only a short time ago, we could with justice repeat Dutroulau's words, "These fevers are a chaos." But those clinical types of subcontinued or remittent fever, as one may say, which deviate so far from the common forms of malarial fever in their course, and in their behaviour when treated with the salts of quinine, &c.—as, for instance, the subcontinued described by Colin, the so-called typho-malarial fevers, Sternberg's adynamic remittent, many of Schellong's remittent, &c.,—these clinical forms no longer appear in the recent descriptions of those who have taken the examination of the blood as their sure guide. Hence the progress now made, lies essentially, not in the increase of the number of clinical pictures of malaria, but in the elimination—guided by the examination of the blood—of all those forms which the insufficiency of means for diagnosis has led many authors, and leads even recent writers, to attribute to this infection.

We now come to the description of the results of our own observations on the clinical course, and on the parasites of the summer-autumn fevers, which we divide, according to the type, into quotidian and tertian.[1]

[1] We tender our best thanks to Dr. A. Ballori for having received us with such courtesy in the Hospital of S. Spirito, and to Dr. Giulio Bastianelli for his kindness in placing at our disposal, for purposes of study, the patients in his wards.

CHAPTER IV.

THE QUOTIDIAN FEVER.

Clinical course of the summer quotidian; mild quotidian and malignant quotidian—Different ways in which the curve of the quotidian becomes irregular—Different ways in which the quotidian gives rise to the subcontinued infections—Regularity of the quotidian type in the relapses of this fever—Amœba febris quotidianæ; *biological and morphological characteristics—Changes in the invaded red blood-corpuscles—Spore formation, normal and premature—Pyrogenic cycle of the amœba in relation to the development and succession of the febrile attacks—Condition of the blood in the irregular quotidians—Instances of irregular quotidian.*

§18. The summer quotidian, which we distinguish from the quotidian of tertian and quartan origin, of which we have already spoken, may have a very regular course, so that the paroxysms resemble each other in the hour of their onset, in their length, in the degree of temperature, and in the symptoms which accompany them.

In the typical quotidian the attack is usually short, lasting for six or eight, rarely for twelve hours, and is caused by a single rise in the temperature without any noticeable oscillations; it is often preceded by a slight elevation of temperature not much above 98·6° F. The rise is generally more rapid and abrupt than the fall of the fever, and as it passes off the temperature, as is well known, sinks very much, usually as far as 96·8° F., and even lower. (See Chart I, tracing 1.)

The summer quotidian may be a very mild fever, and even get well spontaneously; or it may be malignant. The malignant fevers, as well as the subcontinued, we shall consider in the sequel. As for the very mild forms, they seldom show a perfectly regular curve; the paroxysms are for the most part postponing, even for some hours, and as they get weaker they become simply slight rises of temperature. On the other hand, when the fever becomes aggravated, the attacks approximate to each other, and are so prolonged that they join together. In the cases where the attacks are prolonged oscillations are seen in the chart, but are, however, of small importance.

Spontaneous recovery happens for the most part as a consequence of the paroxysms becoming weaker, and this may take place gradually and regularly; for these very mild infections are not always irregular, as we have already remarked, In some cases we notice that the intervals are prolonged, while the paroxysms become shorter, and the elevations in temperature less pronounced; the highest point, however, of the elevations may occur every day at the same or almost the same time. But the paroxysms may cease spontaneously, even when, through their being prolonged and joining together, it would seem that the fever had a tendency to become aggravated. This is a counterpart to what may sometimes be seen in the common tertian; in this, too, spontaneous recovery may take place after a final severe paroxysms.

The most common reason why the quotidian loses its perfectly regular course lies in the fact that the intermissions are, as often happens, incomplete, only reaching to 99·6° or 100° F.; and in the second place, because the attacks have a tendency to be prolonged, or to be anticipating or postponing.

A course which tends to become subcontinued through the paroxysms being prolonged, and following close upon one another, may even take place after the administration of quinine; there are cases in which, although the infection is mild, and correspondingly the parasites are found in but very scanty numbers, the attacks are nevertheless prolonged, the intermissions incomplete, and, in addition, the resistance to the action of quinine remarkable, so that the prolongation and overlapping of the paroxysms is for the most part, but not always, a serious sign. On the other hand, even in the cases in which the paroxysms are quite distinct and regular, the infection may suddenly become aggravated, and that in spite of the action of quinine.

When subcontinued fevers develop from quotidians, they do so in the majority of cases by the prolongation and coalescence of the paroxysms; at the same time the quotidian type may remain clearly discernible in the charts of these cases, because the highest point of the fever takes place every day nearly at the same hour.

The quotidian type is usually less distinct and regular in the original than in the relapsed infections. In the latter the quotidian type is kept either distinctly or less noticeably through one of the modifications above mentioned; but not infrequently the fever is subcontinued in the original infection, and becomes an intermittent quotidian as it relapses or when it recurs.

§ 19. *The quotidian is a fever dependent on the development of an amœba, the life cycle of which is completed in about twenty-four hours.*

Marchiafava and Celli have recently described the condition of the blood in the quotidian, and to their description we now refer.

If the blood be examined while the fever is high, during a paroxysm, we observe the presence of a greater or less number of red corpuscles containing one or more plasmodia [1],[1] with very lively amœboid movement. The same state of things is found in the sweating stage, and in the first hours of the intermission. Besides the forms in motion, which every moment are seen to take successively the strangest shapes, are noticed other motionless forms, discoid or annular in shape. The discoid forms have the appearance of hyaline bodies, more transparent in the centre than at the circumference. The annular forms, enclosing a particle of red blood-corpuscle in their interior, have a bright appearance, as if they were formed of a mass of protoplasm more solid than the former. From this annular, as well as from the discoid form, the parasite may return to that of amœboid movements, or it may also show simple movements of expansion and contraction. The forms which are in amœboid motion never pass with their pseudopodia beyond the edge of the red blood-corpuscle, in which they may be seen, as it were, to swim, and dip down more or less into its substance, in such a way as to become at various moments less or more accessible to view. During the intermissions the plasmodia change; they develop and become pigmented, while their mobility tends to decrease. In this way they turn into bodies endowed with sluggish motion, with very fine granules of pigment at the circumference, to see which sometimes requires careful observation; or else they become motionless forms, of equal smallness, containing one or more particles of hæmoglobin, which, while they are being observed, may be seen to divide into granules and become black. Following on this, the pigment which was at first at the circumference collects together at the centre of the parasite's body in a little heap, or in a mass of granules. These forms with pigment at the centre (or it may also be collected at an eccentric point in their mass) are larger than the preceding forms, and are round and motionless; and

[1] This number within brackets, and others to follow, refer to the numbers in the Appendices.—ED.

sometimes one sees accumulated round them all the remaining hæmoglobin of the red blood-corpuscle, the circumference of which remains discoloured.

As the parasite develops in this way, many of the red corpuscles which contain it undergo a radical change; they shrivel up and contract (to as much as a third of their normal size), and become in colour like old brass (Marchiafava and Celli call these red corpuscles "ottonati," *i. e.* brassy, for shortness' sake); this alteration may be explained as an acute necrosis of the blood-corpuscle dependent on the invasion of the amœba.

When the forms just described are found in the blood, it may be predicted with certainty that a new attack is imminent, *coinciding with the coming to maturity of a generation of parasites.* Indeed, although in the blood of the finger we do not find, except very rarely, forms of fission, nevertheless from the adult forms seen in it (plasmodia with granular pigment, and corpuscles with the pigment collected at the centre) one may infer with certainty that *the fission is just taking place in the internal organs.* This law is proved by examination of the blood taken from the spleen during life, and by examination of the parasitic contents of the various organs after death in cases of malignant infection [2].

The forms which precede the fission are the corpuscles as described, with pigment in the centre, or collected eccentrically in a small heap, or in a mass of granules, which are sometimes in lively oscillatory motion. Around these, by a process analogous to that found in the quartan and tertian, the mass of the parasite divides itself into numerous ovoid or round spores, which give place to the forms represented in the figures. (See Plate I, figs. 50—55.)

Very rarely, in cases of malignant fever, the fission takes place prematurely, that is to say, before the parasite has become pigmented, as we have observed especially in the capillaries of the brain, and sometimes also in the blood of the finger.

When the paroxysm has commenced, the young plasmodia without pigment become again visible in the blood, they increase in number during the attack, and recommence their life cycle as described.

This life cycle of the amœba might be called a *pyrogenic cycle,* because it is directly connected with the development and succession of the attacks of fever; the forms of this cycle disappear when, through the administration of quinine, the fever ceases; they reappear as it relapses. But to the same parasitic variety there belong other forms, the appearance of which does not stand in direct relation to the onset of the febrile paroxysms; these do not disappear, or only do so slowly under the action of quinine, and they continue in the intermission. They belong to the group of Laveran's crescent-shaped bodies (spindle-shaped, ovoid, true crescent-shaped, and round flagellated forms), which we shall discuss later on, after having explained the life cycle of the amœba which is found in the summer-autumn tertian.[1]

§ 20. The pyrogenic cycle of the amœba is in the typical quotidian completed regularly, as we have described. We wish to draw attention to the fact that there is usually no point in the clinical course of this fever which gives a negative result on examination (as may be the case in the summer tertian). At the beginning of the paroxysm it is the adult forms that are found, as we have said (plasmodia with pigment in fine granules at the circumference or at the centre, and similar forms in the so-called brassy red blood-corpuscles); but before these forms have entirely disappeared, there already appears in the blood—at the commencement of the attack—the new generation (amœboid plasmodia without pigment), while in the summer tertian the young forms usually show themselves, as we shall see, only when the attack is in an advanced state.

When the course of the fever deviates from the typical form, it becomes then more difficult to follow the parasites in their development.

Thus if the quotidian tends to become irregular through anticipating or postponing paroxysms, the examination of the blood yields more complex results. At every moment of the fever's course one finds parasites in different degrees of development: those forms, however, which are found in the particular moment of development which corresponds to the phase of the paroxysm are by far the most numerous; that is to say, some hours before and at the beginning of the attack the plasmodia with granular pigment, in red corpuscles either normal or brassy ("ottonati"), prevail, and when the attack has advanced the young plasmodia without pigment, . . . &c., are in the majority. A group of parasites in comparatively small numbers, which are a little behind or a little in advance in their evolution, determines the irregularity of the curve.

When the paroxysms are so far prolonged that no intermediate apyrexia is left, the succession of the forms is found to be the

[1] We shall speak also in the sequel of the action of quinine on this variety of amœba, and we shall set forth minutely the characteristics by which the differential diagnosis between this and the other parasitic varieties may be made.

same as is seen in the typical quotidian, because in this case also there may be in the blood one generation of parasites alone.

We have said that in the quotidian there is, as a rule, no point in the course of the disease when we get a negative result, as may happen in the tertian. An exception to this rule is formed by the very mild quotidians, where examination may give an extremely meagre result; and in some cases also for long intervals, *e. g.* twenty-four hours, the results may be completely negative; but yet in the periods when no parasites are found it may happen *pigmented leucocytes* are seen, though in very scanty numbers.

When spontaneous recovery happens the parasites grow very scarce in the later attacks, and they may be entirely wanting in the last abortive ones. In other cases, with the same conditions, the amœboid forms are replaced by the forms of the crescent-shaped phase.

§ 21. It seems to us unnecessary to give at length instances of typical quotidian; we should have to repeat, as far as regards all about the finding of the parasites, what we have said before on the life cycle of the amœba. We prefer to give some examples of the quotidian which is irregular.[1]

CASE 1.[2]—Morani F—, 23 years old, took fever near Salerno on 2nd August; had it for nine days without intermission (?). After seven or eight days of apyrexia he had again two days of fever, which was cut short by quinine; then he became free from fever until the present. On the evening of the 7th September he was seized with headache, which lasted during the night. On the morning of the 8th he seemed dazed, and in the afternoon the fever became high. On the morning of the 9th there was an intermission and great weakness.

September 9th.—4 p.m., 101°. 8 p.m., 104·4°. 12 p.m., 103·6° F. 3 p.m., blood: moderate number of discoid plasmodia, annular and mobile, diaphanous, all with small granules of pigment at the circumference, some in brassy ("ottonati") blood-corpuscles. 4 p.m., blood: condition as above, *plus* some plasmodia without pigment, very full of motion, and young.

10th.—In the morning the patient says he feels pretty well. 4 a.m., temp. 100·8°. 7.30 a.m., 99·8°. 12 noon, 101·2°. 4 p.m., 104·7°. 8 p.m., 99·8°. 12 p.m., 97·6° F. 9 a.m., blood: a few plasmodia with granular pigment, discoid, annular, and mobile.

[1] See Chart I, tracings 2, 3, and 4.

[2] See Chart I, tracing 3.

A very few younger forms. 10 a.m., blood: condition as above. 3 p.m., vomiting. Blood: a few young annular forms without pigment. 4.15 p.m., blood: numerous plasmodia without pigment, annular, mobile, and discoid. One free specimen with segmentation. White pigmented blood-corpuscles. 5.30 p.m., bimuriate of quinine, 24 grains, by hypodermic injection.

11th.—4 a.m., temp. 96·8°. 7.30 a.m., 97·2°. 12 noon, 98°. 4 p.m., 98°. 8 p.m., 100°. 12 p.m., 98·6° F. 8 a.m., condition good; sulphate of quinine, 16 grains, by the mouth. 8.45 a.m., blood: several discoid plasmodia, annular and mobile, without pigment. Some in brassy ("ottonati") globules. White pigmented blood-corpuscles.

12th.—Without fever; condition good. 9 a.m., blood: a very few plasmodia without pigment and annular. Some white corpuscles with granules and little masses of pigment.

13th.—Complete apyrexia. Blood: result of examination negative.

14th and 15th.—Nothing noticeable.

16th.—About 1 p.m. patient feeling distressed, then slight shivering of short duration, temperature rising rapidly. 3 p.m., temp. 104°. 4 p.m., 103·6°. 8 p.m., 102·6°. 12 p.m., 101·4° F. Blood: several discoid plasmodia without pigment, annular and mobile.

17th.—4 a.m., temp. 99·6°. 7 a.m., 100·4°. 10 a.m., 100·2°. 12 noon, 101°. 4 p.m., 102·7°. 8 p.m., 104·8°. 12 p.m., 103·1° F. 8·30 a.m., blood: moderate number of discoid plasmodia, annular and mobile, with granules of pigment. Some plasmodia without pigment. 9.30 a.m., blood: the same. 3.30 p.m., several plasmodia without pigment. Some still found with granules of pigment, the greater part of them in brassy ("ottonati") corpuscles.

18th.—4 a.m., temp. 100·4°. 7 a.m., 101·1°. 8.30 a.m., 101·3°. 10.30 a.m., 101·8°. 12 noon, 102·2°. 4 p.m., 105·2°. 8 p.m., 103·4°. 12 p.m., 101·4° F. 8.30 a.m., blood: a very few annular plasmodia, rather small with granules of pigment. 10.30 a.m., blood: the same. 3.30 p.m., blood: several plasmodia without pigment. A few white blood-corpuscles with small masses of pigment. 5 p.m., sulphate of quinine 32 grains by the mouth.

19th.—Condition good. Sulphate of quinine 16 grains by the mouth. 9.30 a.m., blood: several plasmodia without pigment as well as some mobile forms.

20th.—9 a.m., sulphate of quinine 16 grains by the mouth. Blood: a very small number of crescent-shaped adult forms and ovoid bodies. The patient gains strength rapidly.

This is a case of quotidian fever, in which both in the primary infection and in the relapse the same febrile type is seen. The relapse occurred four days after the quinine was stopped. The quotidian paroxysms are prolonged in such a way that the greatest decrease of temperature between two attacks keeps somewhere about 100·4° F. *It is a case of a subintrant quotidian caused by the prolongation of the paroxysms.*

CASE 2.[1]—Nannie D—, 24 years old, robust, has had malarial fever for nearly a year: has been in good health since September, 1890. Twenty days ago he was seized with fever near Fiumicino, which lasted four or five days; has been without fever up to last night, when the fever began without shivering. Spleen becoming enlarged.

August 30th, 1891.—4 30 p.m., temp. 104°. 8 p.m., 101·1°. 12 p.m., 102·2° F. The patient complains of muscular pains in the calves of the legs and back; the muscles of the base of the thumb are painful on pressure. 4 p.m., blood: moderate number of discoid plasmodia without pigment, annular and very mobile; some with very fine granules of pigment. 5 p.m., blood: the same.

31st.—4 a.m., temp. 97·5°. 8.30 a.m., 98·6°. 12 noon, 99·4°. 4 p.m., 102·3°. 8 p.m., 100·6°. 12 p.m., 98·7° F. 8.30 a.m., blood: a few plasmodia, discoid and annular, with small granules of pigment. 9.45 a.m., blood: the same. 3.30 p.m., the temperature has risen since midday, unaccompanied by shivering. Blood: several very young plasmodia without pigment, annular and discoid. A very few pigmented plasmodia in brassy ("ottonati") corpuscles.

September 1st.—8 a.m., temp. 98·6°. 12 noon, 98·2°. 4 p.m., 100·4°. 8 p.m., 101°. 12 p.m., 98·2°. 9 a.m., condition good. Blood: a few annular plasmodia with granules of pigment. A very few pigmented white blood-corpuscles. 4 p.m., blood: the same. Some of the white blood-corpuscles contain small masses of pigment.

2nd.—In the morning the examination of the blood gives a negative result. 5 p.m., a very small number of very young annular plasmodia. One form with granular pigment in a brassy ("ottonato") red blood-corpuscle. In the night high fever.

3rd.—In the early hours of the morning the temperature drops to 102·2° F., rises again in the afternoon. 9 a.m., blood: a few discoid and annular plasmodia with granules of pigment in red blood-corpuscles of normal appearance. 3.15 p.m., blood: plasmodia as above, only extremely few in number (a single form

[1] See Chart I, tracing 2.

in one preparation). 4 p.m., blood: a single young annular form without pigment in one preparation. 5 p.m., blood: the plasmodia without pigment increased in number, but still very few.

4th.—In the morning the patient is free from fever; examination of the blood gives a negative result. Patient has a short and slight attack of fever in the evening and night.

5th.—He feels pretty well. He has slight oscillations of temperature during the course of the day. In the blood there are a very few pigmented plasmodia.

6th.—4 a.m., temp. 98·6°. 7.30 a.m., 99°. 12 noon, 101·1°. 4 p.m., 104°. 8 p.m., 102·2°. 12 p.m., 101° F. At the highest point of the fever a very few plasmodia without pigment are found, discoid and transparent; also some white pigmented blood-corpuscles. One crescent-shaped form.

7th.—4 a.m., temp. 99°. 7.30 a.m., 98°. 12 noon, 99·7°. 4 p.m., 103·8°. 8 p.m., 102·2°. 12 p.m., 101·5°. 8 a.m., headache. Blood: several discoid plasmodia, annular and moving slowly, generally without pigment and small in size. Others, a little larger, with pigment. A few crescent-shaped forms and pigmented white blood-corpuscles. 2.30 p.m., blood: condition as above, but the plasmodia remarkably decreased in number. Headache intense. 4 p.m., blood: a very small number of pigmented plasmodia in brassy ("ottonati") red blood-corpuscles. Also a very few plasmodia without pigment, discoid and transparent. A few crescent-shaped forms.

8th.—4 a.m., temp. 103·5°. 7.30 a.m., 100·6°. 12 noon, 103·3°. 4 p.m., 103·5°. 8 p.m., 102·2°. 12 p.m., 98·6° F. 8.30 a.m., intense headache. Sulphate of quinine, 32 grains, by the mouth. 9.30 a.m., blood: a few plasmodia without pigment, or with very fine granules of pigment, discoid and annular. A few crescent-shaped full-grown forms. 3 p.m., depression. Blood: a few plasmodia without pigment, and some full-grown crescent-shaped forms. 5 p.m., sulphate of quinine, 32 grains, by the mouth.

9th.—Patient very weak; free from fever. Blood: a very few plasmodia without pigment in brassy ("ottonati") red blood-corpuscles. Round and crescent-shaped bodies shrivelled and broken up. The patient continues to take quinine.

This is a case of very mild irregular quotidian; the attacks become, without treatment, milder for some days, and then get worse again; and in correspondence with this we find that the parasites are at first but few in number, that then they become extremely rare, and at last disappear for a short space of time.

During the last two days the fever, as shown by the chart, is continued through the prolongation and conjunction of the quotidian paroxysms despite the administration of the remedy. (Continued quotidian through the prolongation and overlapping of paroxysms.)

CASE 3.[1]—Abate P—, 30 years old, took fever in Calabria on August 2nd, when he had continued fever for three days. Sixteen days ago he came to the hospital with a relapse of fever (quotidian). At present he has had quotidian fever for five days, accompanied by shivering, usually between 4 and 5 p.m. In the first attacks and in the first relapsing paroxysm he had no shivering at all.

September 8th.—4 p.m., temp. 104°. 8 p.m., 102·2°. 12 p.m., 101·5° F. 3 p.m., blood: several plasmodia without pigment, discoid, annular, or shaped like small rods, and mobile.

9th.—4 a.m., temp. 100·8°. 7 a.m., 98·8°. 12 noon, 102·2°. 4 p.m., 104·2°. 8 p.m., 103·5°. 12 p.m., 96·8° F. 8.30 a.m., blood: moderate number of discoid and annular plasmodia with granules of pigment; a very small number of younger forms; a very few white blood-corpuscles with granular pigment. 10 a.m., blood: the same, *plus* plasmodia, with granules of pigment in brassy ("ottonati") corpuscles. 11 a.m., blood: the same; the brassy ("ottonati") red blood-corpuscles seem to be increased. 3.30 p.m., a few plasmodia without pigment, mobile, annular, and discoid. 4.15 p.m., several plasmodia without pigment, mobile, annular, and discoid in different sizes; white blood-corpuscles with small clusters of pigment.

10th.—4 a.m., temp. 99·9°. 7.30 a.m., 99·7°. 12 noon, 100·2°. 4 p.m., 103·1°. 8 p.m., 102·2°. 12 p.m., 100·6° F. In the morning the patient feels pretty well. 9 a.m., blood: several discoid and annular plasmodia with granules of pigment, some of them mobile; the forms for the most part are rather small; some are in brassy ("ottonati") red blood-corpuscles. (Some plasmodia appear not to be pigmented.) 10.30 a.m., blood: condition as above. 3 p.m., blood: several plasmodia, annular and very mobile, without pigment; some discoid forms of indistinct outline; a very small number with little granules of pigment.

11th.—4 a.m., 99·7°. 7 a.m., 99·9°. 12 noon, 104·6°. 4 p.m., 102·8°. 8 p.m., 97·7°. 12 p.m., 99° F. 8.45 a.m., blood: moderate number of plasmodia without pigment, annular, discoid, and mobile. The discoid plasmodia with granules of pigment are larger than those seen at first; the annular and mobile forms with pigment are in less numbers. On the whole the large pigmented

[1] See Chart I, tracing 4.

forms are more numerous than the forms without pigment. From 9.30 a.m. till about noon, shivering. 10.40 a.m., blood: small plasmodia without pigment, mobile, a few annular, some in brassy ("ottonati") red blood-corpuscles; the annular and discoid plasmodia with pigment larger. 2.30 p.m., blood: a considerable number of plasmodia without pigment, discoid, annular, and mobile; a few with fine granules of pigment. There are also some rather large plasmodia without pigment. A few pigmented white blood-corpuscles. 4 p.m., blood: condition as above, *plus* a very few crescent-shaped forms. 5 p.m., bimuriate of quinine, 24 grains, by hypodermic injection.

12th.—Without fever. The patient feels pretty well. 9 a.m., blood: several plasmodia without pigment, as well as mobile forms, some of them in brassy ("ottonati") red blood-corpuscles. A few pigmented plasmodia. The patient's temperature rises slightly during the night of September 12-13th, and on the 14th he is quite free from fever. On September 15th, towards midday, he is taken with shivering and high fever. At the highest point of the fever, towards 3 p.m., a few plasmodia without pigment, together with some pigmented white blood-corpuscles and crescent-shaped forms are found in the blood. 6 p.m.: sulphate of quinine, 32 grains, by the mouth. The fever ceases in the night. The patient continues to take quinine during the following days, and makes a rapid recovery.

This is an example of irregular quotidian fever, in which the paroxysms differ in their gravity, and are anticipating (for instance, the third one) by a few hours. There is no complete intermission between the first paroxysms owing to their prolongation, and also because of the fresh paroxysm anticipating (for instance, the third attack in connection with the second). On the administration of a single dose of quinine the relapse follows three days afterwards, during which time abortive attacks take place. The examination of the parasites gives a rather complex result, seeing that it is the forms of a single generation which we always find predominant, although along with these there is often a less number of other forms which are a little forward or backward in development.

CHAPTER V.

THE SUMMER-AUTUMN TERTIAN.

Typical curve of this fever—Differences between the curve of the paroxysm in the mild tertian and the curve in the malignant tertian—Variations in the thermic curve of the paroxysm in the summer tertian—Prolonged paroxysms—Different ways in which the summer tertian becomes irregular: (1) *through modifications in the curve of the paroxysm;* (2) *through modifications in the succession of the attacks*—Amœba febris tertianæ æstivo-autumnalis; *morphological and biological characteristics—The amœba's life cycle at various periods in the clinical course of the fever—Different appearances of the parasites during the paroxysm, and interpretation of the prolonged attack—State of the blood in the very mild tertians—Connection of the crescent-shaped forms with the clinical course of the disease, and pathogenic importance of this phase in the amœba's life—Relapses*[1] *and recurrences*[2] *of fever* (ricadute e recidive)—*Examples of summer tertian.*

§ 22. The tertian type of the summer and autumn differs from the mild or spring tertian in the variety of the parasite; but not only so, it is different also in its clinical course, in its thermographic curve, in its tendency to become aggravated, and in the fact of the paroxysms approaching each other and becoming conjoined, so that in some cases we get a continuous febrile curve. In the simpler and more clearly intermittent cases the characteristics of the curve of fever are as follows:—It begins, as we find in all the malarial fevers, with an abrupt rise, usually to 104° F. or more; then follows a period in which the thermic curve oscillates to an extent perhaps exceeding two degrees. The most important of these oscillations is the one which precedes the crisis (*pre-critical elevation*); in this one the temperature usually reaches its maximum, and, as a rule, it comes after a remarkable fall in the fever, which is attended by a temporary improvement in all the symptoms. In

[1] After two to five days.

[2] After two weeks, or even after months.—Ed.

some cases this decrease in the fever, which is a forerunner of the terminal elevation, is so considerable that it may be mistaken for the real crisis by anyone who is not familiar with this characteristic feature of the fever as found in the summer tertian (*pseudo-crisis*). Hence we may make the following distinctions: *the invasion of the fever, a period of fever,* with oscillations in the temperature sometimes considerable, *a pseudo-crisis, the pre-critical elevation,* and *the crisis.* The whole paroxysm is usually very long; it exceeds, as a rule, twenty-four hours, and may last from thirty-six to forty hours, so that the intermission between two attacks is not longer than from eight to ten hours; and as the headache, the depression, and the gastric and intestinal disturbances remain, the patients believe and assert that the fever has been continuous. This is in the cases which are typically regular, in which the regularity may be so great that the curves of two successive attacks are identical in the hour of the invasion, in the oscillations during the period of fever, in the symptoms which accompany the fever, &c. (See Chart I.)

The differences in the fever curve between this form of tertian and the common tertian are conspicuous at once on examination, and are clearly made evident by our charts (see tracings 5, 6, 7, &c.). They are of such a nature that, if we keep to the classical definition of the tertian, it is impossible for us to give this name to the curve of fever as described. As a matter of fact there is not, on the day that intervenes between one paroxysm and another, that *perfecta integritas* which is often found, but not always[1] on the day free from fever in the common tertian; the attacks are protracted over a great part of the day which lies between the end of one paroxysm and the beginning of the following, so that the day of complete intermission between the two attacks is wanting. But each attack commences every third day (a fundamental characteristic of the tertian type), and is protracted into the following day: hence the summer-autumn tertian is nothing but a tertian with the paroxysms prolonged.

We would observe, further, that the curve we have described may be called typical of the summer tertian, because it is found with its different characteristic stages as we have

[1] According to Antolisei, it is no easy matter to find a case of *pure* spring tertian, that is to say, one without any thermic change on the day of apyrexia. Antolisei mentions, in this connection, that out of the very numerous cases of tertian, the charts of which, giving the temperature every three hours, were collected in the 'Clinica Medica,' only four or five were pure tertian ("Sull' ematozoo della Terzana," 'Riforma Med.,' Gennaio, 1890).

set forth in these cases, which through their clinical course, and through the regular succession of the parasitic forms in the blood, may be considered the simplest. It may, however, happen that we meet with a similar curve also in the common tertian, although under special conditions, and only by way of exception. Thus there has come under our notice a double spring tertian, in which the two paroxysms, instead of following each other, as is the general rule, at an interval of about twenty-four hours, more or less, were so approximated to each other that they were incompletely conjoined; in this way a curve was formed similar to that of a prolonged attack, with two very high elevations of temperature, each of them representing a tertian paroxysm. But in this case the form of prolonged attack resulted from the blending of two paroxysms, and corresponded to the coming to maturity of two generations of parasites which were produced within a few hours of each other; while the curve of the summer tertian, on the contrary, represents a single attack, and corresponds to the coming to maturity of a single generation of parasites, as we have determined.[1] So that we may affirm that *the curve we have described is a typical one for the summer tertian* [3].

When the paroxysm is developed according to the type described, with the different elevations in temperature as set down, the case is often a severe one: an aggravation of the clinical symptoms usually coincides with the beginning of the paroxysm and the pre-critical elevation; but, for the most part, the distress, agitation, and depression of the patient, as well as the clouding over of the sensorium, are at their maximum during the latter, and they have only an incomplete cessation during the following brief intermission. The same curve may, however, take place also in mild infections, where there is the same prolonged paroxysm, the same pre-critical elevation, &c. This form, then, of the thermic curve is connected with the development of the parasite, not necessarily with the fact of the infection taking a serious turn, although in the majority of cases there is the tendency to a progressive aggravation.

In the typical attack the initial and the pre-critical elevations may be alike in intensity; but in other cases, while the initial elevation reaches the ordinary degree of fever temperature as found in these diseases (*i. e.* 104°—104·9°), the pre-critical elevation may touch hyperpyretic temperatures (*e. g.* 106·7°, and even 107·6° F., in the axilla). When the pre-critical elevation is as high as this, it may be preceded by a sensation of cold or even

[1] See preliminary note, 'Rif. Med.,' No. 217, 1891.

by shivering, while the pseudo-crisis which goes before may be accompanied by sweating, which is usually moderate in amount.

The form of the paroxysm, and the complex curve resulting from the succession of the attacks, may vary in many different ways in the summer tertian. Thus it may happen that the initial elevation is wanting, or is but very little marked, so that its own individuality is lost, and it becomes mixed up with the rest of the fever curve. In the same way the pre-critical elevation may be wanting, or may be scarcely noticeable, so that the curve of the paroxysm, through the disappearance of the different oscillations, tends to become continuous, especially when the attack is relatively short. Furthermore, the fall in the temperature which follows the initial elevation may be so considerable as to almost reach normal; for the most part, however, the temperature keeps above 100·4° F. In cases like this the individuality of the attack is almost lost; we seem to have to do with two attacks, while in reality there is but one, as is shown by the study of the parasite's cycle of life. A fact of this sort occurs mostly in the very mild summer tertians, which, as we have said, are only rarely met with. In these cases the oscillations of temperature during the attacks are usually very marked, so that the individuality of the paroxysm is almost lost. At first sight the curve seems to be composed of quotidian attacks, brought together by two and two; but while what we find in the blood clearly shows the tertian origin of this irregular curve, when we come to look into it, we discover that the tertian origin is also demonstrated by the fact that every third day there is a complete intermission, while on the intermediate day the temperature hardly falls to 98·6° F., and that only for a short time, or else it remains somewhat above this. In spite of the pronounced pseudo-crisis, the individuality of the paroxysm can still be perfectly well recognised.

As we have already pointed out, it is to this type of fever that the prolonged paroxysms belong, and they may be observed even when, during the attack, liberal doses of quinine are given. The gravity of the form is for the most part connected with these prolonged paroxysms, and in the second place with their anticipating. This anticipation may be as much as from about eight to ten hours, so that the intermediate apyrexia may be very short, but, although short, complete. But this is not always the case; the prolongation of the paroxysms and their tendency to become blended are not necessarily incidents connected with malignancy in the disease; there are, on the contrary, mild forms of infection, with charts showing paroxysms which are protracted, though but little elevated in temperature. Neither does the anticipation of the paroxysms always coincide with the aggravation of the infection, and this is specially the case when the anticipation is only one of a few hours, and when the anticipating attacks are not at the same time noticeably prolonged.

From all this it results that the thermic curve may be irregular through the anticipation or the prolongation and conjunction of the attacks, not only in the dangerous forms (the subcontinued and malignant); it may also be so in the infections of medium gravity. In the latter, as in the former, we may find in the same chart prolonged or anticipating attacks, and slight elevations of temperature interposed between individual paroxysms in such a way that the interpretation of the charts becomes extremely difficult, and sometimes impossible. But the examination of the blood displays the life cycle of the tertian parasite, and accounts for the irregularity, as we shall see.

There are a number of reasons over and above those deduced from the examination of the blood of which we shall now speak; these assist us to bring back the irregular curves to the type of the summer tertian. The complex chart, or the chart with paroxysms separated by incomplete intermissions, is frequently seen in the primary infections: while it often happens that the fever shows itself regular and typical when it recurs;[1] and it is worth noticing that in this the first paroxysm not infrequently deviates from the type in being shorter and consisting of a single rise of the temperature, and followed immediately by the crisis; but this initial short paroxysm is succeeded by others with the typical curve. The same is also often noticed in the relapse; as well in this as in the recurrence itself, the disease usually begins with some typical paroxysms, after which it often becomes again complicated by one of the modifications already mentioned. In the second place, a fever chart having paroxysms which are prolonged, and sepa-

[1] It is very interesting to quote in this connection Sydenham's words, sect. 1, cap. 2, cited by Puccinotti, 'Opere Mediche,' Milano, 1856:—"Early in the month of July the intermittent autumnal fevers begin, and soon become frequent. They do not immediately assume the genuine type, which is usual in the case of the intermittent spring fevers; but they resemble in all points continued fevers in such a way that, unless you look into both of them with a most searching examination, it is impossible to distinguish between them; and when the impetuosity of the epidemic constitution has been restrained and its force has been checked little by little, they then merge into the regular type." *Vide* Sydenham Society's Edition, 1848, vol. i, p. 37.—ED.

rated only by incomplete intermissions, may become regular, and the paroxysms well individualised, after the administration of a certain quantity of quinine, provided the remedy be not repeated and continued. In the third place, the examination of many thermoscopic tracings demonstrates the fact that there exist all forms of transition between the typical paroxysm and the irregular curves of the dangerous forms on the one hand, or those of the forms of very mild infection on the other, in such a way that it may be maintained that these latter ought to bring us back to the fundamental type of the summer tertian.

Summing up what has been said so far, we arrive at the conclusion that the curve of the summer tertian may become complex, or irregular, or atypic (so to say), in different ways:

1. By modifications in the curve of the attack.

The chief modifications in the curve of the paroxysm are as follows:—The absence of a clearly defined initial elevation, so that the curve rises in a progressive and continuous manner. The exaggeration of the pseudo-crisis, so that the paroxysm tends to lose its own individuality. The prolongation of the paroxysm, which is usually accompanied by an exaggeration of the thermic oscillations of this stage. The absence of a clearly defined pre-critical elevation.

2. By modifications in the succession of the paroxysms.

The modifications in the succession of the paroxysms consist in the anticipation of the paroxysms, which may happen as well in the severe forms as in the mild. The postponement, which may happen also in the severe infections. The prolongation of the paroxysms, through which the intermission becomes incomplete or nearly so. The presence of slight oscillations in temperature during the period which ought to be that of apyrexia. The doubling of the attacks (double summer tertian).

3. The complex or irregular curves may also be produced—

(a) By the presence in the blood of two varieties of parasites (e.g. the mixed infection of the summer and spring).

(b) By the intervention of some therapeutic action (salts of quinine, methylene blue,[1] &c.). It must not, however, be forgotten that the action of quinine may also, in some cases (and we shall see later on in what way), determine the simplification of an irregular or complex curve.

§ 23. *The summer-autumn tertian is connected with the life cycle of an amœba, which is developed within about forty-eight hours.*

[1] Up to twenty-four grains a day in divided doses of medicinal methylene blue, Meister Lucius and Brüning, Berlin.—Ed.

This life cycle is completed in perfect correspondence with the clinical course, as is the case with the other varieties of the malarial parasite. Thus, if the blood be examined at the height of the paroxysm, we find small amœbæ without pigment and without motion, annular or discoid, or furnished with pseudopodia in motion. As the period of apyrexia approaches the amœba begins to be pigmented at the periphery and to increase in size; during the apyrexia it continues to grow larger, and the pigmentation becomes very marked, while the amœba keeps extremely mobile, until just before maturity the movements grow more sluggish, and then cease altogether. The size at this stage may be from a quarter to almost half that of the red blood-corpuscle. During the period which leads up to the new paroxysm there is, as a rule, a noteworthy decrease in the number of the parasites in the blood taken from the finger; and while in the majority of patients the forms of fission, and those which precede the fission, are very rarely found, and almost exclusively in severe cases, instead of these we meet with numerous adult forms enclosed in shrivelled red blood-corpuscles, which have become in colour like brass or old gold (brassy—"ottonati"—red blood-corpuscles); and there are also white blood-corpuscles with granules or masses of pigment, the remains of dead adult forms, or of disintegrated forms of spore formation. The forms which precede the fission are represented by round or ovoid corpuscles, which are in size between a quarter and half that of the red blood-corpuscle, having the pigment collected at the centre or slightly eccentric, in a small mass or in a cluster of granules in motion. The forms of fission vary in size; they may be as large as two thirds of the red blood-corpuscle, and are composed of one or two circles of spores (usually ten or twelve, seldom fifteen to sixteen) [4] arranged round the central mass of pigment. In the tertian as well as in the quotidian the reproductive phase of the amœba is completed by preference in some of the viscera, while those adult forms whose evolution has been arrested continue to circulate for a certain time. Hence it follows that it is difficult in one and the same case to trace the development of the parasite's entire life cycle; it is necessary to construct it by means of observations made on many different patients, taking account also of what we find at autopsies. At the beginning of the paroxysm examination usually yields a very scanty result, and in some cases the parasitic forms even entirely disappear, while the new generation may also, by some hours, delay its appearance within the red blood-corpuscles that have been invaded; then the young plasmodia progressively increase in number step by step with the development of the paroxysm, and recommence the life cycle as described.

Accordingly, from what has been said so far, we may distinguish in the life cycle of this amœba three phases, which pass from the one to the other by a series of modes of transition, with no sharply defined boundaries.

The phase of the young forms is represented by hyaline plasmodia, without pigment, diaphanous, generally rather large, in size from a fifth to a fourth of that of the red blood-corpuscle; there may also be found along with these, amœbæ of very small dimensions, not larger than a third of the former. These forms, which, as in the quotidian, may be annular and discoid in shape, or display lively movements, are contained, for the most part, in red blood-corpuscles [5] of normal aspect: nevertheless in some the hæmoglobin takes a deeper colour than usual, the corpuscle itself tending to become smaller.

This phase of life commonly has a long duration, and lasts during the whole, or almost the whole, of the paroxysm. Then the outline of the amœba grows somewhat indistinct, without, however, the granules of pigment becoming discernible on the margin so modified, even if we make the most careful observation; or in other cases the amœba encloses some particles of red blood-corpuscle, in which the colour of the hæmoglobin goes on changing under the eyes of the observer.

These are the appearances that precede the phase of pigmentation. This phase is represented by amœbæ which vary in size from a fourth to a third of that of the red blood-corpuscle, with very fine granules of pigment, generally arranged on the edge of the amœba, but sometimes also scattered about in the protoplasm of the parasite. Forms are found as well whose size is considerably less than that of the preceding. Although the granules of pigment are, as a rule, without motion, they may happen to display a movement and oscillation like the pigment of the amœba in the common tertian,—and this is specially so in the larger forms. After pigmentation the amœba may take the same forms that it assumes in the preceding phase; it may be annular, discoid, or mobile. The discoid forms frequently have, as it were, a wavy outline; the annular forms are large, have a shining appearance, and are capable of returning to motion; the mobile forms often assume strange shapes,—for instance, dendritic. The blood-corpuscles which contain the pigmented amœbæ are of normal size and aspect; but much more frequently than those blood-corpuscles which contain younger plasmodia, they display a darker colouring than usual, which tends to take a brassy tint. And when (as we have already remarked) the end of the apyrexia approaches, and the new paroxysm is shortly to begin, this change in the red blood-corpuscle goes on till it is completely shrivelled up; at the same time the pigmented amœba loses its power of motion, and ceases to grow larger.

After this phase come the modifications which prepare and complete the fission. By a process analogous to that which is seen in the other varieties of malarial parasites, the pigment collects into a group of granules at the centre, or a little outside the centre, these granules are sometimes mobile and oscillating, and they may form into a single mass with very sharply defined outline, or again they may form two small masses.

As we have said, the size of these bodies varies from a fourth to a half of the red blood-corpuscle; as a rule it is about one third. It is possible to find also smaller forms, which we have seen in two cases of malignant tertian. The red blood-corpuscle containing these bodies is seldom of normal size; it is generally shrunken, frequently atrophic, and of the colour of old brass.

The fission is not completed in all the corpuscles that have central pigment. Many are swallowed up together with the red blood-corpuscles by leucocytes; others may be seen free in the plasma, and in these is sometimes noted a process by which they tend to form vacuoles, and evidently in this way they degenerate and die.

The forms in which the fission is completed are always found in red blood-corpuscles radically changed [6]; they occur in red blood-corpuscles shrivelled up and brassy in colour, and in red blood-corpuscles entirely discoloured and dried up, or else they are free in the plasma. The general appearance of the forms ready for extruding the spores is more bulky than that of the corresponding forms with central pigment (see Figs. 1—45, Plate II).

§ 24. This life cycle of the amœba takes place in close connection with the various phases of the paroxysm and with the succession of the paroxysms in the way described. There are, however, other facts worth noticing to which we shall now direct attention.

As we have said, during the first hours of the paroxysm of fever the adult forms gradually decrease until they disappear, so that the result of the examination of the blood may be negative for some hours—that is to say, until the moment when the new generation shows itself.

But there are cases in which some adult forms (*i. e.* large pigmented plasmodia, and bodies with pigment at the centre in brassy red blood-corpuscles) continue to be seen in the blood during a great part of the paroxysm. Usually these forms are rare, but sometimes (and this usually happens by preference during the course of the prolonged paroxysms) the adult pigmented forms remain in the blood in considerable numbers, and only when the paroxysm is far advanced do they slowly give up the field to the young plasmodia. In some cases this is so pronounced as to make one believe that the coming to maturity of the parasitic forms, takes place in groups during the attack, in such a way that an elevation in the temperature corresponds to the maturation of each group (sporulation), while the pre-critical elevation is correlated with the delayed sporulation of the last group.

It may also happen that some adult forms reappear in the blood when the paroxysm is in an advanced stage, they having disappeared—at least from the blood of the finger—at its beginning. In the same way the forms in which the process of fission has already begun may do the same thing, as well as the bodies which have already completed spore formation. In the fevers of medium gravity and in the mild ones they are either not found at all or else very rarely, and only at the beginning of the paroxysm, and for the most part in company with forms less advanced in development (amœbæ with granules of pigment at the circumference). Whereas in severe cases, and especially when the paroxysms are prolonged, they may continue to be seen throughout the paroxysm and even up to the pre-critical elevation. Nevertheless the forms of fission which may be found in the blood of the finger when the attack is far advanced are always extremely few in number. This completion of the maturation or spore formation of the amœba in a rather long period, and in successive groups, is probably the chief cause of the prolonged attack; indeed, in the quartan and tertian we see the attack, which is usually of short duration, renewed simultaneously with the reproduction of the amœba, which takes but a short time to accomplish; whereas in the prolonged paroxysms of the summer tertian the observer may frequently convince himself of the fact that the reproduction takes place not only at the beginning of the paroxysm, but continues to go on after it has reached an advanced stage, as we have seen. If, as appears more than probable, a certain quantity of pyrogenic matter is liberated in the blood by the act of the parasitic reproduction, the observation we have related gives sufficient reason for the prolongation of the paroxysm.

The new generation (plasmodia without pigment) generally

appears when the paroxysm is advanced; the first young forms make their appearance, as a rule, during the first six hours of the paroxysm, and reach their maximum in point of number towards its close, after the pre-critical elevation. They begin to become pigmented during the intermission, but while in some cases the pigmentation in a certain number of forms is backward, so that even eight or ten hours before the new attack young plasmodia without pigment are seen in the blood, in other cases it is premature, and we accordingly see the amœba develop and become pigmented, even before the paroxysm is finished, during the pre-critical elevation and the crisis. This development takes place more rapidly than usual when the paroxysms tend to be anticipating.

We have stated that during the six hours which precede the attack (and sometimes also for a longer time—ten or twelve hours) it is the adult pigmented forms which, as a rule, are exclusively found in the blood (these are the plasmodia with granules of pigment, and the forms with small masses at the centre). Nevertheless the development of a certain number of parasitic forms may be delayed, so that even from eight to ten hours before the expected paroxysm a few plasmodia without pigment may be found in the blood along with the adult forms; these then gradually decrease in number, while the adult pigmented forms increase. On the other hand, the sporulation in a small number of forms may precede the attack by some hours; in one case, indeed, a very small number of fissions were observed by us about twelve hours before the paroxysm. These facts, these deviations from the law, may be easily explained. Thus we may obviously suppose that the coming to maturity of a certain number of parasitic forms is necessary for the production of the paroxysms; while, if the amount of fissions fall below a certain limit, which of course cannot be determined with exactness, then the paroxysm does not take place.

All this, however, does not invalidate the law which establishes the connection between the life cycle of the parasite and the clinical evolution of the fever. This law may be formulated as follows:—*The return of the paroxysms is determined by the fact, that the parasites set free in the blood a certain quantity of pyrogenic material, in the act of their reproduction.*

In the very mild fevers the results of the examination of the blood are usually extremely meagre, so much so that one cannot succeed in following the life cycle of the plasmodium. Seeing that in these cases we usually get a negative result at the beginning and in the first hours of the paroxysm, and that the new generation appears only when the paroxysm has become advanced, it follows that the relatively larger number of parasitic forms occurs during the intermission. In the mildest fevers of all, which are often irregular through the presence of abortive or incomplete attacks, which lend themselves with difficulty to be studied, it may be impossible to find plasmodia in the blood even for twenty-four hours and more; while, if the plasmodia be wanting, there may be found in circulation a very few pigmented white blood-corpuscles.

§ 25. As in the quotidians, so in the summer tertian, one of the life phases of the amœba is represented by Laveran's so-called crescent-shaped bodies. The question of the connection of these forms with the life cycle of the amœba and with the clinical evolution of the fever has been recently investigated by Bignami and Bastianelli; our own latest researches have furnished us with no new elements likely to help towards the solution of the difficulty, which concerns the biology and the meaning of these forms, and which has been so much discussed.[1]

Bignami and Bastianelli, in their investigations of the fevers belonging to this group (the quotidians and the tertians taken together), have established the following facts:

1. "On the seventh or eighth day of the disease there are found in the blood extracted from the spleen, and exceptionally also in the blood of the finger (*i. e.* in cases where the parasites are extremely numerous), endoglobular pigmented corpuscles, ovoid or spindle-shaped, the evolution of which may be traced up to the adult crescent-shaped form. During the first paroxysms the blood of the spleen, especially if it be taken near the beginning of the paroxysm, usually shows the presence of round corpuscles within the red blood-corpuscles, with central pigment, in some of which the formation of spores may be seen to be proceeding; but after a variable number of paroxysms, a certain number of corpuscles with central pigment, instead of advancing to sporulation, take the ovoid or spindle-shaped form, and develop into the falciform body."

"The presence of these corpuscles, as soon as they can be differ-

[1] For the various opinions expressed on this subject see Bignami and Bastianelli, "Osservazioni sulle Febbri Malariche Estivo-Autunnali," 'Riforma Med.,' 1890. On the morphology of the crescent-shaped forms see Antolisei, "Intorno alla Classificazione dei Parassiti della Malaria," 'Rif. Medica,' Aprile, 1890, and Celli e Guarnieri, "Sulla Etiologia della Infezione Malarica," 'Arch. per le Scienze Mediche,' 1889. Here we devote our attention solely to the connection between this phase in the amœba's life and the clinical evolution of the fever.

entiated, may be generally apparent about the seventh day from the beginning of the infection; but in some cases they have been found on the fifth or sixth day on examination of the blood of the spleen: in severe infections, when the corpuscles were in great abundance, they have even been detected in the blood of the finger at that date. If we only study the blood of the finger, instead of that of the spleen, it frequently happens that we find bodies of the crescent-shaped phase only on the eighth or ninth day; but in these cases we have nearly always to do with bodies which are already well developed."

"After the formation of the young crescent-shaped forms has thus commenced, on an average towards the seventh or eighth day of the disease, their production continues with each successive paroxysm, so that after a series of attacks the blood contains an accumulation of crescent-shaped forms. Excepting, however, those cases in which the parasites are very numerous, such as the severe subcontinued and malignant fevers, it is always difficult to find in the blood of the finger the young endoglobular crescent-shaped forms."

"Thus in all the fevers of this group, which have been studied for a sufficiently long time without therapeutic interference, we are able to trace the development of the plasmodia, on the one hand up to the corpuscle with central pigment, and its fission, and on the other hand up to the young endoglobular crescent-shaped form; and the conclusion we arrive at is that the amœba of the summer-autumn fevers (the *Amœba præcox* of Grassi and Feletti) and the crescent-shaped body are two forms of one and the same parasite, and not two different parasites."[1]

2. Whether the fever ceases spontaneously, or this be brought about by the action of quinine, the crescent-shaped forms continue to be seen in the blood for one or two weeks; as a rule, after nine or ten days of freedom from fever they diminish considerably in number, and then disappear in a few days.

In this interval there are usually seen in the blood crescent-shaped forms becoming vacuolated and disintegrated, and from time to time also young crescent-shaped forms; but we cannot succeed in tracing a progressive development of these bodies up to the paroxysms of the recurrence of the fever, which generally ensue after a period manifestly equal to the time of the malarial parasite's incubation (for the most part a little less than two weeks).

3. On the recurrence of the paroxysms the development of the

[1] Loc. cit.

amœbæ is completed just as in the fevers of the original infection, and the life cycle is certainly not slower and different from the former, as other writers have maintained.

Bignami and Bastianelli base their argument on these facts, and also on the fact that they have never succeeded in finding forms of spore formation or fission belonging to the crescent-shaped bodies, and this "not only after systematically examining the blood of the spleen during the different periods of the infection, but also not even after studying the fresh organs in cases of malignant fever in which, throughout all their stages of development, bodies of the crescent-shaped phase were accumulated in very large numbers." Hence they formulate with reserve the hypothesis that the crescent-shaped bodies represent sterile forms of the parasites belonging to this group of fevers.[1]

The question is certainly still far from being solved. At present we shall confine ourselves to a statement of the facts resulting from observations which have recently been carried out in a series of fifty-nine cases in which only the blood of the finger was examined; and we shall concern ourselves exclusively with the points of connection between the clinical development of the fever, and the presence in the blood of these parasitic forms, at the same time abstaining from a discussion of the hypotheses that have been put forward concerning their morphology and significance. If our latest results be compared with those of Bignami and Bastianelli, which we have already mentioned, it is necessary to bear in mind an observation which these writers have made, namely, that the administration of quinine may exert an influence on the crescent-shaped forms, and cause their appearance to be more or less delayed; thus if quinine, for instance, be given at once from the beginning of the fever in sufficiently large doses, the crescent-shaped phase of the parasite may be entirely wanting, and it may only appear in the recurring attacks. The recurrence takes place after a

[1] Kruse also seems to accept the opinion that the crescent-shaped bodies have no phase of sporulation.

"The crescent-shaped bodies" (he says), "although the contrary may be believed, are not capable of a progressive development, but frequently turn into spindle-shaped bodies, either ovoid or round, which may be flagellated. The fact that there may be in the blood a considerable number of adult crescent-shaped forms without fever being caused, weighs against the possibility of their having a progressive development; and the facts which are known in relation to the analogous forms of the other blood-parasites bear the same testimony."—D. W. Kruse, "Der gegenwärtige Stand unserer Kenntnisse von den parassitären Protozoen," 'Separatabdruck aus der Hygien. Rundschau, 1892, No. 9 (pp. 39, 40).

period of time, usually a little less than a fortnight, equally in these cases as in those in which, after some paroxysms of the primary infection, the forms of the crescent-shaped phase made their appearance in the blood. We now give the results of the most recent researches. We have found no crescent-shaped forms in twenty-eight cases of primary infection; that is to say, in seventeen cases of summer tertian, in nine cases of quotidian or tertian subcontinued fever, and in two cases of quotidian. In these cases we continued our researches, as a rule, till the fifth, sixth, and seventh day of the disease, rarely till the ninth, and in one instance until the twelfth day. We must, however, remark that in many of these cases quinine was given from the fourth or fifth, sometimes from the third day of the fever, and in large doses, and this may influence the appearance, more or less rapid, of the crescent-shaped forms, as Bignami and Bastianelli have observed. In the second place, the fact also determined by Bignami and Bastianelli must not be forgotten, namely, that the appearance of the crescent-shaped forms in the blood of the finger may not be observed till some days after these forms have already been found in the spleen. All our observations have been made with the blood of the finger.

Among the different cases there was one of comatose malignant fever which deserves mention. In this instance death supervened on the ninth day of the disease, the treatment with quinine having been only commenced on the fifth day. No crescent-shaped forms were found even in the viscera, and in the spleen alone were seen some small ovoid forms within the red blood-corpuscles, which possibly might be explained as young crescent-shaped forms.

The crescent-shaped bodies were found in thirteen cases of primary infection, usually between the seventh and eighth day of the disease, rarely as soon as on the fifth day, and rarely also later than on the tenth, twelfth, and fourteenth day. The crescent-shaped forms were often only found when, after the first doses of quinine had been given, the infection passed away. In one case, simultaneously with the appearance of the crescent-shaped forms the infection became milder of itself, and then disappeared.

From these facts we conclude (as Bignami and Bastianelli have already done from their observations) that during the first paroxysms of fever the crescent-shaped phase of the parasite does not occur; that it appears only after several paroxysms, and in some of the viscera, such as the spleen and the bone marrow, before being visible in the blood of the finger. If quinine be administered from a very early stage the infection may pass away (excepting the chance of a recurrence later on) before the formation of the bodies of the crescent-shaped phase has taken place. On the other hand, if quinine be not given till a later stage, it almost seems as if the transition of the parasite into this phase of life is thereby promoted and furthered; for the crescent-shaped forms appear and continue in the blood of the finger, while the other parasitic forms disappear.

In the recurrences, just as in the original infections, the crescent-shaped forms were found from the sixth to the eighth day of the disease, rarely on the fifth day,—always, be it understood, in the blood of the finger. The same fact was observed as well in the quotidians as in the tertians, as well in the cases where we were dealing with a first as in those of a second and third recurrence.

The crescent-shaped forms, then, become visible in the fevers which recur only after some paroxysms have run their course, as Bignami and Bastianelli have remarked.

There were only eight cases of the recurring infection in which no crescent-shaped forms were found, although they were observed up to the fifth and sixth day. We must, however, bear in mind that some of these patients took quinine on the fourth day of the disease, while with others the infection was extremely mild, and only a very small number of parasites were found,—facts which may serve to explain the late appearance of this phase in the life of the plasmodium.

Among these cases we had instances of tertian, of quotidian, and of subcontinued fever, in some patients the second recurrence was observed, but in the greater number the first, and in one case the fourth.

In our opinion these observations also allow us to draw the conclusion which we have expressed on this subject in our preliminary publication. The development of the fever, alike in the summer tertian as in the quotidian, is in intimate connection with the evolution of the amœba's life cycle, and this not only in the original infections, before the crescent-shaped forms have appeared in the blood, but also in the recurrences of the fever when these forms have become visible; and therefore we consider it inexact to say that these fevers owe their origin to falciform hæmatozoa. It is not the crescent-shaped body, but the amœba that has the greatest pathogenic importance,—the amœba which passes through a developmental cycle with every paroxysm of fever.

§ 26. *Relapses and recurrences of fever.*—All medical men know that almost all the fevers belonging to this group are liable to recurrences—frequently obstinate ones. We have drawn attention to the fact that the recurrence of the fever takes place for the most part after intervals of variable length of freedom from fever, lasting, where the infections are not of very old standing, about a fortnight, usually a little less; and that if the infections continue a long time, and through their long duration become milder, then the intervals are somewhat longer. We have also noted that these intervals are generally equivalent in their length to the time of incubation of the malarial parasite—a fact which has been determined by Antolisei's, Gualdi's, and Angelini's experimental inoculations on the human subject.

During this period of natural temperatures the examination of the blood gives, in a number of cases, a completely negative result, while in others it discloses the presence of parasitic forms belonging to the group of crescent-shaped bodies. If the apyrexia be complete, no forms belonging to the pyrogenic cycle of the amœba are found in the blood; in those cases in which from time to time a very small number of amœbæ appear in the blood, the patients usually have slight elevations of temperature, reaching to about 100·4° F. in the evening or during the night.

We wish now specially to draw attention to the fact that very frequently the fevers that recur are made up of groups of paroxysms which are much more regular and distinctly intermittent than those of the primary infection. For instance, one may see a typical summer tertian in the recurring fever, while in the original infection the fever was irregular or subcontinued. But it is the quotidians especially which, in the majority of cases, are observed to be distinctly intermittent in their form only in the relapses. Perhaps it may be true to suppose that this peculiarity of the fevers stands in connection with the way in which, in the two cases, the infection arises. In the original fevers the infection comes from the surrounding atmosphere, and, as everything would lead us to believe, from the actual inhalation of the air. From this it will be understood how in a large number of cases parasites must be found in the blood in different stages of development, and, *considering that a periodic series of paroxysms corresponds to the evolution of a single generation of parasites*, how it is that the fever in these cases is irregular or complex. In many cases the curve becomes regular without any therapeutic treatment being employed; and we may suppose that this occurs because the predominant generation of parasites continues to develop, and thus determines a series of periodic paroxysms, while the parasitic groups or colonies of secondary importance become exhausted, cease to develop, and finally disappear.

On the other hand, in the recurrences, the fever is determined by the fact that parasitic forms, which have remained during the whole of the apyrexia in a condition of latent life, after a fairly constant period of time begin again to develop in the blood, and to complete their normal life cycle. It is more than probable that these forms, which thus persist, are represented by a certain number of spores deposited in the spleen and in the bone marrow during the acute infection before they have given place to the development of young amœbæ; from these would be evolved, after a period corresponding to the time of incubation, the new parasitic colony which determines the recurring fever. And also in those cases where the original infection was determined by more than one generation, and where in consequence the fever was complex or irregular, the relapsing fever on the other hand, arising in an entirely special manner, would be frequently determined by a single generation of amœbæ; whence the greater regularity and simplicity of the fever.

It is necessary to distinguish the recurrences from the relapses of fevers. These latter are often separated from the group of paroxysms of the first infection by only a short interval (that is to say, three, four, or five days), and occur usually when an insufficient quantity of quinine has been given, or when it has not been continued long enough. In this case the actual infection has not entirely exhausted itself, and the interval which lies between the first and second group of paroxysms cannot be considered as a real period of latency. As a matter of fact the apyrexia, for the most part, is not complete, but is interrupted by abortive paroxysms, which often pass unobserved both by patients and physicians unless thermometric observations be made frequently. Some amœboid forms may also be found from time to time in the blood, but in such small numbers that it is impossible to follow their life cycle until the relapse of the fever suddenly appears with its usual parasitic characteristics (see Chart II, tracing 14).

§ 27. We shall only give here in detail a few cases of summer tertian as an illustration of some of the facts mentioned by us, and we would remark that each of these cases must be considered as an example of a group of similar ones which we have observed.

CASE 4.[1]—Saverio B—, 37 years old, a carter, able-bodied,

[1] See Chart I, tracing 5.

coming from Storta. Has had fever in the beginning of August from the 8th to the 12th; the fever appears to have been incessant all that time except during brief intervals; the patient cannot specify the type. There have also been recurrences, the date and duration of which he is unable to determine. He has now had fever for four days, and says that the fever is severe on one day, diminishes or ceases on the following, only to increase again on the day after that, without shivering. He complains of abdominal pains and diarrhœa. Spleen very large.

On September 2nd the patient says that he had high fever.

September 3rd.—10 a.m., blood: many discoid and annular plasmodia; *large-sized* ones in motion, with small granules of pigment at the circumference, some of which are in movement. 3.30 p.m., blood: as above, but the quantity of parasites considerably decreased. Some white blood-corpuscles with little masses of pigment. 5.15 p.m., blood: a few annular and discoid plasmodia, with small pigmented granules, found in brassy red blood-corpuscles. A very small number of white blood-corpuscles with little clusters of pigment. 12 noon, temp. 97·5°. 4 p.m., 101·5°. 6 p.m., 104°. 8 p.m., 102·2°. 12 p.m., 102° F.

4th.—8.30 a.m., the fever continues high. Blood: a few discoid and annular plasmodia without pigment. 2 p.m., profuse sweating; the headache, hitherto intense, decreases. Blood: there are still some discoid plasmodia without pigment, also mobile and annular ones. 4.30 p.m., blood: many plasmodia without pigment, as above. 4 a.m., temp. 102·2°. 8 a.m., 101·4°. 12 noon, 104·6°. 4 p.m., 100·9°. 12 p.m., 96·8° F.

5th.—Intermission; patient feeling well; has appetite. 8.30 a.m., blood: many discoid plasmodia, annular and mobile, with granules of pigment; the *large-sized* mobile forms are predominant. 9.45 a.m., blood: as above; in addition, several pigmented plasmodia in brassy red blood-corpuscles. 3.30 p.m., the temperature has already risen. The patient states that he began to feel ill towards 2 p.m., with a sensation of heat; no shivering. Blood: a very few pigmented plasmodia in brassy shrivelled red blood-corpuscles. 4.30 p.m., the fever is already very high. No young forms are found in the blood as yet. 4 a.m., temp. 96·8°. 7 a.m., 97·2°. 12 noon, 98·6°. 4 p.m., 104°. 8 p.m., 103·8°. 12 p.m., 103·6° F.

6th.—The fever continues. Towards 8.30 a.m. there is a slight sweating. Blood: a rather scanty number of discoid and annular plasmodia with pigment. A very few adult crescent-shaped forms. Many white blood-corpuscles with small masses of pigment. 3.30 p.m., the fever has become slight. Blood: a moderate number of plasmodia without pigment, discoid, annular, and mobile—some with indistinct outline. The adult crescent-shaped forms very rare. Several white blood-corpuscles with little masses of pigment. 4 a.m., temp. 102·2°. 8 a.m., 103·1°. 12 noon, 103·6°. 4 p.m., 101·5°. 8 p.m., 98·6°. 12 p.m., 96·8° F.

7th.—Intermission in the morning. 10 a.m., blood: several *large-sized* plasmodia, annular, discoid, and mobile, with small pigmented granules (in size from a third to a fourth of the red blood-corpuscle); a few are found in blood-corpuscles which are tending to become brassy. 2.30 p.m., intermission; condition good. Blood: as above; in addition, some white pigmented blood-corpuscles with needles of pigment. 4.30 p.m., the fever begins. Blood: only a very small number of pigmented plasmodia. 6 p.m., sulphate of quinine, 32 grains, by the mouth. Temp., 4 a.m., 96·1°. 7 a.m., 96·8°. 12 noon, 96·5°. 4 p.m., 100·4°. 8 p.m., 101·3°. 12 p.m., 100·9° F.

8th.—Intermission. Patient very weak. Sulphate of quinine 24 grains by the mouth. 9.30 a.m., a very small number of plasmodia, without pigment, in motion; some with very fine granules of pigment. The crescent-shaped forms are extremely rare, and likewise the pigmented white blood-corpuscles. The patient continues to take quinine during the day. Temp., 4 a.m., 99·4°. 7.30 a.m., 100·2°. 12 noon, 99·2°. 4 p.m., 99·5°. 8 p.m., 97·9°. 12 p.m., 97·4° F.

9th.—The natural temperature continues. In the blood there are only a very few adult crescent-shaped forms, and a small number of pigmented white blood-corpuscles. The patient improves rapidly during the following days, continuing to take quinine.

This is a case of summer tertian. The biological cycle of the parasite is developed typically, the microbes decreasing in a remarkable manner at the beginning of the paroxysm, and increasing during the intermission while the new paroxysm is in course of preparation. In the first paroxysm there is a strong pre-critical elevation, which is but little marked in the second.

The sulphate of quinine, which was given when the temperature began to rise in the third attack, caused the paroxysm to become abortive; only an extremely small number of plasmodia developed, giving a correspondingly small number of young forms.

Case 5.[1]—The following is a characteristic example of summer

[1] See Chart II, tracing 8.

tertian, not only owing to the regularity of its curve, but also because of the uniform succession of the different phases of the parasite's life.

Torretta F—, 42 years old, able-bodied. Has had malarial fever last year, with recurrences up to April of this year. He works near Storta, where he contracted fever again on September 6th. On that day the fever began towards noon, and lasted till midnight; on the 7th it commenced, according to the patient, at noon, and ceased the morning after; the third attack was short, lasting from 2 to 7 p.m. After this the disease became aggravated; from September 11th onwards the fever was continued.

12th.—11 a.m., slight fever. Blood: a moderate number of plasmodia without pigment, discoid, annular, and mobile, some with granules of pigment. Towards 1 p.m., shivering. 2.45 p.m., the fever high. Blood: several plasmodia without pigment, discoid and annular; with very lively movement, and young; several with fine granules of pigment, discoid in shape. 4.30 p.m., blood: as above, there are some pigmented plasmodia in brassy blood-corpuscles. The fever ceased spontaneously in the night. Temp., 11.30 a.m., 101·3°. 2.45 p.m., 105·8°. 4 p.m., 107·2°. 8 p.m., 102·8°. 12 p.m., 99° F.

13th.—Free from fever in the morning; the patient feels well. 8.30 a.m., blood: moderate number of plasmodia with small granules of pigment, discoid and annular in shape, moving slowly, of medium size. A very inconsiderable number of small annular plasmodia without pigment. Some white blood-corpuscles with granules and small clumps of pigment. 9.30 a.m., blood: there are only annular and discoid plasmodia, pigmented and in motion; white blood-corpuscles as above. 3 p.m., the patient begins to feel ill. Blood: many plasmodia, with fine granules of pigment, annular and discoid in shape, in motion, but the greater part of them *without motion*—of medium and also large size (some almost as much as a half of the red blood-corpuscle). There are many in brassy red blood-corpuscles—one round form in a brassy red blood-corpuscle with the pigment collected towards the circumference. Some white blood-corpuscles with small masses of pigment.

3.45 p.m., intense shivering. Blood: same as above. The brassy red blood-corpuscles have increased in number. There is one form with a small clump at the centre. 4.30 p.m., the shivering has ceased. Blood: the condition is as above, but the forms are somewhat less in number. Some brassy red blood-corpuscles are very much shrivelled up. *No young forms are observed.* Temp., 4 a.m., 97°. 7 a.m., 96·8°. 12 noon, 97·3°. 4 p.m., 103·3°. 8 p.m., 104·2°. 12 p.m., 104·5° F.

14th.—The high fever continues; the patient is quiet. 8.45 a.m., blood: a few young amœboid forms. 9 a.m., blood: plasmodia as above. Many white blood-corpuscles with small masses of pigment. 3 p.m., blood: several plasmodia without pigment, or with very fine granules of pigment, discoid and annular in shape, and in motion. There are still many white blood-corpuscles with little masses of pigment, and a single young crescent-shaped form. 4 p.m., blood: the same; in addition, one specimen with small mass at the centre *in the act of sporulation.* The fever completely passes away in the night. Temp., 4 a.m., 102·6°. 7.30 a.m., 102·6°. 12 noon, 101·6°. 4 p.m., 105·8°. 8 p.m., 102·2°. 12 p.m., 98·1° F.

15th.—8.30 a.m., intermission; condition of patient good. Blood: many *large-sized* plasmodia, discoid and annular in shape, with sluggish movements; all with granules of pigment. A few pigmented white blood-corpuscles. 8 a.m., sulphate of quinine, 32 grains, by the mouth. 3 p.m., blood: the same as above; in addition some pigmented plasmodia in brassy red blood-corpuscles. Towards 5 p.m. there is profuse sweating, with normal temperature. Temp., 4 a.m., 96·8°. 7 a.m., 97°. 12 noon, 98°. 4 p.m., 98°. 8 p.m., 100·4°. 12 p.m. 102·4° F.

16th.—A mild and delayed attack of fever followed after the administration of quinine. 9 a.m., a few white blood-corpuscles, with granules and small masses of pigment. 4 p.m., the blood is in the same condition. Temp., 8 a.m., 100·6°. 12 noon, 100·6°. 4 p.m., 101·1°. 8 p.m., 99·5°. 12 p.m., 97·2° F. The normal temperature continues.

In this case, as we have remarked, the curve of the tertian was typical. As regards the parasites found in the blood, it is to be noted how one fissional form is found near the time of the pre-critical elevation; which fact harmonises with what we have said about the interpretation of the prolonged attacks. The expected attack is delayed and rendered abortive by the administration of quinine some hours before; the new generation does not develop completely, and the freedom from fever continues, although no more quinine is given.

Case 6.[1]—The following is another example of a typical attack of summer tertian:—Pelliccioni P—, 28 years old, works at Magliana; has malarial fever for the first time. For four days

[1] See Chart I, tracing 7.

he suffered from headache, but says that he has only had fever since July 31st. He enters the hospital on August 1st, and is put in the Lancisi Ward, No. 54.

August 1st.—4 p.m., headache and profuse sweating. Blood: a moderate number of amœboid plasmodia without pigment. 5 p.m., blood: the same. Temp., 5 p.m., 101°. 8 p.m., 98·6°. 12 p.m., 99° F.

2nd.—8.30 a.m., intermission; condition perfectly good. Blood: a moderate number of *large-sized* plasmodia, discoid in shape and in motion, with granules of pigment on the circumference. 11 a.m., blood: the same. The plasmodia are large-sized, discoid in shape, and sluggish in movement. The fever begins with shivering towards midday. 3.30 p.m., high fever. Blood: only pigmented forms in brassy red blood-corpuscles. 5 p.m., blood: there are still a few pigmented plasmodia in brassy red blood-corpuscles; and a very small number of young forms, small and annular in shape. Temp., 4 a.m., 96·8°. 8 a.m., 98°. 12 noon, 102·4° (with shivering). 4 p.m., 104·2°. 8 p.m., 104° (with sweating). 12 p.m., 103·8° F.

3rd.—The fever, which continued all night, tends to decrease in the morning. Intense headache. 8.30 a.m., blood: there are still some pigmented plasmodia in brassy corpuscles, and a few young amœboid forms with very lively movements; the discoid forms are a little larger than before. 10.30 a.m., shivering. Blood: there are still discoid forms with little granules of pigment; but the young forms, annular in shape, and in motion, dominate. There are also several pigmented white blood-corpuscles. 3.30 p.m., the fever is still high. Blood: an extremely large number of discoid and annular plasmodia in very lively motion; they are not pigmented, and almost all are very small (even two or three in a single red blood-corpuscle). A very limited quantity of *large-sized* discoid plasmodia with fine granules of pigment at the circumference. 6 p.m., the high fever continues; headache and depression. Sulphate of quinine, 48 grains, by the mouth. Temp., 4 a.m., 102·2°. 8 a.m., 101·1°. 11 a.m., 105·4°. 12 noon, 106·3°. 4 p.m., 103·1°. 8 p.m., 97·3°. 12 p.m., 98·1° F.

4th.—8 a.m., intermission. Sulphate of quinine, 32 grains, by the mouth. 9.30 a.m., blood: several plasmodia without pigment, and some in very lively motion. A few *large-sized* plasmodia with pigment at the circumference; also a few pigmented white blood-corpuscles. 5 p.m., patient in good condition. Blood: several discoid and annular plasmodia, some pigmented in brassy blood-corpuscles; a very small number without pigment, and in motion. In the night the fever returns. Temp., 4 a.m., 97°. 8 a.m., 96·8°. 12 noon, 97°. 5 p.m., 97·1°. 10 p.m., 103·1° F.

5th.—8.30 a.m., the fever tends to diminish. Blood: a very scanty number of annular plasmodia of very small dimensions. 5.30 p.m., blood: examination gives a negative result. Temp., 2 a.m., 102·2°. 8 a.m., 101·1°. 12 noon, 101·1°. 4 p.m., 99·9°. 8 p.m., 99·7°. 12 p.m., 100·4° F. After midnight the temperature becomes normal; the patient continues to take quinine.

During the paroxysm the parasitic forms are not all found in the same stage of development; the pigmented adult forms continue during the whole length of the paroxysm. The coming to maturity of the different parasitic forms is completed in a rather long period, which explains the lengthy duration of the paroxysm. Large doses of quinine do not prevent an abortive paroxysm.

Case 7.[1]—Beaujean, an able-bodied man, middle-aged, has had malarial fever in Africa three times at different intervals, but for the last three years he has been free from it. He has now had fever for a week with intermissions, which, he says, have been irregular; there has been little or no shivering. The paroxysms have become constantly stronger, and from the morning of July 13th up to the present (the 14th) the fever has lasted without intermission.

July 14th.—4 p.m., profuse sweating. Blood: a considerable number of plasmodia without pigment. There is one tertian (spring) form of medium size. 5.30 p.m., discoid and annular plasmodia without pigment in great numbers. There are no pigmented leucocytes. The profuse sweating continues during the night. Temp., 5 p.m., 102·9°. 8 p.m., 99·5°. 12 p.m., 97·7° F.

15th.—8.30 a.m., no fever. A considerable number of plasmodia without pigment, and also with very fine granules of pigment (these latter are in the majority), also large forms, discoid and annular in shape, in red blood-corpuscles, mostly deeper in colour than usual, and a few in brassy blood-corpuscles. No pigmented white blood-corpuscles are observed. 4.30 p.m., the temperature has risen, accompanied by slight shivering. Blood: the parasites have much decreased in number; a few plasmodia are seen with pigment at the circumference. 6.15 p.m., blood: result of examination is negative. The fever continues during

[1] See Chart I, tracing 6.

the whole night. Temp., 4 a.m., 97·7°. 12 noon, 99·7°. 4 p.m., 104·6°. 8 p.m., 102·9°. 12 p.m., 103·5° F.

16th.—8 a.m., the fever continues high. Blood: a few plasmodia without pigment. 10.30 a.m., blood: plasmodia without pigment, as above. Some pigmented white blood-corpuscles with small masses of pigment. One adult tertian (spring) form! 4 p.m., sweating commences; the headache with which the patient has been tormented has ceased, but the fever continues. Blood: a considerable number of plasmodia without pigment, with very lively motion, and a few with very fine granules of pigment at the circumference. 5 p.m., profuse sweating. 6 p.m., blood: as above; in addition, a young form of spring tertian. A very few pigmented white blood-corpuscles. Temp., 4 a.m., 103·4°. 8 a.m., 102·5°. 12 noon, 104·6°. 5 p.m., 102·2°. 8 p.m., 98·6°. 12 p.m., 98·6° F.

17th.—Intermission; and condition good all through the night. 8 a.m., a moderate number of plasmodia without pigment, and also with very fine granules of pigment at the circumference (the pigmented forms are also in the majority). They are mostly very mobile, and larger than on the evening of the 16th. A few pigmented white blood-corpuscles. 3.45 p.m., the patient has had slight shivering and headache for the last half-hour. The temperature has risen. Blood: a very small number of forms with pigment at the centre (there is one spring tertian free form, larger than a red blood-corpuscle, apparently belonging to those which end by forming vacuoles). Several pigmented leucocytes. The plasmodia in motion with pigment at the circumference are no longer to be seen, as in the morning, and the number found has considerably decreased. 5.45 p.m., high fever. Blood: in one preparation not a single parasite! In another, one annular form of very small size without pigment. Temp., 4 a.m., 99·5°. 8 a.m., 97·5°. 12 noon, 98·3°. 4 p.m., 105·2°. 8 p.m., 102·2°. 12 p.m., 103·8° F.

18th.—The fever has been maintained during the whole of the night, and still continues. 8.30 a.m., blood: a few plasmodia without pigment, small and annular in shape. Some pigmented white blood-corpuscles. 10.30 a.m., blood: the same. 4 p.m.: still a few plasmodia without pigment. Some pigmented white blood-corpuscles. Some spring tertian forms, in size from one third to two thirds of the red blood-corpuscle. 4.45 p.m.: sulphate of quinine, 32 grains, by the mouth. Temp., 4 a.m., 101·5°. 8 a.m., 100·7°. 12 noon, 100·9°. 4 p.m., 104·2°. 8 p.m., 100·2°. 12 p.m., 97·4° F.

19th.—Intermission; condition good. 8.30 a.m., blood: a few plasmodia without pigment. A very small number of developed crescent-shaped forms. Several pigmented white blood-corpuscles. 10 a.m., sulphate of quinine 24 grains by the mouth. 5.30 p.m., examination of the blood gives a negative result. The intermission lasted the whole day; the patient felt well. During the following days a few crescent-shaped forms continue to be seen in the blood. The patient recovers strength, and leaves the hospital on July 27th. This is a typical instance of summer tertian.

It is worth noticing that the presence of a very small number of spring tertian forms, so few are they that it is impossible to follow their development, does not in the least modify the characteristic chart of the summer tertian.

Case 8.[1]—Merbetti G—, 23 years old, comes from outside Porta Salara. He has had fever since September 5th; after five days of illness he was cured by treatment with quinine. The recurrence of fever began after about twelve days of apyrexia, so that he has now suffered from paroxysms for three days. In the recurrence the paroxysms have been milder than they were in the original infection.

He entered the hospital on September 26th in a seriously anæmic condition. 10.30 a.m., blood: a few plasmodia with granules of pigment at the circumference. The patient has a sensation of cold about 11 a.m.; at 4 p.m. this cold feeling still continues. 4 p.m., blood: there are still plasmodia with small granules of pigment, and some are in brassy red blood-corpuscles. There is a moderate number of young plasmodia, annular in shape and mobile. Temp., 12 noon, 100·4°. 4 p.m., 105·6°. 8 p.m., 103·1°. 12 p.m., 101·1° F.

September 26th.—The patient is almost completely free from fever, feels well, and has no headache. 8.30 a.m., blood: several plasmodia, discoid and annular in shape and in motion, of medium size, with very fine granules of pigment. 11 a.m., blood: the same; several of the pigmented plasmodia are found in brassy red blood-corpuscles. 2.30 p.m., the temperature begins to rise. Blood: the number of parasites has much decreased; the same pigmented forms are found in red blood-corpuscles, both normal and brassy. In these latter some forms are also mobile. 4.30 p.m., high fever. Blood: there are still a few forms with small pigmented granules in red blood-corpuscles, both normal and brassy. A very scanty number of bodies with a small mass of pigment at the centre. Young forms are found, annular and discoid in shape,

[1] See Chart II, tracing 14.

and in motion. Temp., 4 a.m., 99·5°. 7.30 a.m., 99·1°. 12 noon, 99·3°. 2 p.m., 100·8°. 4 p.m., 101·6°. 8 p.m., 103·8°. 12 p.m., 103·1° F.

27th.—The fever continues, but is diminishing; the patient is quiet; there is slight bleeding at the nose. 9 a.m., blood: several plasmodia, discoid and annular in shape, and in motion; for the most part with very fine granules of pigment, some in brassy red blood-corpuscles. A few pigmented leucocytes. 10 a.m., the temperature is increasing. Blood: several discoid plasmodia, of medium size, mobile and with small granules of pigment, some in brassy red blood-corpuscles. There is a very small number of annular plasmodia in motion, without pigment. Towards 3 p.m. the patient has a feeling of cold. 4 p.m., high fever. Blood: there are still rather large plasmodia with granules of pigment; they are discoid and annular in form, and are found also in brassy red blood-corpuscles. Several annular plasmodia, mobile and without pigment; also some very young ones, small and annular in shape, as well as leucocytes containing small masses of pigment. Slight but frequent headache. 5 p.m., bimuriate of quinine, 32 grains, by hypodermic injection. Temp., 4 a.m., 97·6°. 7.30 a.m., 99·3°. 12 noon, 98·8°. 4 p.m., 99·3°. 8 p.m., 101°. 12 p.m., 102·2° F.

28th.—The patient is free from fever and feels well. Sulphate of quinine, 16 grains, by the mouth. The patient has fever during the night which continues by day.

29th.—10 a.m., blood: there are a few plasmodia with very fine granules of pigment and in brassy corpuscles. 4 p.m., blood: the same.

30th.—Incomplete intermission. Blood: a very small number of adult crescent-shaped forms. The patient is cool till October 3rd.

October 3rd.—In the morning the patient complains of headache, and after this the temperature gradually rises. 3 p.m., high fever. Blood: a very limited number of plasmodia without pigment, and a few adult crescent-shaped forms. Temp., 10.30 a.m., 101·5°. 12 noon, 102·4°. 4 p.m., 103·2°. 8 p.m., 102°. 12 p.m., 100·1° F.

4th.—In the morning the patient is cool, complains of slight headache. 10 a.m., blood: several plasmodia with granules of pigment, discoid and annular in shape, mobile, and of medium size; some have only an indistinct outline, and the granules of pigment are not clearly defined. 3.30 p.m., the patient complains of severe headache. Blood: condition as above, but the plasmodia are much reduced in numbers; there are also a very few adult crescent-shaped forms. Temp., 4 a.m., 99°. 8 a.m., 97·5°. 12 noon, 99·4°. 4 p.m., 101·6°. 8 p.m., 103·1°. 12 p.m. 102·6° F. Towards 10 p.m. there is sweating.

5th.—The fever continues. 10 a.m., blood: annular and discoid plasmodia in sluggish movement (dendritic forms) with little granules of pigment. A very small number of large amœboid forms with indistinct outline. Several crescent-shaped forms, some in process of disintegration. A few pigmented white blood-corpuscles. 3.15 p.m., high fever. Blood: there are still a few plasmodia with small granules of pigment; also a few young plasmodia without pigment. Temp., 4 a.m., 101·2°. 7 a.m., 101·6°. 12 noon, 102·6°. 4 p.m., 103·6°. 8 p.m., 100·6°. 12 p.m., 99·4° F.

6th.—The patient is almost completely free from fever, and feels well. 10 a.m., blood: several plasmodia with little granules of pigment, discoid and annular in shape, of medium size and also small, some in brassy red blood-corpuscles and in those tending to become brassy. Several adult crescent-shaped forms, with flagella. A few pigmented leucocytes. 3.30 p.m., fever; a few discoid plasmodia with granules of pigment, some in brassy red blood-corpuscles. Several crescent-shaped forms, ovoid and round. Temp., 4 a.m., 99·2°. 7.30 a.m., 98·6°. 12 noon, 97·6°. 4 p.m., 101·8°. 8 p.m., 102·2°. 12 p.m., 101·8° F.

7th.—Patient says that he felt very ill in the night. The fever continues. 9 a.m., blood: several discoid and annular forms with granules of pigment. A few young annular forms without pigment. There are endoglobular crescent-shaped forms, and also round free forms, as well as pigmented leucocytes. 5 p.m., blood: the same. Sulphate of quinine, 32 grains, by the mouth.

8th.—Cool. Condition good. The patient continues to take quinine.

This is a case of summer tertian in which, when quinine was administered, a period of incomplete absence of fever supervened, followed soon after by a recurrence. The tertian type is more clearly defined in the recurrence than in the original infection, in which the interval without fever is very short and incomplete. (The minimum temperature is 99·2°.) The long duration of the paroxysms is explained by examination of the blood. In reality we find that the parasites develop in groups in such a way that during the paroxysm there are almost always adult forms (*i. e.* plasmodia with granules of pigment) and young forms (*i. e.* plasmodia without pigment) at one and the same time. Nevertheless during the period without fever preceding the paroxysms only adult forms in normal or brassy corpuscles are seen in the blood—a fact which bears witness to the presence of a single parasitic generation.

CASE 9.[1]—Giulio M—, very able-bodied, comes from outside Porta Portese. Has had fever since August 18th; it began with shivering, according to the statement of the patient, towards 10 a.m., and continued without intermission until his admission into the hospital (10 a.m. on August 19th).

August 19th.—10.30 a.m., blood: several small plasmodia without pigment, mobile; in shape annular and discoid. 3 p.m., blood: many annular and discoid plasmodia without pigment, in motion, and of different sizes; there are also some rather large ones. Temp., 12 noon, 105·4°. 4 p.m., 104°. 8 p.m., 100·2° F.

20th.—The fever has decreased during the night, without, however, complete defervescence occurring. The patient feels a little better, but the headache continues. 8.15 a.m., blood: a moderate number of plasmodia of medium size, discoid and annular in shape, with granules of pigment; some in red blood-corpuscles which are tending to become brassy. 10 a.m., the temperature rises again unattended with shivering. Blood: a few plasmodia with granules of pigment, almost all in brassy corpuscles; one form with a small mass of pigment at the centre. An extremely scanty number of very young plasmodia without pigment, in motion (two in one preparation). 3 p.m., high fever, headache. Blood: still a very small number of plasmodia with granules of pigment. 4 p.m., blood: a very limited number of plasmodia without pigment, in motion. 5.30 p.m., the plasmodia without pigment have increased in number; they are annular and discoid in shape, and are in motion. Temp., 4 a.m., 101°. 8 a.m., 101·3°. 12 noon, 103·1°. 4 p.m., 104·6°. 8 p.m., 103·7°. 10.30 p.m., 101·7°. 12 p.m., 103·7° F.

21st.—The patient has constant fever in the night, with headache. 8 a.m., blood: a few plasmodia without pigment, discoid and annular in shape, also mobile; some discoid forms are observed with indistinct outline, in which the pigmentation appears to have begun; some are in blood-corpuscles which are tending to become brassy. There are several pigmented white blood-corpuscles, also with small masses of pigment. 8.30 a.m., the patient is troubled with a sensation of cold. 9.30 a.m., blood: condition as above; in addition there are some plasmodia

[1] See Chart II, tracing 11.

with very fine granules of pigment in red blood-corpuscles tending to become brassy. 3 p.m., blood: condition as above; the forms are for the most part small, but there are some of medium size with granules of pigment; also a few pigmented white blood-corpuscles, in one of which there is a form with pigment at the centre. 4 p.m., blood: condition as above. The pigmented white blood-corpuscles have become numerous, and most of them contain small masses of pigment. Temp., 4 a.m., 105·1°. 8 a.m., 104·9°. 9.30 a.m., 104·7°. 12 noon, 105·1°. 4 p.m., 102°. 8 p.m., 98·6°. 12 p.m., 99·5° F.

22nd.—During the early part of the morning the patient feels pretty well, but the headache, although not severe, continues. 8 a.m., blood: a moderate number of plasmodia, discoid and annular in shape, and mobile (though their movement is sluggish); all of them pigmented. As a rule they are rather large, but there are also some small ones, about a third of the former in size. A very small number of young annular plasmodia without pigment. 9.45 a.m., blood: there is nothing abnormal to be seen but plasmodia with granules of pigment at the circumference, in less numbers than at the first examination. Some are in brassy red blood-corpuscles; there are also a few pigmented leucocytes. 3.30 p.m., blood: a very few pigmented plasmodia in brassy red blood-corpuscles, also a small number of very young plasmodia, annular and discoid in shape, without pigment, and many white corpuscles with little masses of pigment. Temp., 4 a.m., 98·3°. 8 a.m., 99·7°. 12 noon, 101°. 4 p.m., 101°. 8 p.m., 101·3°. 12 p.m., 102·7° F.

23rd.—8 a.m., blood: a moderate number of young plasmodia without pigment, in motion, and discoid and annular in shape; only a very few have a somewhat indistinct outline. 10 a.m., there are many plasmodia without pigment, and also with granules of pigment of medium size, annular and discoid in shape, and mobile, some in red corpuscles which are tending to become brassy. Between 10.30 a.m. to 3 p.m. the patient was given 48 grains of sulphate of quinine by the mouth. 3 p.m., the fever has already considerably decreased. Blood: there are many plasmodia without pigment, and also with granules of pigment of medium size, for the most part annular and discoid; the forms with granules of pigment or with granules of hæmoglobin are in the majority. Temp., 4 a.m., 103·1°. 8 a.m., 102·2°. 12 noon, 101·5°. 4.30 p.m., 101·1°. 8 p.m., 98·1°. 12 p.m., 96·8° F.

24th.—Condition favorable. 10 a.m., blood: a few plasmodia in motion, discoid and annular in shape, mostly without pigment, but some with very fine granules of pigment. Also pigmented leucocytes. 3 p.m., the patient was given 16 grains of sulphate of quinine by the mouth. Blood: a very few plasmodia without pigment, or with little granules scarcely visible, in red blood-corpuscles which are brassy or tending to become so; also motionless forms, annular and discoid in shape. Temp., 4 a.m., 97·4°. 8 a.m., 99·9°. 12 noon, 101·7°. 4 p.m., 103·6°. 8 p.m., 102·6°. 12 p.m., 102·2° F.

25th.—8 a.m., the fever is decreasing. 24 grains of sulphate of quinine given by the mouth. 9.30 a.m., blood: there are still a very small number of plasmodia with and without granules of pigment. 10.45 a.m., blood: a single plasmodium without pigment found in one preparation. Temp., 4 a.m., 99·5°. 8 a.m., 100·6°. 12 noon, 99·7°. 4 p.m., 101°. 8 p.m., 99·9°. 12 p.m., 97·9° F.

Continues without fever during the following days, excepting slight and short elevations in the temperature which do not reach 100·4° F. The patient continues to take quinine.

On August 27th a few adult crescent-shaped forms are found in the blood, and a very small number of pigmented leucocytes, some also with small masses of pigment.

On the 29th the examination of the blood gives a negative result.

This is a case of summer tertian with prolonged paroxysms, in which we may see set before us one of the ways by which the fever can become subcontinued. Between the first and second paroxysms there is no interval without fever, the minimum temperature being only 100·4°. Between the second and third paroxysms the apyrexia is incomplete and very short, the temperature scarcely touching 98·6° F. Owing to the action of 48 grains of quinine, taken during the third paroxysm, there is a complete intermission between the third and fourth paroxysms. The examination of the blood shows the existence of a single generation of parasites.

Case 10.[1]—Angelo B—, 28 years old, day labourer, had malarial fever for seven or eight months, eight years ago. He comes from outside Porta S. Pancrazio, where he has been for a week. On August 15th he had slight fever with headache; on the 16th the fever increased; on the 17th, towards 6 a.m., he had shivering and high fever; and to-day the fever has lasted since the morning. The spleen is becoming enlarged.

August 18th.—10 a.m., blood: some rather small annular plasmodia with granules of pigment; a few with a small mass

[1] See Chart II, tracing 9.

of pigment almost in the centre, and many in brassy red blood-corpuscles. 3 p.m., blood: the parasites are as above, only more scanty; there are a very few forms with a small mass and granules of pigment at the centre, in size from a sixth to a fourth of the red blood-corpuscle. The temperature rises rapidly without shivering. 4 p.m., blood: the number of parasites continues to decrease; in a preparation there are only two plasmodia with a small mass of pigment at the centre, one of which is in a brassy red blood-corpuscle. 5 p.m., blood: condition as above; in addition there is a very limited number of very young plasmodia, annular and discoid in shape. The fever continues all through the night. Temp., 11 a.m., 100·7°. 12 noon, 100·7°. 4 p.m., 104·4°. 8 p.m., 103·3°. 12 p.m., 103·6° F.

19th.—Headache intense. Blood: a few plasmodia without pigment; the annular and discoid forms are in the majority. In some plasmodia very fine granules of pigment begin to be visible; also some white blood-corpuscles with small masses of pigment. 9.45 a.m., blood: the plasmodia without pigment have increased, and some very small annular forms are visible, otherwise the condition is as above. 3 p.m., high fever; the patient is in a state of agitation. Blood: a moderate number of plasmodia without pigment, of small size, the greater number annular in shape. 4.30 p.m., blood: several discoid plasmodia without pigment, and a few with very fine granules of pigment; also pigmented white blood-corpuscles. Temp., 4 a.m., 102·2°. 8 a.m., 104·5°. 12 noon, 105·6°. 4 p.m., 104°. 8 p.m., 103·1°. 12 p.m., 99·2° F.

20th.—No fever. The patient feels much better. 3.15 a.m., blood: many pigmented plasmodia, discoid and annular in shape, with small granules at the circumference; some are in sluggish motion: for the most part they are of medium size; some are in red blood-corpuscles which are tending to become brassy. Also a very small number of pigmented white blood-corpuscles. 10.45 a.m., blood: there is a remarkable decrease in the number of the parasites; otherwise the condition is as above. The paroxysm begins towards midday without shivering. 3 p.m., blood: there are still a few plasmodia with little granules of pigment, annular and discoid in shape, in normal and brassy blood-corpuscles; also a few white blood-corpuscles with pigment in needles and small masses. 4.30 p.m., blood: there are only white blood-corpuscles with small masses of pigment. From 6 p.m. onwards the patient was given 48 grains of sulphate of quinine by the mouth. Temp., 8 a.m., 98·1°. 8 a.m., 98·1°. 12 noon, 101·5°. 4 p.m., 104·4°. 4 p.m., 104·2°. 12 p.m., 104° F.

21st.—The patient feels better, the headache has decreased, and the fever tends to grow less in the morning. Sulphate of quinine, 16 grains, is administered by the mouth. 8.45 a.m., blood: a few discoid and annular plasmodia without pigment; also some pigmented white blood-corpuscles with little masses. 3 p.m., intense headache. Blood: condition as above; some of the plasmodia are in brassy blood-corpuscles. Sweating sets in, and the fever ceases in the night. Temp., 4 a.m., 103·3°. 8 a.m., 101·4°. 12 noon, 104·4°. 4 p.m., 102·2°. 8 p.m., 100·4°. 12 p.m., 99·4° F.

22nd.—Complete freedom from fever. In the blood there is nothing abnormal except several white blood-corpuscles pigmented and with small masses of pigment. The patient continues to take sulphate of quinine.

This is a summer tertian with a typical curve and a typical parasitic cycle. When the paroxysm is far advanced its curve is not modified by the administration of quinine. After the remedy has been given there appear in the blood a very small number of young parasites, which do not develop further. The pigmented white blood-corpuscles, and specially those which contain small masses of pigment, showing that the forms producing spores have become disintegrated, display a marked increase in number after the patient has been treated with quinine.

CHAPTER VI.

DIFFERENTIAL DIAGNOSIS OF THE PARASITIC VARIETIES AND THE MIXED INFECTIONS.

Differences between the quotidian amœba and the amœba of the summer-autumn tertian—Differences between the amœba of the spring tertian and that of the summer tertian—Distribution of the parasitic forms in the blood in the different types of fever—Instances of mixed malarial infection (summer and tertian—summer and quartan).

§ 28. The points of resemblance between the amœba of the summer-autumn quotidian and that of the summer-autumn tertian are very numerous, at the same time their differences are considerable; both the former and the latter are shown in Figs. 34 to 55 (Plate I) and Figs. 1 to 45 (Plate II), and we may therefore be allowed to dispense with a lengthy description.

The differences are biological and morphological.

Let us say at once that the chief difference exists in *the duration of the cycle of development*, which in the quotidian is completed in about twenty-four hours, while in the summer tertian the period is forty-eight hours, more or less. Both this and the other differences have been pointed out in the description of the two varieties which we have given above; but it may be worth while to repeat them here in the form of a brief summary.

Differences in the pigmentation.—As Marchiafava and Celli have long since noticed, in the quotidian the sporulation on rare occasions is completed before the amœbæ have become pigmented; whereas in the summer tertian we have never observed this fact. Further, the pigment, which is in fine granules at the circumference of the tertian amœba, is sometimes seen to be endowed with oscillatory movements; this we have not once noticed in the quotidian.

Differences in the size of the amœba.—The tertian amœba is usually larger than the quotidian at an equal stage in the development. In the tertian the adult pigmented forms may be as much as one third of the size of the red blood-corpuscles, and the forms of fission may be as large as one half or two thirds of it. The corresponding forms in the quotidian are considerably smaller.

Differences in the amœboid movements.—In the tertian these movements are maintained longer, even in the pigmented adult forms; moreover the motion is more lively, and the amœba is wont to assume different strange shapes, through the rapid projection and retraction of the pseudopodia; whereas the movements of the little quotidian amœba during the pigmented phase are less active and lasting.

Differences in the duration of the various life-phases in connection with the fever cycle.—The duration of the non-pigmented amœboid phase in the tertian is very long, and may exceed twenty-four hours. Further, the forms of the young generation in the summer tertian usually appear in the blood several hours after the beginning of the paroxysm,—that is to say, much later than in the quotidian.

The points of resemblance between these two parasitic varieties are so many that it becomes very difficult to make a differential diagnosis; and this is only possible with the adult forms, especially during the period of intermission, when the new paroxysm of fever is being prepared. As we have already pointed out, the amœba of the summer tertian affects the red blood-corpuscle in the same way as the amœba of the quotidian does,—that is to say, they both alike cause it to shrink, shrivel up, and waste away, while the colour of the hæmoglobin becomes deeper than the normal. Further, the forms of the crescent-shaped phase are found in both varieties.

§ 29. The points of difference between the amœba of the common or spring tertian, and the amœba of the summer-autumn tertian, are much more prominent than those which distinguish the amœba of this last-mentioned clinical form from that of the quotidian.

The differences are comprised under the following heads:

(1) *The size of the parasitic forms.*—The amœba of the summer tertian, in corresponding stages of development, is always smaller than the amœba of the common tertian.

(2) *The appearance of the parasitic forms.*—The summer amœba often takes the annular shape, which is not the case with the other, and has, moreover, a more clearly defined outline, so that it shows more distinctly than the other on the background of the red blood-corpuscle.

(3) *The characteristics of the pigment.*—In the spring tertian the pigment is abundant, and almost always in motion; but in the

summer tertian it is in very fine granules, and relatively speaking scanty in quantity, and arranged for the most part at the extreme edge of the amœba; it is, moreover, seldom mobile.

(4) *The changes produced in the invaded red blood-corpuscle.*—In the spring tertian the corpuscle swells and grows pale rapidly, while in the other tertian, as we have stated more than once, it tends to shrink and shrivel up, while the hæmoglobin becomes more deeply coloured than in its normal state.

(5) *The forms of segmentation.*—The process of fission is similar in the two tertians; but the spores of the summer tertian are smaller, and, generally, less numerous than those of the common tertian.

(6) In the common tertian there are very often seen, especially near the beginning of the paroxysm, flagellated forms developing from the large round pigmented bodies of which we have spoken (see p. 10), but crescent-shaped bodies are never found.

On the contrary, the bodies which belong to the group of the crescent-shaped forms (spindle-shaped bodies, round bodies with pigment shaped like a crown, crescent-shaped forms properly so called) represent a phase in the life of the amœba of the summer tertian, in which the flagellated forms develop from the round bodies of this group.

Another series of differences between the group of the summer-autumn fevers and the mild winter-spring fevers (quartan and tertian) arises from the varied distribution of the parasitic forms in the blood as it circulates during the different periods of the life-cycle. The amœbæ of the quartan complete their whole life-cycle in the blood as it circulates, without accumulating by preference in the vascular system of some of the viscera.

In the spring tertian, throughout the entire phase of life in which the parasite is endoglobular, there are no noteworthy differences to be observed—as far as the amœbæ are concerned—between the blood of the finger and that of the spleen; on the other hand, at the beginning of the paroxysms of fever, the adult forms, which have radically altered the red blood-corpuscle, the free pigmented bodies, and the forms of fission tend to accumulate in the spleen, as Bastianelli and Bignami have noticed.[1]

This accumulation is, however, not so great as not to allow one easily to trace the complete life-cycle of the amœba, even if only the blood taken from the finger be studied.

Lastly, this tendency of the adult and fissional forms to accumulate in the vascular system of some of the viscera is one of the

[1] "Sulle febbri malariche primaverile," 'Rif. Med. Giugno,' 1890.

most salient facts in the summer fevers. We[1] have always drawn attention to this as explaining the great difficulty encountered in the study of these varieties of parasite; and as establishing a clear difference between this group of fevers on the one hand, and the quartan and tertian on the other. If, for instance, the blood of a quartan patient be observed shortly before and during the paroxysm of fever, one is surprised to see that the young amœbæ are always relatively few in number in comparison with what would be expected from the large amount of spore-producing forms found.[2] Whereas, in the summer tertian, while during the course of the attack the amœbæ without pigment are as a rule extremely numerous, the forms producing spores, which may be found by studying the blood of the finger, are always remarkably scanty, and sometimes they are entirely wanting. The reason of such a fact as this we have already discussed.

§ 30. The above analysis leaves no doubt on the discovery that the amœba of the summer tertian represents a variety of parasite which is totally distinct from the amœba of the common tertian. On the other hand, the points of resemblance which we have noticed between the quotidian amœba and the amœba of the malignant tertian, which are so remarkable, make it very difficult to solve the question whether we have to do with different sorts of parasites in the strict sense of the term, or with one and the same parasite which varies greatly in the time of its development, so that between the two extremes—twenty-four hours (for the quotidian) and forty-eight (for the tertian)—there are all the intermediate degrees. If this theory be followed out, it becomes easy to ascribe the morphological differences which we have explained to the varying length of the cycle of development. But to this hypothesis the following facts are opposed. In the first place, the two clinical types of the quotidian and tertian are clearly distinct from each other, and have a certain stability which is maintained in the relapses and recurrences. In the second place, we have never met with intermediate clinical forms which could not be referred to one or other of these two types; neither have we ever seen forms of fever which could be interpreted as constituting a transition stage between the quotidian and tertian, forms of transition which would be required by the second hypothesis as a logical necessity. Only, as we have already remarked, it may be a very difficult matter to interpret some of the irregular fevers. In any case, granting that the

[1] Marchiafava e Celli, "Sulle febbri malariche predominanti nell' estate e nell' autunno in Roma," 'Atti Accad. Med. di Roma,' 1890.

[2] See Antolisei, 'L' emat. della quartana.'

question cannot at present be solved definitely, when we remember that the *typical* forms of the quotidian and summer tertian are attended by clinical and parasitological characteristics which have been clearly determined, we are inclined to adopt the view that the amœba of the quotidian and the amœba of the summer tertian are closely related varieties of one and the same parasite.

The same great resemblance is also seen between the quartan amœba and that of the common tertian; but, for the reasons we have already set forth, this does not interfere with the fact that they ought to be considered as distinct parasitic varieties. Between the quartan amœba, which completes its life cycle in three days, and that of the quotidian, which develops in about twenty-four hours, there lies the group of tertian amœbæ which complete their cycle in forty-eight hours, more or less. This group of amœbæ comprises two varieties, one of which is connected by morphological and biological characteristics with the quartan amœba, while the other bears in the same way a very close resemblance to the quotidian amœba, with which it constitutes the parasitic group of the summer-autumn fevers.

We have seen that both in the quotidian and in the summer-autumn tertian there occurs a biological phase of the amœba which is represented by the crescent-shaped bodies; but this fact stands in no opposition to the theory above expressed, according to which the quotidian amœba and the amœba of the summer-autumn tertian would be varieties closely connected, but still distinct, of a single parasitic species. The analogy which exists on the one hand between the sterile forms of the summer-autumn tertian and the quotidian—to which we have referred—exists also on the other hand between the degenerative forms of the quartan and the tertian. If our hypothesis be correct, the former are represented by the bodies of the crescent-shaped phase, the latter by the large pigmented bodies which differentiate themselves from those that are approaching the spore-forming phase, and which become first vacuolated and then disintegrated into small hyaline fragments. For the rest, it is well known that all these degenerative or sterile forms have certain final phases in common,—that is to say, they may all emit gemmules, they may all become vacuolated and disintegrated, and they may all turn into flagellated forms.

§ 31. By means of the facts ascertained it is possible to make a differential diagnosis of the manifold varieties of malarial parasites; but not only so, it is also possible, solely by examination of the blood, to determine whether we have to do with a simple or complex fever, to foresee the approach of a fresh paroxysm, and, up to a certain point, to foretell the gravity of the different cases. For this purpose it is necessary to take account of the number of parasitic generations present in the blood, of the phase of life in which each colony of parasites is found, and of the greater or less amount of amœbæ discovered.

But while it is a simple matter to form a judgment on these facts in the case of the quartan and tertian, in the summer fevers it is rendered more difficult by the necessity of taking account of all the possible different forms or phases of amœbæ found at the same time in correlation with the development of the fever. To these varieties we have already drawn attention. It is only long practice that can give to the judgment of the observer the desirable certainty and precision.

The same difficulty is met with in the study of the mixed malarial infections caused by the summer-autumn amœba and the quartan amœba together, or by that of the common tertian. In these cases, just in proportion as the study of the parasites yields a complex result, so also is the course of the fever complex and irregular. Here it is easy to predict the possibility of a very large series of combinations, caused by the number of the parasitic colonies, by the way in which their life cycles are, so to say, interwoven, &c.; so that, as a resultant therefrom, the fever takes the most different courses—from the irregular intermittent fevers on the one hand, to the subintrant and subcontinued on the other. We will give as examples only two cases of this sort, in one of which quartan and summer parasites are found together, in the other spring tertian and summer amœbæ.[1]

[1] Among the *composite intermittent* fevers the ancients attached great importance to Galen's *semi-tertian* or ἡμιτριταῖος. This form of fever is described by him as resulting from the union of an *intermittent tertian* with a *continuous quotidian.* It is well known that the theory regarding the origin of the ἡμιτριταῖος has been considerably modified by different writers. Thus, for instance, Torti supposes that the ἡμιτριταῖος arises from a multiplex intermittent tertian (loc. cit., p. 290); others speak of continued tertian or of continued tertian accompanied by an intermittent quotidian, &c. Among the mixed infections which we have studied we have not met with any thermic curves to which, if we follow Galen's description, the name of semi-tertian could be given; all the curves we have traced belonging to this series of cases are irregular. As regards the curve proper of the summer tertian which we have described, this could only be mistaken for a composite intermittent, and consequently set down as similar to Galen's ἡμιτριταῖος by falling into the error of supposing that the different oscillations of the curve of a paroxysm represent different paroxysms which have come closer together. We have already shown how it is that this interpretation cannot be admitted.

CASE 11.[1]—Fontana G—, 19 years old, able-bodied, has recurring malarial infection. He came into the hospital on the third day of the recurring fever; he states that he has fever every day without shivering. He was at work at Assalone. He is very pale and the spleen is becoming enlarged.

September 18th.—Temp., 5 p.m., 102·4°. 8 p.m., 101·5°. 12 p.m., 99·9° F. 4 p.m., blood: some quartan plasmodia as large as two thirds of the red blood-corpuscle; also others from one third to one half of the red blood-corpuscle. In addition there are summer annular plasmodia without pigment.

19th.—Temp., 4 a.m., 100·4°. 7.30 a.m., 99·6°. 10 a.m., 98·3°. 12 noon, 99·2°. 2.30 p.m., 98·3°. 4 p.m., 103·7°. 8 p.m., 102·7°. 12 p.m., 102·2° F. 9.30 a.m., blood: several summer plasmodia, discoid and annular in shape, with granules of pigment; some in brassy blood-corpuscles (forms of summer tertian). There are a few quartan forms almost as large as a red blood-corpuscle—a few also in the act of forming spores; in addition some pigmented white blood-corpuscles. 2.30 p.m., sensation of chill. Blood: a few adult quartan forms, and one quartan producing spores; also a few summer plasmodia with granules of pigment, and a very few pigmented white blood-corpuscles.

20th.—Temp., 4 a.m., 100·4°. 8 a.m., 99·7°. 12 noon, 101·1°. 4 p.m., 103·3°. 8 p.m., 99·4°. 12 p.m., 97·7° F. 9 a.m., a very few quartan forms, in size from a fourth to a half of the red blood-corpuscle; also a very small number of summer plasmodia without pigment. 3.30 p.m., the patient feels ill and is agitated. Blood: condition as above.

21st.—Temp., 4 a.m., 97°. 7 a.m., 97·5°. 12 noon, 97°. 4 p.m. 100·8°. 8 p.m., 105·3°. 12 p.m., 103·5° F. 9.30 a.m., blood: several summer plasmodia, discoid in shape and of medium size, with granules of pigment; also pigmented white blood-corpuscles. 2.30 p.m., blood: condition as above, *plus* a free pigmented sphere of quartan origin.

22nd.—Temp., 4 a.m., 101°. 7 a.m., 100·6. 12 noon, 99·7°. 4 p.m. 104·4°. 8 p.m., 98·6°. 12 p.m., 102·2° F. 10.30 a.m., blood: a very few mature quartan forms; also pigmented white blood-corpuscles. No summer plasmodia are seen. 3.30 p.m., the patient appears distressed, and complains of headache. Blood: several amœboid forms without pigment, annular and discoid in shape. One quartan form in the act of spore production. Sulphate of quinine, 32 grains, administered by the mouth.

23rd.—Without fever in the morning. 10 a.m., blood: some

[1] See Chart III, tracing 19.

annular plasmodia without pigment, also some in red blood-corpuscles which are tending to become brassy. In the afternoon the patient has slight fever. He is free from fever till September 26th, the day when he leaves the hospital.

This is a case of mixed infection caused by the parasites of the summer tertian and of the quartan. The result is an irregular fever which tends to become subcontinued during its last days when the treatment by quinine intervened. The matter becomes clear if it be observed that before the fever produced by the parasitic generation of summer tertian ceases the formation of spores of the quartan forms begins.

CASE 12.[1]—Luigi B—. This patient had malarial fever some years ago, and now has had, according to his own statement, continuous fever for four days.

September 12th.—4.45 p.m., blood: several discoid and annular plasmodia without pigment and in motion, many of medium size. A few mature tertian forms; also a few pigmented white blood-corpuscles. Temp., 1 p.m., 105·1°. 4 p.m., 105·5°. 8 p.m., 103·5°. 12 p.m., 100·4° F.

23rd.—Temp., 4 a.m., 99·5°. 7.30 a.m., 99·2°. 12 noon, 97·6°. 4 p.m., 98·1°. 8 p.m., 99·9°. 12 p.m., 104° F. 9 a.m., blood: several discoid and annular plasmodia in motion, with very fine granules of pigment. (As a rule they are of medium size, and are clearly summer forms.) A very few forms with pigment collected together eccentrically. Also a small number of plasmodia in brassy corpuscles, and a few tertian forms (spring), in size between one third and two thirds of the red blood-corpuscle. 10 a.m., blood: the parasites are the same as above, but less in number. 3 p.m., blood: the same; also a very few white blood-corpuscles with small masses of pigment.

24th.—Temp., 4 a.m., 102°. 7 a.m., 102·4°. 12 noon, 101°. 4 p.m., 99°. 8 p.m., 101·3°. 12 p.m., 99·4 F. 8.30 a.m., headache. Blood: a few amœboid forms annular in shape, in motion and without pigment, both of medium size and small. 3 p.m., the fever tends to decrease, and the patient feels better. Blood: there are plasmodia without pigment, annular in shape and in motion. Some, which are also in motion, display granules of hæmoglobin as well as very fine granules of pigment. Several pigmented white blood-corpuscles.

25th.—Temp., 4 a.m., 102°. 7.30 a.m., 99°. 12 noon, 100·6°. 4 p.m., 104·7°. 8 p.m., 104·5°. 12 p.m., 102·2° F. 8.30 a.m., the patient feels better. Blood: a moderate number of discoid

[1] See Chart III, tracing 20.

plasmodia in motion, with granules of pigment at the circumference (summer tertian forms); there are also tertian forms (spring tertian), as large as two thirds and more of the red blood-corpuscle. They are but few in number. 3.30 p.m., a small number of plasmodia with granules of pigment at the circumference (summer tertian forms). 4 p.m., blood: a few pigmented discoid plasmodia. Also similar forms in brassy blood-corpuscles, and several very young annular plasmodia in motion. In addition tertian forms (spring) almost mature, and several pigmented white blood-corpuscles. Sulphate of quinine, 32 grains, administered by the mouth.

26th.—Temp., 4 a.m., 101·8°. 7.30 a.m., 100·3°. 12 noon, 100·8°. 4 p.m., 101°. 8 p.m., 99·9°. 12 p.m., 99·9° F. 8 a.m., sulphate of quinine, 16 grains, administered by the mouth. 10 a.m., blood: several plasmodia without pigment, annular and discoid in shape, and *endowed with very rapid motion;* also pigmented white blood-corpuscles. 3 p.m., blood: a few plasmodia without pigment, for the most part in brassy blood-corpuscles; also pigmented white blood-corpuscles.

27th.—The patient is free from fever and very weak. He continues to take quinine.

This is a case of mixed summer and spring infection (there are spring tertian forms), and it will be seen that the intervals between the paroxysms are not complete during the period from the 24th to the 25th of September. The parasites are found to be composed of a generation of summer plasmodia together with a few forms of spring tertian. Bearing in mind this complex state of things, and this tendency of the periods of intermission to become badly marked, we may suppose that if the remedy had not been given the fever would have become really subcontinued.

CHAPTER VII.

MALIGNANT FEVERS.

The most frequent forms of malignancy in the Roman Campagna—Classification of the complicated (comitatæ) *malignant infections according to the type of fever—Malignant paroxysm (complicated), short and protracted—Subcontinued malignant infections, and their origin from the summer tertian and from the quotidian—Condition of the parasites in the malignant fevers; malignant infections determined by one or by more generations of amœbæ—In the malignant fevers the examination of the blood never gives a negative result—There are no constant differences between the complicated and the subcontinued infections as far as regards the condition of the parasites—Causes of malignancy inferred from examining into the biological condition of the parasites—Abundance of parasitic forms in the malignant fevers—Activity of reproduction, and toxic properties in the summer-autumn amœbæ—Varied resistance of the parasites to the action of the salts of quinine—Elements for forming the prognosis in the severe fevers drawn from the examination of the blood—Distribution of the parasitic forms in the vascular system of the different viscera in fatal cases—Pathogenesis of certain malignant symptoms, and specially of coma; anatomical and pathological lesions of the brain in the comatose malignant infection of the intestines in choleraic malignancy, &c.—The changes of the blood in the malarial hæmoglobinuria—Examples of the principal forms of malignant fever.*

§ 32. The group comprising the malignant malarial fevers may be studied from the point of view of the culminating symptom which gives to the clinical picture its characteristic aspect, or they may be studied from the point of view of the course which the temperature takes, or from that of the parasites as found in the blood. The classification of malignant fevers according to the culminating symptom, as determined by Torti, has been adopted by almost all writers, and he remains entirely unsurpassed in the clearness of his descriptions, and in the acumen and exactness of his clinical observation. It will be found in the short historical sketch with which this work is prefaced.

The clinical forms of the malignant fevers which are most often met with in medical practice in Rome belong to the group of Torti's "complicated" fevers (*comitatæ*), and it is precisely with these that our observations, in the majority of cases, have to do.

All physicians know, and it is in accordance with the statements of many authors (Colin may be taken as an instance), that it is the "complicated" fevers with cerebral symptoms that are the most frequent. Thus we not infrequently see in our hospitals the *lethargic and comatose "complicated"* fevers with all the intermediate gradations between lethargy and profound coma; after these the *delirious fevers*, the *bulbar*, the *convulsive*, the *hemiplegic*, the *tetanic*, &c.; and in the second place the algid, then the choleraic "complicated" fevers, the *cardialgic*, and after these the *hæmorrhagic*, the *hæmoglobinuric*, &c. We shall see how this prevalence of cerebral symptoms in the malignant fevers can be satisfactorily explained in the greater number of cases by pathological anatomy.

It is also a well-known fact that the *course of the temperature* in the "complicated" malignant fevers *may be very varied*; and just as there are cases in which the *malignant symptoms* continue, and even become aggravated after the fever has ceased (see Case 15), so we also find instances where the fever is [illegible] [illegible] *malignant fevers*), although the symptoms of infection in general, and the cerebral symptoms in particular, may be most serious (see Case [illegible], hemiplegic malignant fever). In these cases the appearances found in the blood do not differ from those which are seen in the ordinary "complicated" fevers. But there are also cases of malignant infection which are deceptive in their course, and in which [illegible] [illegible] [illegible], the fever may be [illegible] [illegible] the gravity of the infection, especially in old people. Among these [illegible] infections may occur and the greatest danger may be [illegible] [illegible] examination of the blood, showing the presence of parasites in great quantities, while the clinical [illegible] [illegible] [illegible] a certain time [illegible] [illegible] [illegible] [illegible] suddenly the condition of the patient becomes worse and death ensues after a short [illegible] of lethargy or coma. [illegible] a certain analogy [illegible] between the course of malignant fevers [illegible] [illegible] other infections [illegible] —e.g. [illegible] (see Case [illegible]).

As regards the type of fever, all the malignant cases which up to the present have been studied belong to the group of the summer-autumn fevers, which is divided into two types, the quotidian and the tertian; hence it would appear natural to arrange the "complicated" fevers in two classes, as follows:

(a) The malignant tertian.

(b) The malignant quotidian.

We may add that the *majority of malignant* fevers must be ascribed to the summer-autumn tertian, and only a few to the quotidian.

The duration of the malignant paroxysm may vary: it may be (a) *short*, and within certain limits nearly the same length as the typical paroxysm, tertian or quotidian; (b) *protracted* for two or three days with continued fever, the chart of which shows remittent periods more or less pronounced. In this case, after the intermission, the malignant paroxysm (*e. g.* the comatose) appears, and the fever with coma lasts two or three days. The issue may be favorable as well in the first as in the second case; on the other hand, it is well known that the intermittent malignant fevers may be fatal during the first paroxysm, while, in other cases, different malignant paroxysms follow each other at short intervals without making recovery impossible; as, for instance, a case of quotidian which we shall mention, with two malignant paroxysms, ending in recovery (see Case 23).[1] There is, however, a series of cases which must be carefully distinguished from that group of the "complicated" malignant fevers in which both the symptom that stamps the disease as malignant and the fever lasts for some days. We refer to those instances in which a malarial fever without clear periods of intermission grows progressively worse, and presents a complex picture of symptoms, among which one or more of those symptoms that characterise the "complicated" fevers may be more or less marked, without at the same time any single one of these predominating to such an extent as to constitute by itself alone the clinical characteristic of the case. (This is *Torti's "simple" malignant fever—" solitaria."*)

It is well known that in this series of cases the malarial fever may begin as subcontinued (*subcontinua d'emblée, i. e.* subcon-

[1] We refrain here from giving descriptions of the clinical forms of malignant fevers because this constitutes no part of the plan of our work; moreover in the series of cases which are given at the end of the present chapter the most common forms are recounted in detail.

tinued at the first onset), the parasites being found in a complex condition, or else it may become subcontinued gradually as the periods free from fever become badly marked; while as regards the parasites we find that the state of things which was at first simple now grows complex.

We shall briefly consider the course of the temperature in these cases, and parallel with this the condition of the parasites.

It seldom happens that we who possess the specific remedy for malaria can observe typical and prolonged curves of malarial fever in which the individual paroxysms are not separated by complete intermissions. This is because these fevers are generally serious, and compel the physician to administer quinine promptly. In spite of this dearth of material we can still form an idea of the way in which the malarial fevers become continued if we observe how the paroxysms in fevers of medium gravity are characterised, and how they succeed each other; we have already noted the tendency the paroxysms have in these fevers to become anticipating and prolonged.

We have mentioned above that there are cases of subcontinued fever (though they certainly are not frequent) which belong to the group of spring fevers; but these, notwithstanding the course of the temperature, are never so serious and fraught with danger as the summer-autumn subcontinued ones, nor have we ever met with a single case of the former which has terminated in death.

But we shall only now consider the summer-autumn subcontinued fevers, and especially those which have their origin in the summer tertian. It is precisely because the subcontinued fevers of this group are usually malignant that they have their place in this chapter.

The summer tertian may assume the form of a continued fever in many different ways.

We have already drawn attention to the prolonged paroxysms and to their probable origin. *If these paroxysms are so far protracted that they become conjoined the fever will become continued.* In this case it often becomes difficult, if the thermic curve alone be examined, to determine the fundamental type of the fever, and to separate from each other the individual paroxysms, in which it is often impossible to distinguish the initial from the pre-critical elevation. Here also we are helped by an examination of the blood. But even in these cases where the original infection is accompanied by fever *which is subcontinued through the prolongation and conjunction of the paroxysms,* in the recurrence the fever may be simplified and become clearly tertian.

In the second place, the paroxysms may become *prolonged and anticipating to such an extent that one begins before the other has finished*. Both the thermic curve and the condition of the parasites are usually complex in a case of this sort. The curve generally shows a series of elevations occurring near together (three and even four in twenty-four hours), and we must interpret these as the thermic oscillations of a single paroxysm, such as are commonly found in the typical chart of the summer tertian. The results obtained from the examination of the blood are opposed to the hypothesis that each elevation of temperature represents a fresh paroxysm. *The beginning of every paroxysm is in reality to be discerned by the prevalence in the blood of the mature parasitic forms.*

These fevers which become continued *through subintrant paroxysms* may be very severe and malignant, just as those in which the subcontinuity is produced by other means.[1]

[1] The distinction of the *subintrant* from the *subcontinued* fevers is traceable, as is well known, back to the old writers, and Torti insists much on the importance of it. However, this excellent observer, as we have remarked in the historic sketch, while admitting that the subintrant fevers may "*progredi ad malignitatem essentialem atque periculosam*," nevertheless maintained that the *subcontinua*, that is to say, the fever, "*quæ continuitatem acquirit simul atque acutiem*," becomes such "*per viam paroxysmorum subingredientium.*" It was the gravity of the symptoms more than the course of the fever which gave the stamp of malignancy to the subcontinued fevers. The onset of the subintrant paroxysms takes place in the summer-autumn fevers just as in the quartan and spring tertian. In these latter the subintrant character is clear on the most simple clinical examination through the alternate succession of the symptoms which characterise the different stages of the single paroxysm of fever, such as shivering, sweating, &c., and there is no malignancy; so that in these subintrant attacks we have to do with Torti's *benigna continuitas.* Whereas in the summer-autumn fevers the subintrant paroxysms, which are both prolonged and anticipating, are not often capable of being recognised, inasmuch as the symptoms characteristic of the various stages of the attack may be entirely wanting; so that these paroxysms become recognisable solely from a combined study of the temperature chart and of the parasites found in the blood. These subintrant fevers, unlike those in the quartan and spring tertian, may be *malignant*, and Torti put them among the malignant subcontinued fevers, as is shown by the cases cited by him. Owing to these considerations and the difficulties which arise in practice when we wish to distinguish the various ways by which continuity is established in the group of the summer-autumn fevers, we proposed in our preliminary monograph to call all the fevers of this group subcontinued in which the intermittence was lost, however this may have originated and whatever the gravity of the fevers may have been, notwithstanding that several authors maintain that the subintrant fever is always a mild one, and the subcontinued always malignant. But we cannot help repeating that, as far as all the facts which we have observed and explained lead us, this distinction between the sub-

In the third place, the subcontinued fever may arise from the *doubling of a summer tertian*, two parasitic generations or colonies appearing in the blood. If we remember the long duration of the paroxysm in the summer tertian, it is easy to understand how it is that the attacks in these cases are subintrant or overlapping, and the type of fever difficult to recognise. As a rule, the fever grows rapidly worse, so that it is impossible to follow its development except for a short period.

The *mixed tertian and quotidian infections* lead to the same result. Two parasitic generations are sufficient, the one developing in forty-eight hours, the other in about twenty-four; for *then* every interval without fever between the paroxysms disappears. In these cases also the thermic curve is difficult to interpret.

It follows from what has been said that, in the greater number of cases, the doubling of the summer tertian (the presence of two generations of parasites) is sufficient to produce a subcontinued fever. This is almost always seen in the so-called "comitatæ" malignant fevers, in which the course of the fever becomes subcontinued, through the presence of more than one parasitic generation, and, *in the vast majority of cases, of two generations alone.* In these instances the thermic curve shows a series of elevations, varying in number, during the twenty-four hours, on account of which it often becomes impossible to recognise the fundamental type of the fever.

To sum up the preceding, the summer tertian may become continued (tertian subcontinued fever) in various ways:

(1) By the prolongation of the paroxysms.

(2) By anticipating and subintrant paroxysms.

(3) By the doubling of the paroxysms (double tertian), without the attacks losing their individuality and becoming unrecognisable.

(4) By the multiplication of the paroxysms due to the presence of more than one parasitic generation, *generally two*; by

continued and subintrant fever from the point of view of malignancy does not, as a matter of fact, correspond to the reality. *It is necessary to take account of the parasitic varieties, and to draw a distinction between the subintrant fevers which belong to the quartan and tertian group and those which belong to the group of the summer-autumn fevers.* The subintrant fevers of the first group (*i.e.* the quartan and tertian) are mild, *those of the second* (the summer-autumn fevers) *may be malignant.* If the simple intermittent fevers in the summer-autumn group may be malignant (*malignant quotidian and malignant tertian*) it is incredible to suppose that an intermittent belonging to this group, having subintrant paroxysms, cannot be in its turn malignant. For the rest facts prove that this can be so.

this process we get double tertians in which the attacks have lost their own individuality by being prolonged and overlapping.

(5) By mixed infection—tertian and quotidian. The *quotidian fever*, in the majority of cases, loses its intermittence by the prolongation of the paroxysms.

Now if we consider, on the one hand, that the malignant infections may be attended by intermittent, subintrant, and subcontinued fevers, in an order of frequency which rises from the intermittent to the continued fever, and if we remember, on the other hand, that the same types of fever are found in non-malignant infections, we must conclude that there is no type of fever which is necessarily malignant (and this agrees with what is known of all the other infections, in which there is no thermic curve existing to distinguish the serious and fatal forms from those which are less serious and not fatal). This, however, does not prevent our having to rank the subcontinued fevers, in order of frequency, among those which are highly dangerous; and this is especially true of those subcontinued fevers which are produced by more than one parasitic generation. It is precisely these forms of subcontinued fever which Baccelli has thrown light upon, and to which we have called attention at the beginning of this work.

§ 33. In order to interpret the complex curve of these fevers, it is necessary to make an accurate examination of the parasitic cycle. Inasmuch as there is a direct correspondence between the development of the life cycle of the amœba, and the changes in the fever, it follows clearly enough from what has been said with regard to the way in which the fevers become complicated, and as regards the different fluctuations of the temperature, in the malignant infections, that the condition of the parasites ought also to vary. And so it does in point of fact.

In the malignant infections which are accompanied by an intermittent fever, quotidian and tertian, the examination of the blood shows the presence of a single generation of amœbæ: cases of this sort are not frequent, and we have observed only a few instances. (See Case 17.) But that such cases do exist has been proved by examination carried out on all the organs, in examples of malignant fever terminating fatally, and where, consequently, the investigation could be made in the most thorough way. However, in the vast majority of cases we have to do with more complex conditions, and we may divide them into three groups. (1) We find a single generation of parasites, in which the development and especially the sporulation of the forms take a period of many hours to complete, while there is at the same time not such a distance between the more advanced parasitic forms and those less forward in development as to warrant us in admitting the existence of more than one generation; or (2) we find two generations of parasites, whose life cycle may be clearly followed; or (3) we meet with amœbæ in different degrees of development at different periods in the fever, in such a way that it becomes impossible to distinguish the various groups or colonies and trace their growth. Judging from our experience during the last few years, cases belonging to the second group would appear to be the most frequent.

We will now briefly illustrate these points.

We have already spoken of the so-called *prolonged paroxysms*, and have endeavoured to determine their origin. Now these are precisely the cases in which the examination of the blood makes us suppose that the evolution of the adult forms takes place successively, in groups, and not in a short period of time, as happens in the typical attacks of fever. Nor is it possible to speak of the presence of more than one generation of amœbæ, because the intervals between the initial and deferred sporulation last but a short time, and all this takes place during the course of a single paroxysm.

An instance of subcontinued fever caused by a single parasitic generation, in which the multiplication occurs successively, during a period of several hours (even twelve), is found in the *subcontinued by prolongation of the paroxysms*.

On the other hand, we speak of two generations of parasites, only when, on the blood being examined, it is possible to follow two groups of forms, which mature (or sporulate) successively, but with rather long intervals, and in two distinct groups, in such a way that the two life cycles may be clearly recognised and traced out,—as happens, for instance, in the double tertian. It must be remembered that even in the typical summer tertians the adult pigmented forms sometimes continue to be seen in the blood, during the whole course of the paroxysm, along with the forms of the young generation; but during the apyrexia the position becomes simplified, and in the six or twelve hours which precede the new paroxysm only adult forms are found (*i. e.* plasmodia pigmented at the circumference and corpuscles with pigment collected at the centre). This fact shows that there was only one colony of parasites involved, in which, however, both anticipating and deferred sporulations took place. The same thing is seen in the prolonged paroxysms, although more pronounced. Now the first accompaniment of the complication of the fever curves is the combined presence of young forms (plasmodia without pigment) and adult forms in the incomplete apyrexia which precedes a paroxysm.

Under these circumstances the periods of apyrexia are usually incomplete and short, and the fever tends to become subcontinued through the presence in the blood of two generations of parasites.

Of the two generations one is frequently preponderating in quantity, and then the fever curve has a clear resemblance to that of the typical cases, and it is easy for a period of continued fever to be followed by one in which the paroxysms are distinctly intermittent. This may occur spontaneously, when the generation of parasites is scanty and disappears; or it may be determined, artificially, when the amœbæ disappear under the action of quinine. On the other hand, it more frequently happens that the two parasitic colonies develop vigorously in two distinct groups, in such a way that when one group is approaching sporulation, the other is composed of young amœbæ in process of growth. The two colonies may belong to the same parasitic variety or to two different ones (for instance, to that of the tertian and of the summer quotidian).

Bignami[1] has already drawn attention to this fact,—that is to say, to the presence of parasites in different stages of development in the majority of cases of malignant fever, and he connects it with the extreme gravity of these infections, and with the subcontinued course of the fever. The cases which we detail in the sequel only confirm this opinion afresh. If we bear in mind what has been said about the curve of the summer tertian and the life cycle of the tertian amœba, it is easy to understand how the presence of two generations of amœbæ in this group is more than sufficient for the fever to become subcontinued. The matter is otherwise in the group of spring fevers. Thus, for instance, it is not difficult to perceive (as Antolisei has observed) how in the subcontinued fever of quartan origin there might be seen forms *in all stages of development* in one and the same preparation of blood. It is clear that here we have to do with subcontinued fever, in the strict sense of the term, caused by multiplication of the paroxysms, as proved by Baccelli.

Similar to the preceding should be counted those cases which we have classed under the third group, and which always belong to the summer-autumn fevers; we mean those malignant fevers

[1] "Anat. patol. delle Pernic.," p. 54 of the extract, 'Atti della Accademia Medica di Roma,' 1890.

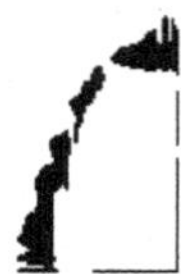

in which the examination of the blood shows the presence of parasites in all phases of life, during the various moments in the development of the fever, while at the same time it is impossible to trace out different groups quite distinctly, and determine their life cycle. The fever accompanying these infections is of course subcontinued.

§ 34. It follows, as a consequence from all we have said, that in these complex fevers, whether caused by two or more parasitic generations, or by one alone (in which case the adult forms usually continue to multiply for a rather long period) there are, as a rule, not even short intervals in which the condition of the blood is negative; unlike the typical summer tertian, where, from what we have seen, this may occur. The knowledge of this fact enables us to assert that the microscopic diagnosis of malaria is much more certain in serious cases than in those of medium gravity and where the fever is regular.[1]

[1] NOTE.—During the summer in Rome cases of severe infection may be observed with symptoms which are for the most part cerebral, and which are even now regarded by nearly all physicians as cases of malaria, and named in different ways, *e.g.* lethargic or delirious malignant fevers, subcontinued fevers, &c. The clinical study of these cases is incomplete; in those observed by us the disease has run a short course—a week or a little more. The fever continues, but with noteworthy remissions, or even with real but short intermissions; the cerebral symptoms, which are serious from the first beginning of the disease, consist in some cases in an incoherent delirium accompanied by great agitation which lasts till death; in others we find a state of lethargy or coma; the spleen is generally not so much enlarged that the swelling can be clinically diagnosed; the abdomen is usually flattened. The urine may be albuminous. The examination of the blood shows that the malarial parasites are wanting as well as the melaniferous leucocytes. If these symptoms persist death ensues, the patient being in a state of collapse. Now, both because some of these cases come from places which are intensely malarial, and because the clinical examination points to the improbability of a typhoid infection, a meningitis, &c., many physicians find the idea of a malignant malarial infection so suggestive, owing to the aspect of the patients, the symptoms, &c., that they do not abandon it, although the salts of quinine are manifestly useless, and the examination of the blood gives a negative result. During the last few years Marchiafava has made autopsies of some such patients in the hospital of San Spirito; and this year two post-mortem examinations have been carried out by Professor Ferraresi and Bignami in the hospital of San Giovanni on women brought from Dr. Pelizzari's division.

It is noteworthy that one of these came from a house outside Porta San Giovanni, the other from Pratica di Mare, a place intensely malarial. The autopsy showed in these cases a cerebral hyperæmia of varied intensity without lesions of the meninges; the heart flabby, with the ventricles dilated and full of fluid blood; bilateral pulmonary hypostasis; the liver of

§ 35. If after this we take the facts which have been determined with regard to the condition of the parasites in the malignant infections and attempt to put them in connection with the various clinical forms, at the same time keeping to the classical grouping of these fevers, we cannot avoid the conclusion that, from the point of view of the parasites as we find them, there does not exist any sharply defined boundary between the so-called "complicated" malignant infections and those that are subcontinued in Torti's sense.

As we have said, there are certain "complicated malignant" intermittent fevers in which enormous quantities of parasites are found, all in the same stage of development in the blood of the living person, and after death in the spleen and bone marrow. But in a large number of the "complicated malignant" fevers (*e. g.* the comatose, the delirious, the bulbar, the choleraic, &c.) we find in the blood two, and rarely more than two generations or colonies of amœbæ—that is to say, the very same state of things as constantly occurs in the subcontinued fevers. Therefore one of the fundamental facts, and probably one of the factors which are of the greatest importance in determining the malignancy, is common to the two classical divisions of malignant fevers. This explains, in our opinion, why it is that in so many cases the "complicated malignant" infections are attended with a continued fever, and why the malignant subcontinued infections show in their turn, in a more or less pronounced manner, one or more of the symptoms characterising the "complicated malignant."

In a word, this classification is very useful for nosography and for practice, although, as Torti himself admits, it leans a little on the scholastic exigencies of the time,[1] but it does not corre-

normal size and flabby, the sectional superfices being of a yellowish-grey colour and dried-up appearance; the spleen a little enlarged; the kidneys with signs of cloudy swelling of the cortical substance; the serous cavities normal; the pharynx, the larynx, the stomach, and the intestines in normal condition, except that in some parts there was hyperæmia of the mucous membrane and a slight degree of catarrh; so that not only the examination of the blood in life but also the anatomical and pathological condition in these cases exclude the possibility of malarial infection. Everything leads one to suppose that here we have to do with an acute infection about which we as yet know nothing. Hitherto we have had no opportunity of making bacteriological researches, as we have been unable to carry out the autopsies under favorable conditions. We wish, however, here to draw attention to these facts, which owing to their obscurity are the cause of frequent mistakes of diagnosis in malarial countries.

[1] Torti, i, p. 273.

spond, as we have seen, to etiological data, except imperfectly and incompletely.

§ 36. It remains then to inquire what elements these data furnish us with in view of the judgment we may be able to make concerning the causes of the malignancy of these malarial infections, and, in the second place, what elements we obtain from them as a help towards forming a prognosis of the serious fevers.

From what we have already said, certain facts connected with the condition of the parasites are made clear—facts which must be considered as factors in the serious course these fevers take, and which, from the etiological point of view, account for the phenomena of malignancy. First and foremost in the cases which have been studied up to the present we see that malignancy coincides *with an exceptionally abundant quantity of parasitic forms*, a quantity much more abundant—where the cases terminate fatally—in the blood of the viscera than in the blood of the finger. Bignami has already drawn attention to the fact that "the contradiction so often found in life between the number of parasitic forms, the gravity of the disease, and the degree of anæmia, disappears in the vast majority of cases, when all the organs can be examined at the autopsy."

Secondly, we must bear in mind the fact constantly confirmed by fresh experience which proves that the malignant infections are for the most part produced *by two* and rarely *by a larger number of parasitic colonies* that give place, in a relatively short space of time, to invasions of young amœbæ which succeed each other, and draw nearer and nearer to each other; here we have a cause of the progressive course of the infection and of the insufficiency in many cases of the specific remedy which, as clinical experience teaches us, is not equally active against the different phases of the parasite's development. We know, however, that this fact of successive invasions of young amœbæ, tending to approximate to each other—invasions which are caused by the presence in the blood of two or more parasitic generations—may occur also in the group of fevers which we have named spring, "*a potiori*" without these fevers ever becoming malignant. Hence, as far as the origin of malignancy is concerned, this circumstance is only of importance in the group of summer-autumn fevers, from which, exclusively, the malignant infections arise.

It is in the biological properties of the amœbæ of this last group that we must unquestionably look for the fundamental facts which are the cause of the malignant course of the disease; and two of these biological properties strike us at once if we compare them with what is seen in the common quartan and tertian; we mean *the greater activity in propagation and the higher degree of virulence.*

The greater activity in multiplication. As a matter of fact, in the majority of the malignant infections an enormous invasion of parasites takes place, whereby the capillaries of certain organs, *e. g.* the brain, are so filled with amœbiferous red blood-corpuscles that often none but a few normal ones can be found, and this sufficiently proves the prodigious power of propagation which the parasites of this group possess. Moreover, in the infections of medium gravity the attention of the observer is immediately attracted by the great quantity of young amœbæ which invade the blood at every attack of fever after the fission of the adult forms has taken place; a quantity which has no counterpart in what the vast majority of quartans and tertians have to show. Hence the chief cause of the rapidly progressive course of these infections must undoubtedly be attributed to the great biological activity displayed by the summer-autumn amœbæ.

In spite of this remarkable reproductive energy every one knows who has studied these fevers that it always remains difficult to find forms of fission in the blood of the finger, especially in the fevers of medium gravity. Indeed this is the reason why the reconstruction of the life cycle of this variety of hæmatozoon has been accomplished with such difficulty, and it has only been successful when the examination of the blood in life has been combined with the study of the different viscera in cases of fatal malignancy. It may be said that only in the serious infections does it happen that a few rare sporulating forms are found in the blood of the finger. To explain this fact it is necessary in the first place to bear in mind the mechanical reasons owing to which the adult forms and those in a state of fission tend to accumulate in the vascular network of certain viscera; and, secondly, we must suppose that this variety of hæmatozoon requires but a very short period of time for the completion of that series of intimate processes whereby the fission is accomplished, as well as the separation of the clusters of spores which are shed abroad in the blood-plasma; the time is certainly shorter than that which the same processes need in the other varieties of the malarial amœba. Everything leads to the belief that to this fact more than to any other must be assigned the reason why forms in the act of fission so rarely appear in the blood of the finger; and hence arises the great difficulty of studying this phase in the life of the amœba belonging to the summer-autumn fevers.

The higher degree of virulence. This second characteristic may be inferred from many facts, but especially from the rapid change which the red blood-corpuscles undergo in these fevers. In the quartan and tertian fevers, when the red blood-corpuscle has been attacked by the amœba, it is slowly destroyed little by little as the parasite increases, until it is completely invaded, and almost all the hæmoglobin changed into melanin; whereas in the summer-autumn fevers the red blood-corpuscle is early altered; it shrivels up and its colouring is modified, even when only from a fifth to a third of its mass is filled by the parasite. The change of colouring in the whole blood-corpuscle (*brassy red blood-corpuscles*) resembles that which the particles of hæmoglobin pass through when they are enclosed in the actual body of the amœba, before being transformed into black pigment. Seeing that this rapid necrosis of the blood-corpuscle is not brought about by a progressive increase in the amœba, it must, in all probability, be considered as the result of acute poisoning. All this is not seen in the quartan, and is only very exceptionally observed in the common tertian. Considering that all the malarial parasites determine the fever in and by the act of their multiplication, we may obviously suppose that in this phase of their life they evolve *a pyrogenous virus;* and if no one as yet has affirmed this, it is because in the present state of our knowledge no direct proof of the hypothesis can be given. But the facts above described make it sufficiently clear that even during the development of their endoglobular life the amœba of the summer fevers evolve a substance or substances endowed with properties which have a fatal effect on the red globules; a peculiarity which, up to a certain point, would appear to be characteristic of the summer amœbæ, in contradistinction to those of the quartan and common tertian. Other facts, leading to the same conclusion, are furnished by the results of anatomical and pathological examination of the malignant infections. Thus Bignami has drawn attention to the extensive necrosis of the renal epithelium, especially in the convoluted tubules which are not infrequently seen in the malignant fevers; the cause of these necroses cannot be found in changes of the vascular walls directly produced by the parasites, so that he (Bignami) attributes their origin to poisoning.

Another proof of the greater virulence of the summer-autumn parasites is afforded us by the malarial hæmoglobinuria, which, if we may trust the observations hitherto collected, is determined solely by the parasites of this species and never by the tertian and quartan amœbæ. We do not in this connection speak of the interpretation of other malignant symptoms, *e. g.* the coma, the choleraic diarrhœa, &c., because in all likelihood the origin of these must be sought for in another class of facts. But in support of the theory of malarial poisoning we may mention those morbid states which are developed after the malarial (parasitic) infection has passed away; for instance, the post-malarial fever, the delirium, the post-malarial hæmoglobinuria, &c., to which we shall have occasion to return.

It is also well known, and Dionisi[1] has proved, that the anæmic conditions which follow the summer-autumn fevers are more slowly and with greater difficulty overcome than those which succeed the other malarial infections. Whether this difficulty in recovering depends alone on the fact that the states of anæmia induced by the summer amœba are more serious in kind than the others, and the lesions of the hæmatopœtic organs, which occur during the acute infection, deeper; or whether, on the other hand, it must be attributed to the persistence of a condition of post-infective poisoning, we cannot now decide. It is sufficient here to call attention to the fact itself.

Fourthly, we must take account *of the varying resistance the parasites offer to the action of the salts of quinine.* Without leaving the group of summer-autumn fevers we meet with cases of obstinate infection, which persist, notwithstanding the administration of large doses of quinine; while other cases, even where the infection is serious, *e. g.* the true subcontinued, yield quite readily to the action of the specific remedy. But there are fevers in which, when the blood is examined, the impending outbreak of a malignant paroxysm can be foreseen, and, although the remedy is promptly and energetically used, the malignancy develops and the life-cycle of the parasites is completed, and this even till the patient dies. We shall illustrate these instances when we speak of the action of quinine on this group of fevers; for the present we confine ourselves to establishing the principle that this resistance of the parasite—varying as it does within rather extended limits—must be considered as one of the factors of the malignant infections.

Another series of factors of malignancy must be looked for *in the varying resistance of the individual to the infection*—a circumstance which applies not only to malaria but to all infectious diseases. Thus, for instance, it is well known that the severe continued and malignant fevers seize those who are not accli-

[1] Dott. A. Dionisi, "Variazioni numeriche dei globuli rossi e bianchi nell' infezione malarica, in rapporto coi parassiti," 'Sperimentale,' 1891.

matised more frequently than the natives of malarial districts (see Colin and others), and seldom attack chronic sufferers from malaria or cachetic persons, &c. Some important facts from this point of view have been brought to light by anatomical pathology. For instance, several cases of malignant infection on which we have held an autopsy were found to be in subjects of arterial sclerosis and in individuals suffering from interstitial nephritis in a more or less advanced stage, or having arterio-sclerotic changes in the heart. If we bear in mind the fact that acute dilatations of the heart take place during the malignant fevers (as clinical study shows), and also that a rapid change for the worse usually follows the enfeeblement of the myocardium, it will be understood how it is that the lesions of which we have spoken, easily involving, as they do, the weakening of the heart, must have an important influence on the issue of the serious malarial infections.

§ 37. It is from the examination of the parasites that we can draw materials which enable us to form our prognosis of the dangerous fevers. From what has been said it is clear that the elements for such a prognosis cannot be entirely deduced from the clinical observation of the fevers, they being too variable. Indeed, between the so-called "masked" malignant infections, on the one hand—where the fever is entirely wanting, or only transient and slight elevations of temperature exist—and certain cerebral malignant fevers, which are attended with hyperpyrexia, on the other hand, we find all possible curves and all possible intermediate forms.

But clinical observation in the malignant infections furnishes the data for forming a judgment, especially through the study of the circulatory and nervous functions, and if this be reinforced and supplemented by examining into the condition of the parasites, we are in a position to affirm, as far at least as our experience proves it, that the opinion arrived at respecting the gravity of the patient's condition gains much in certainty and exactness. In some cases it is the only means of avoiding mistakes; for example, we give an instance of malarial infection in an epileptic person who was found in a state of coma during a paroxysm of fever. The examination of the blood, while it showed the existence of a malarial infection, showed also that it was a mild one, and hence it was possible to determine the nature of the coma as not malarial, but epileptic, although it was not known that convulsive attacks had previously occurred (see Observation 13). The facts which characterise the condition of the parasites in the malignant infections have been already described (see the preceding paragraph); but in order to judge of the gravity of the infection, and to form a prognosis of its progressive aggravation, what must rather be relied on is, as may be *a priori* foreseen, *the presence in the blood of numerous forms ripe for multiplication* (corpuscles with pigment at the centre).

When this is the case, even though there be no malignant clinical symptoms, one may with certainty predict that the infection will grow rapidly worse. (See Case 27.) But it is of more importance here to determine the way in which the amœbæ behave in cases of fatal malignancy after the administration of strong doses of quinine. Two facts may be noticed which are illustrated by the examples given below: (1) either the parasitic generations continue to develop up to the time of death until the blood as a whole is filled with amœbæ in different degrees of development; or (2) after the remedy has been energetically administered the parasites become progressively fewer and fewer, while the large phagocytes, which enclose small masses of pigment, amœbiferous red corpuscles, spore-forming bodies, &c., increase in number, very often enormously; and although the parasites thus progressively diminish, the clinical symptoms may grow continually worse till death takes place. Of these two possibilities the first is observed for the most part where the malignant infection runs a short course, the second where it is protracted, also in cases of three or four days' duration. (See Case 27.) This progressive decrease of the plasmodia in the blood of the finger may take place even when *the post-mortem examination reveals the presence of numerous plasmodia and fissions in the cerebral vessels and in the spleen, or, it may be, only in the brain.* But there are cases in which all the viscera contain but a scanty number of parasites, or they may even have entirely disappeared. In some of these latter the cause of the fatal issue is found in the existence of serious alterations in the endothelium of the cerebral vessels and of many punctiform hæmorrhages, owing to which the endocranial pressure may be considerably increased; in some, on the other hand, the anatomical and pathological examination shows no sufficient reason. In these last cases, whatever be the cause of the persistent coma and of the fatal result, it can only be investigated by way of hypothesis. Thus, for instance, it is not an improbable supposition that there are certain nutritive changes produced in the nervous elements by the progressive invasion of the parasites; changes that in many cases are beyond the reach of the anatomical and pathological examination, while in others they are shown by clearly marked histological alterations in the nerve cells. Marchiafava[1] has lately illustrated an instance of this sort which occurred in a bulbar malignant infection.

§ 38. It follows from the foregoing that it is impossible to form an exact conception of the invasion of the parasites in the blood of patients suffering from malignant infections without studying the different organs in fatal cases. We shall here briefly set forth the knowledge we possess on this subject, as it provides us with materials by which we may explain the pathogenesis of some of the malignant symptoms.

After the recent acquisitions in the etiology of malaria, Guarnieri[2] and Bignami[3] turned their attention to these histological researches, and the latter, after studying the different organs in twenty cases of malignant infection, obtained the following results.[4] We pass over the macroscopic changes in the various organs (the brain, the spleen, the liver, the bone marrow, the kidneys, the intestines, &c.) ; these are now sufficiently well known, and we shall consider solely the alterations which examination by the microscope reveals. In the comatose malignant fevers the capillaries of the *brain*, and especially the grey matter, are found to be injected with an immense quantity of red blood-corpuscles loaded with plasmodia. As a rule one may say that the vessels of larger diameter contain a smaller number of parasites. The amœbæ are found for the most part in the different phases of their life cycle, but generally one special phase is predominant. The pigmented adult forms and those in the act of forming spores are seen by preference within the capillaries, while the young forms without pigment preponderate in the small veins and arteries. In rare cases it happens that the parasites are not visible in very large quantities, but the traces of a preceding parasitic invasion are nevertheless manifest in the masses of free pigment, in the endothelia which are swollen and loaded with pigment, and in the leucocytes which are full of red blood-corpuscles and pigmented.

In the *spleen* appearances are usually observed which prove the phagocytosis of the pigment, of the parasites, and of the necrotic red corpuscles. The pulp is invaded by a number of

[1] See 'Atti del Congresso di Medicina interna,' Ottobre, 1890.
[2] Guarnieri, 'Atti della R. Accademia Medica di Roma,' 1887.
[3] Bignami, ibid., 1890.
[4] These have now been confirmed by the researches made in the malarial season of 1891.

red blood-corpuscles, containing to a large extent parasites, which separate the elements of the pulp. In some cases the pigmented forms prevail, in others those producing spores. The crescent-shaped figures are seldom wanting altogether, but they are generally less in number than the other parasitic forms. But our attention is attracted much less by the parasites in the cells of the pulp than by the large white cells which contain pigment in smaller or larger masses, in small rods, and in granules, as well as discoloured red blood-corpuscles loaded with plasmodia or those brassy in colour; sometimes also complete forms with spores are found in these cellules. In contrast to the pigmentation of the pulp stand the Malpighian follicles, the lymphocytes of which never contain pigment. While the capillaries abound in parasites the splenic veins contain but few, and sometimes none at all. In the first case the red blood-corpuscles, full of parasites, and the macrophagi, containing pigment and fragments of red blood-corpuscles, are next the delicate venous walls, whereas the normal red blood-corpuscles are found collected in the centre of the blood-vessel.

By studying the spleen we are better enabled to see the way in which the blood gets rid of the parasites. This is principally effected by the amœbæ being enclosed in the large phagocytes, and, in a secondary way, through the agency of the endothelia, and not only of the adult pigmented forms and entire sporulations, but even of the small endoglobular parasites, when the red blood-corpuscles, which contain them, are struck by premature necrosis.

Guarnieri's observations on the changes in the *liver* in the malignant infections, which have been to a large extent confirmed by Bignami, prove the presence of macrocytes loaded with pigment, which occasionally close the lumen of the intralobular capillaries, the pigmentation of the endothelium, and of Kupfer's stellated cells. The parasites are generally scanty in the liver, and more numerous in the portal ramifications and in the capillary net than in the sublobular veins, where the melaniferous leucocytes are predominant.

Along with these changes in the vessels and connective tissue we find also alterations of the hepatic cells, in the form of cloudy swelling, atrophy, isolated or extended necroses, and signs of fresh cellular formation; and, moreover, Bignami has proved that many hepatic cellules contain masses of hæmoglobin and fragments of brassy red blood-corpuscles, which give an iron reaction. This condition of things explains how the liver is the instrument by which is effected the elimination of the colouring matter of the amœbiferous red blood-corpuscles which are prematurely dead; hence the bilious condition which is so frequent in the malignant fevers, and the jaundice which accompanies certain severe forms of malarial infection.

In the *lungs* the capillary net of the alveoli is found full of phagocytes pigmented and loaded with red blood-corpuscles, which often show signs of degeneration. These phagocytes are observed in the veins, in great masses, clinging to the walls of the blood-vessels, of which, in the transverse sections, they appear to occupy almost a third. As regards the forms of the parasites, one may say that, as a rule, those forms prevail which in individual cases are found in large numbers in the brain. Pigmented endothelia in the capillaries and in the small veins are only rarely to be seen, and still more rarely pigmented leucocytes inside the alveoli. If cases of pneumonia or of broncho-pneumonia come under observation in infections of long duration it is a remarkable fact that there is no excretion of pigmented leucocytes in the interior of the alveoli, the exudation being composed of the ordinary polynucleated leucocytes.

In the *kidneys* the number of endoglobular parasites, as well as those within the white cells, is generally small in comparison with that in the other organs. They are seldom met with in the small vessels of the glomerulus, while they are easily detected in all stages in the intertubular capillaries; in the large veins they are very rare. On the other hand the glomeruli are usually pigmented, and the pigment is found collected, sometimes in large white cells which obstruct the lumen in the loops of the glomeruli, sometimes in the endothelium of the glomerulus. As regards the extra-vascular changes, in addition to the pigmentation of the endothelium which we have mentioned, there is the desquamation and degeneration of the endothelium of Bowman's capsule, and the necroses of the epithelium, especially of the convoluted tubules. These alterations are probably of toxic origin.

In the *intestines* the parasites are found in the same condition, and there is the same quantitative relation between the parasitic contents of the capillaries and those of the larger vessels as in the other organs. In one case of choleraic malignant infection the mucous membrane of the stomach and of the small intestine was found to be intensely hyperæmic, with punctiform hæmorrhages and swelling of the lymphatic follicles. Examination by the microscope revealed an enormous accumulation of parasites in the vessels of the mucous membrane, on the superficial part of which there was an extensive necrosis, and consequently parvicellular infiltration.

The marrow of the flat bones (ribs) is of a reddish-brown colour, that of the long bones (the femur) is for the most part reddish brown in the two upper and lower thirds, while in the middle third it has a yellowish, jelly-like appearance. Its consistence is usually very soft, indeed it is almost fluid. The endoglobular parasitic forms generally fill up the lumen of the blood vessels of the bone marrow; the adult forms and those sporulating are the most common; in some cases also the crescent-shaped forms preponderate. Besides this we find parasitic forms outside the blood-vessels, where, nevertheless, the most prevalent shapes are, as in the spleen, the large phagocytes, mostly in a state of necrosis. In some cases the vessels of the marrow contain great quantities of the nucleated red blood-corpuscles, in which parasites are never found.

The principal facts relating to the varied distribution of the parasites may be summed up as follows:—The parasites are always found in remarkably greater numbers in the small arteries and capillaries than in the larger vessels and veins, where the blood-corpuscles that are loaded with amœbæ are always mixed with no small number of normal blood-corpuscles. The adult forms, as well as those in process of forming spores, tend to accumulate in some of the capillary networks, especially in that of the brain, where, owing to the very small lumen, the circulatory resistance is great. From the point of view of the frequency of the forms of sporulation the brain contains the largest number, then come in order the lungs, the spleen, the osseous marrow, the liver, and the intestines; but in some cases the intestines have a greater quantity than the organs last mentioned. The other forms, the crescent-shaped and the ovoid, are more abundant in the spleen and bone marrow than in the viscera. Lastly, in the spleen, in the bone marrow, and in the liver the forms which are enclosed in the white blood-corpuscles, that act as phagocytes, are usually predominant.

§ 39. These facts, disclosed by pathological anatomy, make us reconsider the interpretation of certain symptoms observed in the malignant fevers. Among these it is the coma and the cerebral phenomena in general which have attracted the greatest attention, and the attempt has been made to explain their origin in various ways.

Frerichs has described (as is well known) the accumulations of pigment in the small vessels of the brain, and has stated further that there are not infrequently also to be found, in the cerebrum of those who have died from a malignant infection, certain stoppages of the vessels produced by a species of *white coagula*, not unlike those of the fibrin. He maintains, moreover, that the mechanical alteration of the circulation might involve the laceration of the vascular walls, and lead to the formation of capillary apoplexies. With regard to the causal connection of these lesions with the cerebral clinical symptoms, Frerichs expresses himself with great reserve; he notes especially that cases have been observed in which the cerebral symptoms were wanting, but yet the brain was found to be melanotic; and, on the other hand, cases in which there were cerebral disturbances, without any pigmentation of the brain being afterwards found at the autopsy. This last fact was observed by Frerichs six times out of twenty-eight cases of cerebral intermittent fever. These phenomena lead him to the conclusion that the above-mentioned cerebral symptoms may, without doubt, occur in fevers without melanæmia, and that therefore there are other causes besides this latter which are capable of producing them; and, lastly, he supposes that a study of the chemical products, which are set free in the circulation by the disintegration of the red blood-corpuscles, will bring us nearer to a knowledge of these facts.

Laveran recognised the parasitic nature of the pigmented bodies, and attributed the origin of the cerebral phenomena, and especially of the coma, to their accumulation in the cerebral capillaries; in his opinion, these bodies obstruct the capillaries and produce parasitic vascular thromboses.[1] This theory answers some of the objections made to the hypothesis of the emboli and thromboses of the pigment; the fact that the obstruction of the cerebral vessels is produced not by an inert substance (the black pigment), but by living parasitic elements, accounts (if we follow Laveran) for the rapidity of the disappearance of the cerebral symptoms which is seen in many cases, and explains the wonderful effect of the salts of quinine.

It is, however, evident that even this way of considering the matter does not remove all the difficulties which Frerichs himself set up against his own hypothesis.

In our opinion, recent researches allow a different view to be taken of the mechanical theory of the cerebral symptoms in malignant infections; these investigations have placed on a firm foundation the doctrine of *the endoglobular position* of the *parasites*, and have made manifest the degenerative changes of the red blood-corpuscles. Owing to these alterations, those of them which have

[1] 'Traité des fièvres palustres,' pp. 482, 483.

been invaded by the parasite offer greater resistance to the circulation than the normal ones, whence it happens that they accumulate towards the circumference of the larger vessels, and their circulation is either stopped or retarded in certain portions of the capillaries, in which the degenerative changes of the endothelium, induced by the defective circulation, constitute a fresh cause for stagnation. When the comatose malignant infections are submitted to anatomical and pathological examination, we generally find an increase of the endocranial tension, and an intense hyperæmia of the cerebral substance,—a hyperæmia which is always caused *by the accumulation in the cerebral vessels of red blood-corpuscles loaded with amœbæ,* while a greater quantity of normal red blood-corpuscles is found in the larger vessels; the blood which circulates in the very fine vascular network of the brain is always more changed than that which we find in other viscera, for instance the lungs, and, generally speaking, in vessels of medium and large size. Now it seems to us that no other explanation of these facts can be given, except that which is based on the mechanical alterations in the circulation, of which we have spoken.

Another fact leads to the same conclusion. It has been observed that in the capillary apoplexies almost all the extravasated red blood-corpuscles are without parasites, while the cerebral vessels contain amœbiferous red blood-corpuscles in immense numbers. This stagnation of blood-corpuscles loaded with amœbæ ought accordingly to furnish a reason for the intense hyperæmia of the grey matter, for the increase of the cerebral tension, for the capillary apoplexies, &c. Only exceptionally do we find in the cerebral vessels accumulations of small masses of free pigment (thromboses of pigment) or masses of melaniferous leucocytes (thromboses of phagocytes), and rarely also free adult parasitic forms, or accumulations of free spores (parasitic thromboses in the proper sense of the term). Hence, in determining the morbid symptoms, much less importance must be attached to these facts than to the stagnation of the altered blood-corpuscles which we have mentioned. It is not unlikely that this retarding of the circulation, and this stoppage, in the brain, of the blood-elements in a completely altered condition, are the cause of functional changes, and, in some cases, even nutritive alterations of the nervous centres.

Recent researches allow us also to answer the well-known objections brought against the theory of the emboli or thromboses of pigment. First, in forming a judgment on cases in which the autopsy reveals cerebral melanoses, although there had been no coma during life, we must take into consideration the varying intensity of the melanosis, and also distinguish the melanosis of the vascular walls, which is the after-effect of preceding parasitic invasions, from the actual accumulation of parasites within the vessels, and further, it is needful to bear in mind the rapidity with which the parasitic invasion is completed. The effects on the cerebral functions ought indeed to be very different, according as the invasion, for instance of red blood-corpuscles containing mature parasites—as happens at the beginning of a paroxysm—is completed in a short period (whence the fulminant coma), or slowly and by degrees, as there is reason in some cases to suppose. Secondly, when we judge of cases in which death took place during coma, without the post-mortem examination showing any cerebral melanosis, it is necessary to keep in remembrance the fact which we have ascertained,[1] namely, that sometimes the cerebral vessels are found full of red blood-corpuscles, all or almost all of them containing non-pigmented amœbæ, of which, moreover, the fission may be in process of accomplishment, or may have already taken place. Nor ought we to forget those cases of malignant infection where the course is protracted, and in which the coma persists, and death ensues, when the parasites have entirely, or almost entirely, disappeared from the blood, without the effects of the preceding invasion being removed. We have already considered instances of this sort.

Such being the state of the question, we can maintain that the facts brought to light by the anatomical and pathological examination furnish a sufficient explanation of the cerebral symptoms of the malignant infections, such as the lethargy, the coma, the convulsions, the delirium, &c.; symptoms pointing to localisation, such as the aphasia, the hemiplegia, the bulbar symptoms, &c.; while we must admit, on the other hand, that we possess no facts capable of sustaining the hypothesis of the poisonous origin of phenomena like these. There is no doubt that poisonous products are formed during the malarial attack, yet no one has adduced facts in support of the view that they are formed to the extent of producing the effects described; so that, at present, the chemical theory of the cerebral symptoms cannot be maintained, except by way of exclusion,—that is to say, by showing that the anatomical and pathological changes, which

[1] Marchiafava e Celli, "Nouvelles études sur l'infection malarique." 'Arch. ital. de Biologie,' 1887.

we have explained, do not form a harmonious group of facts sufficient to explain the phenomena, and this is, in our opinion, impossible at the present moment.

In addition to the above-mentioned alterations in the brain, the most considerable part of which may be said to be intravascular, it is not an unusual thing to find punctiform hæmorrhages in the nervous centres, just as they are seen in life on the skin of the face and in the retina. These are sometimes only few and scattered; sometimes, on the other hand, they are so numerous, and so blended together from close proximity, as to give a red colouring to the cerebral substance.

Bastianelli and Bignami have recently given us their views on the pathogenesis of these punctiform hæmorrhages, and they have noted the following facts:

1. These hæmorrhages are always met with in the white substances of the hemispheres and the bulb; more rarely on the boundaries between the white and grey matter, in which latter they are not usually found.[1]

2. The hæmorrhages are composed of normal red blood-corpuscles, even in cases where the capillaries are entirely filled, both with red blood-corpuscles loaded with parasites, and with free parasites.

3. They are generally found surrounding the finest arteries, and often surrounding the small thrombosed vessels, in which the endothelium is altered by the parasitic thrombosis.

From these facts they draw the conclusion that the punctiform hæmorrhages are probably caused by diapedeses through the altered walls of the small capillary arteries, in which a stagnation, and in some cases a real thrombosis, is produced by the slowness of the circulation, which is greatest in the white substance, where the capillary network is less abundant and the lumen of the vessels smaller than in the grey substance.

These lesions account for certain clinical facts, *e.g.* for the persistent coma, in spite of the decrease in the number of the parasites, and for the hard and full pulse already noticed by Torti in some of the lethargic malignant infections.

The changes in the mucous membrane of the stomach and of the intestines, consequent on the invasion of the capillaries by the parasites, make very clear the pathogenesis of the choleraic malignant fevers, &c.

But other malignant phenomena, those, for example, of the algid

[1] In a solitary case observed by Dr. Bastianelli and ourselves numerous punctiform hæmorrhages even into the grey matter were seen.

malignant infections, the cardialgic, the hæmorrhagic, &c., cannot up to the present time be solved by any interpretation based on sufficient observation, for these forms of malarial infection are in our country very rare.

The acute swelling of the spleen is determinined by various factors, that is to say, by the accumulation in it of a considerable quantity of changed red blood-corpuscles, of pigmented leucocytes loaded with red blood-corpuscles and plasmodia, of endothelial cells, of necrotic leucocytes, and of parasites both endoglobular and free, young, adult, and in process of forming spores. Accordingly, while we infer the purifying activity of the splenic pulp from this last element, the others previously mentioned lead us to consider this acute swelling as chiefly spodogenous.[1] Moreover, both in the pulp and in the Malpighian follicles we often find many of the elements in a state of karyokinesis.

§ 40. We shall not return to the alterations in the red blood-corpuscles, after all that has been said as to the endoglobular development of the parasites; we only wish to insist on a fact on which too little stress has been laid; we mean the separation of the hæmoglobin from the discoplasm; in some cases the hæmoglobin does not turn into melanin, but is dissolved in the plasma, and produces the hæmoglobinæmia, which, if it exceeds certain proportions, becomes hæmoglobinuria.

Rossoni, Bignami, and Bastianelli have lately given their attention to the malarial hæmoglobinuriæ.

Marchiafava has observed a case of hæmoglobinuric malignant infection, with all the characteristic renal lesions; the patient was a traveller, who had already suffered from the disease on the Congo. He showed all the signs of chronic malarial infection, with the spleen enormously enlarged; the disease was overcome by liberal doses of quinine, which was also administered by hypodermic injection, but it left a very serious anæmia, recovery from which was slow and difficult.

During the hæmoglobinuric paroxysm there was jaundice, together with enlargement and pain in the liver and spleen; the hæmoglobinuria lasted a little more than twenty-four hours after it was first treated with quinine. The state of the urine was such as is seen in all the hæmoglobinuriæ, that is to say, there is hæmoglobin, albumen, and hæmoglobinic, granular, and epithelial cylinders. When the hæmoglobinuria has passed away, the albumen and the cylinders generally still persist, but on the third day the urine is normal. In all the cases observed by us and by Bastianelli, as

[1] Σποδός, literally ashes of the dead; hence necrotic débris, &c.—Ed.

we have explained, do not form a har[illegible] of Rossoni, the
sufficient to explain the phenomena, and [illegible] the blood has been
impossible at the present moment. [illegible]gnami have found

In addition to the above-mentioned [illegible] condition, being
the most considerable part of which [illegible]rpuscles; they have
vascular, it is not an unusual thing to fi[illegible] in the macrocytes
in the nervous centres, just as they ar[illegible] size, of which they
the face and in the retina. These [illegible]ne blue, they have
scattered; sometimes, on the other [illegible]ing to Ehrlich, would
and so blended together from clo[illegible]plasma.
colouring to the cerebral substance [illegible]globinuriæ in malaria,

Bastianelli and Bignami have r[illegible]hrough a predisposition
the pathogenesis of these punctifo[illegible]ure necrosis of the red
noted the following facts: [illegible]oss of the hæmoglobin,

1. These hæmorrhages are [illegible]hat this is the case even
substances of the hemispheres [illegible]ave not been invaded by the
boundaries between the white [illegible] of poisonous substances
they are not usually found.[1] [illegible] cases of malarial hæmo-

2. The hæmorrhages are [illegible]blood-corpuscle is accom-
corpuscles, even in cases whe[illegible] is to say, either (1) by the
both with red blood-corpusc[illegible]elanin; or (2) by the pre-
free parasites. [illegible]rpuscle (brassy red blood-

3. They are generally [illegible] of the hæmoglobin from the
and often surrounding the [illegible]ccurs extensively in all the
endothelium is altered by [illegible] also the third in a more

From these facts they [illegible] is not uniformly observed,
hæmorrhages are prob[illegible]s dissolved in the blood when
altered walls of the sma[illegible] Ponfick), and it is not elimi-
and in some cases a [illegible] of the bilious condition which
ness of the circulation [illegible] of the jaundice with which
where the capillary ne[illegible]
the vessels smaller th[illegible]ions to the Società Lancisiana

These lesions acc[illegible], Bignami and Bastianelli
persistent coma, in [illegible]nuria, in one of which the condi-
parasites, and for [illegible] was negative as regards the
Torti in some of th[illegible]nting signs of a very recent

The changes in [illegible]ther only those parasitic forms
the intestines, con[illegible] fever could be determined with
parasites, make ve[illegible] served as evidence of precedent
nant fevers, &c. [illegible]inuria of this sort they place in

But other ma[illegible]mena.

[1] In a solitary [illegible]acts, we would remark that under
punctiform hæmor[illegible]omena we refer to those morbid

[illegible] been verified, not only after the cessa- [illegible] even when the parasites, especially the [illegible] no longer met with in the blood. In [illegible]larial fevers, there are individual cases of a [illegible] condition, which must be put by the side of [illegible] after other infectious diseases (typhoid, pneu- [illegible], &c.).

[illegible] we find states of anæmia, of acute delirium, [illegible]obinuria, which develop in cases where the acute [illegible] has passed away along with the disappearance [illegible] from the blood; these phenomena are post- [illegible]rbid manifestations, and we must distinguish them [illegible] delirious, anæmic, and hæmoglobinuric malignant fevers. [illegible] just as certain groups of complex nervous symptoms, [illegible] remind us of bulbar paralysis, of disseminated sclerosis, and [illegible] psychoses, constitute in certain cases the symptoms belong- [illegible] a malignant malarial infection, as Marchiafava, Torti, [illegible] Angelini have recently observed; so, on the other hand, the [illegible] symptoms may be developed after the cessation of the [illegible] infection, as is proved by instances which Bignami, Bastia- [illegible]nelli, and Marchiafava have lately described.

The distinction between post-malarial phenomena, as being post-infective facts, and the phenomena of the malignant infections, in the proper sense of the term, is of importance from the point of view both of therapeutics and of prognosis.

In point of fact, while we sometimes see the most serious nervous phenomena—for instance, a hemiplegia, symptoms of acute bulbar paralysis—disappear in a short time under specific therapeutic treatment, this does not take place, as far as our experience goes, when the case is one of post-infective phenomena, which may last even weeks and months. Hence, it is obvious that an examination of the blood is indispensable in cases of this sort, especially in the masked forms, in order to arrive at a differential diagnosis.

§ 41. The cases of malignant fever now to be described are given chiefly with the aim of demonstrating what we have stated with reference to the condition of the parasites. Some of them, and especially those of cerebral malignant fever, must be taken as examples of a series of similar cases observed by us during the last few years.

well as in one case which came under t[illegible]
existence of summer-autumn parasitic [illegible] [illegible]rson.
verified. Furthermore, Bastianelli [illegible]
numerous parasitic forms in an app[illegible] [illegible]onio C—, 33 years
perhaps enclosed in decolorized red [illegible] [illegible]elo, has had fever
also detected a considerable macro[illegible] [illegible]ning, and ceases in
and in many red blood-corpuscles [illegible] size, and becoming
had made a preparation coloured [illegible]
seen spots of blue colouring, wh[illegible] [illegible]rature is 104·7°. On
represent degenerative changes [illegible] [illegible]ber of young plasmodia

As regards the pathogenesi[illegible] [illegible]nnular in shape, and in
everything points to the conc[illegible] [illegible]mber of pigmented white
in the individual varying in [illegible] in addition some rather
blood-corpuscles takes pla[illegible] The fever ceases spon-
after the invasion of the p[illegible]
in those red blood-corpus[illegible] several large discoid plas-
amœbæ, perhaps throu[illegible] 10.15 a.m., condition the
(Bignami, Bastianelli). [illegible] hæmoglobinic granules are
globinuria the destr[illegible] [illegible]ature 101°. Small plasmodia,
plished in three dif[illegible] [illegible]so forms with a very minute
conversion of the [illegible] a small number of brassy
mature necrosis [illegible] [illegible]ented white blood-corpuscles.
corpuscles), or (3 [illegible] [illegible]ering; prostration of patient.
discoplasma. O[illegible] [illegible]ministered by the mouth.
severe summer [illegible] [illegible]ent falls into a state of lethargy.
limited degre[illegible] [illegible] state, and showing great
the reason [illegible] with much difficulty and with
it does not [illegible] [illegible]equent, and soft. Respiration
nated by t[illegible] [illegible]mp. 99·7°. Quinine, 32 grains,
is seen i[illegible] [illegible]ection; also hypodermic injections
many of [illegible] [illegible]ood is found a very small number

In [illegible] [illegible]lso a few white blood-corpuscles,
('Ri[illegible] [illegible]pigmented. 10.30 a.m., blood as
men[illegible] [illegible]hargy continues. The right angle
tio[illegible] [illegible]ips dry; in the urine there is no
pa[illegible] [illegible]ment. 12 noon, temp. 99·9°. During
pa[illegible] [illegible]rises to a maximum of 101·6° F.
([illegible] [illegible]s above. Blood: a few plasmodia
c[illegible] [illegible]shape, and motionless; they are a little
[illegible]. There are no pigmented white
[illegible]dermic injections of quinine (16 grains
[illegible]ulants administered subcutaneously.
[illegible]hree or four plasmodia found in one

[illegible] ient, on being shaken and called with a loud [illegible] and gives very faint answers to questions. [illegible] complete helplessness, with the muscles more [illegible] right side of his body than on the left; he cannot [illegible], and there is a quivering of the eyelids. From [illegible] however, he wakes up spontaneously, and asks for [illegible] things; occasionally, also, he raises himself so as to sit [illegible] of his own accord. An abundant quantity of urine [illegible] during the last twenty-four hours (above 64 oz.); it is [illegible] coloured.

[illegible]—Morning: the patient has a little headache, but otherwise feels well. He states that he has had on other occasions attacks like the preceding, attended with epileptic symptoms; he remembers having felt the preliminary sensations of a convulsive attack during the night before. 8.30 p.m., natural temperature. Blood: examination gives a negative result. Nothing noteworthy on the following days.

We have here the case of an epileptic person, as is shown from the recollection of the patient. He had an attack during the malarial fever, an attack of which the nurses—it being in the night—were not aware. When seen on the following morning in a condition of post-epileptic lethargy, he appeared, at first sight, to be suffering from the effects of a severe malarial infection. The examination of the blood, however, did not support this view of the case, and accordingly indicated the way to reach the real diagnostic interpretation.

2.

A Prolonged Paroxysm of Fever.

CASE 14.[1]—Giuseppe T—, able-bodied, coming from Bracciano, has had fever since midday on August 10th; the shivering persisted for a long time, and, according to the patient, the fever has lasted continuously up to the present. The spleen is a little enlarged, but does not project beyond the ribs.

He entered the hospital on August 11th, 4 p.m. Sweating begins. Temperature 100·4°. Blood: there are many plasmodia without pigment, large in size, discoid and annular in shape, and in motion. The sweating continues during the night. 4 p.m., temperature 100·4°. 8 p.m., 100·4°. 12 p.m., 101°.

August 12th.—Temperature: 4 a.m., 101·2°. 8 a.m., 99·9°. 10 a.m., 99·4°. 12 noon, 99·7°. 4 p.m., 100·8°. 8 p.m., 101·8°.

[1] See Chart II, tracing 10.

12 p.m., 103·5° F. 8 a.m., blood: an immense number of very large plasmodia, some almost one third of the red blood-corpuscle in size; they are discoid and annular in shape; they display movement, and all of them have granules of pigment at the circumference. Patient complains of slight headache. 10 a.m., the condition of the parasites is as above; in addition, there are several pigmented plasmodia in brassy red blood-corpuscles. Bimuriate of quinine, 32 grains, administered by hypodermic injection. 3 p.m., patient has headache, and is a little lethargic. Blood: condition as above; the brassy red blood-corpuscles have increased in number, and besides these some discoid forms are seen with the pigment collected at the centre, or else eccentrically, in a group of granules or formed into a small mass. The temperature rises unaccompanied by shivering. 4 p.m., blood: nothing but brassy red blood-corpuscles are seen, in large quantities, containing parasites with granules or small masses of pigment.

13th.—Temp., 4 a.m., 103·1°. 8 a.m., 102·4°. 7.30 a.m., 103·3°. 4 p.m., 105·4°. 8 p.m., 105·4°. 12 p.m., 105·6° F. 8 a.m., blood: a few plasmodia with granules of pigment, or with a small collection at the centre enclosed in brassy red blood-corpuscles, or in corpuscles tending to become so; also white blood-corpuscles with small masses of pigment. 9.30 a.m., condition the same. *No young forms are found.* 2.30 p.m., blood: there are still a few forms having a small central mass of pigment. *No young forms are visible.* 4.30 p.m., blood; there are still a very few forms with small central collections of pigment; also *several plasmodia without pigment,* in motion, and discoid or annular in shape; in addition, some pigmented white blood-corpuscles with small masses of pigment. 6 p.m., the patient is depressed and agitated. Bimuriate of quinine, 32 grains, administered by hypodermic injection.

14th.—Temp., 4 a.m., 102·7°. 8 a.m., 100·8°. 12 noon, 99·6°. 4 p.m., 98·5°. 8 p.m., 98·1°. 12 p.m., 98·1° F. 8.15 a.m., the state of depression continues. Blood: a rather scanty number of plasmodia without pigment, some in brassy red blood-corpuscles. A few white blood-corpuscles containing small masses of pigment. Sulphate of quinine, 16 grains, administered by the mouth. 3.15 p.m., blood: condition as above; in addition, a very small number of plasmodia with granules of pigment in brassy red blood-corpuscles, or in corpuscles tending to become so. 5 p.m., blood: condition the same, but the parasites are much decreased in number,—in fact, they are extremely scanty.

15th.—Complete absence of fever ensued. The condition of the patient is good; in the blood there are only a very few motionless plasmodia without pigment.

On the 16th, examination of the blood gives a negative result; the patient continues to take sulphate of quinine, and rapidly recovers strength.

In this case a tertian paroxysm is protracted, while preserving its own proper form of curve, in spite of strong doses of quinine. As regards the parasites, only a few develop up to the point of producing the young forms of the new generation, which appear very slowly in the red blood-corpuscles,—almost twenty-four hours after the beginning of the paroxysm of fever. This may be explained if we allow that the quinine, when present in the blood in sufficient quantity, hinders the young forms from invading the red blood-corpuscles; whereas, if the remedy be withheld, and there be no longer a sufficient amount of it in the circulation, then the invasion takes place. This accounts for the delayed appearance of the young plasmodia and for the prolongation of the paroxysm.

3.

Malignant Infection with Lethargy and Delirium.

CASE 15. The Lancisi Division, No. 12.—B—, a man from outside the Porta Cavalleggeri, where he took the fever, has suffered from it for four days.

He entered the hospital on July 25th at 5 p.m.: he is lethargic, gives answers with great difficulty, and remembers nothing about his illness. Blood: there is an abundant number of parasites—many plasmodia without pigment, or with granules of pigment at the circumference, almost all of them in brassy blood-corpuscles; also many forms with pigment at the centre; endoglobular spindle-shaped forms of different sizes, with pigment along the axis; endoglobular round forms, with pigment dispersed in different parts; adult crescent-shaped forms, and also adult round forms in a state of disintegration. In addition, brassy red blood-corpuscles in a disintegrated condition; the hæmoglobin is collected in masses, one of which surrounds the parasite, leaving part of the blood-corpuscle discoloured; pigmented white blood-corpuscles, some of necrotic appearance. Soluble hydrochlorate of quinine, 32 grains, administered by hypodermic injection.

July 26th.—The patient's general condition is slightly improved. Blood: 11 a.m., condition as above; but the forms of the crescent-shaped phase, both free and endoglobular, are less

12 p.m., 103·5° F. 8 a.m., blood: an immense num
large plasmodia, some almost one third of the red bl
in size; they are discoid and annular in shape;
movement, and all of them have granules of pigme
cumference. Patient complains of slight headac
the condition of the parasites is as above; in add
several pigmented plasmodia in brassy red bl
Bimuriate of quinine, 32 grains, administered
injection. 3 p.m., patient has headache, and is
Blood: condition as above; the brassy red blood
increased in number, and besides these some
seen with the pigment collected at the centre, or
in a group of granules or formed into a small ma
ture rises unaccompanied by shivering. 4 p.m
but brassy red blood-corpuscles are seen, i
containing parasites with granules or small ma

13th.—Temp., 4 a.m., 103·1°. 8 a.m.,
103·3°. 4 p.m., 105·4°. 8 p.m., 105·4°.
8 a.m., blood: a few plasmodia with granules
a small collection at the centre enclosed in br
puscles, or in corpuscles tending to become
corpuscles with small masses of pigment.
the same. *No young forms are found.* 2.30
still a few forms having a small central
young forms are visible. 4.30 p.m., blood;
few forms with small central collections of
plasmodia without pigment, in motion,
in shape; in addition, some pigmented whi
small masses of pigment. 6 p.m., the
agitated. Bimuriate of quinine, 32 grai
dermic injection.

14th.—Temp., 4 a.m., 102·7°. 8 a.m.
4 p.m., 98·5°. 8 p.m., 98·1°. 12 p.m.
state of depression continues. Blood:
plasmodia without pigment, some in bra
few white blood-corpuscles containing
Sulphate of quinine, 16 grains, admini
p.m., blood: condition as above; in a
of plasmodia with granules of pigme
puscles, or in corpuscles tending to
condition the same, but the parasi
number,—in fact, they are extremely

15th.—Complete absence of fever

the blood of the finger the majority of the red blood-corpuscles contain plasmodia without pigment, and some even two or three parasites; there are a few forms with pigment at the centre, and many pigmented white blood-corpuscles. High fever (between 102·2° and 104° F.).

July 31st.—In the night the fever decreases; the state of lethargy continues in the morning. The most striking feature is the very grave anæmic condition. The hæmoglobin is only 34 to 35 per cent. (Fleischl). In the blood (at 9 a.m.) the quantity of the parasites is still very abundant; the same forms are seen as on the preceding day, and in addition there are endoglobular crescent-shaped forms.

Treatment.—From 2 a.m. on the 30th till 9 a.m. on the 31st, 96 grains of bimuriate of quinine are administered by hypodermic injection. At 12 noon on the 31st about 120 cubic centimetres[1] of defibrinated blood are injected by Ziemssen's method into the subcutaneous tissue of the thighs. At 4 p.m. the general condition has improved; the patient replies to questions, he remembers nothing of the journey from Foggia to Rome. Temp. 99·6°. Pulse 120. At 5 p.m. the hæmoglobin is 35 per cent. (Fleischl). In the blood there is still a considerable number of plasmodia without pigment; also a very few with pigment at the centre, and white blood-corpuscles with black or rusty-coloured pigment.

Treatment.—Bimuriate of quinine, 24 grains, given by hypodermic injection.

On August 1st skin cool, and a remarkable improvement. The hæmoglobin is 36 per cent. (Fleischl). The parasites show a marked decrease; there are plasmodia without pigment, or with granules of pigment at the circumference, for the most part in brassy red blood-corpuscles, the forms of the crescent-shaped phase being less common; besides these, many macrocytes and microcytes are found, as well as many pigmented macrophagi. Bimuriate of quinine, 32 grains, administered by hypodermic injection during the day.

On August 2nd the improvement continues. In the blood there is nothing visible but pigmented white blood-corpuscles, and a very small number of crescent-shaped forms.

3rd.—The hæmoglobin is 35 per cent. (Fleischl). Blood: as above. In addition there are nucleated macrocytes and microcytes.

4th.—As above.

5th.—The patient says that he feels well; he eats largely (three

[1] Say 4¼ oz.—Ed.

and a half pints of milk in the day, half a chicken, soup, &c.). He takes Baccelli's mixture[1] of iron, arsenic, and quinine. Blood: the crescent-shaped forms are rare, but there are enormous macrophagi with masses of pigment, some having a necrotic appearance; also macrocytes and red blood-corpuscles with mobile protuberances (poichilocytes).

6th.—The improvement goes on. The parasites are decreasing in number; at the same time a few young plasmodia without pigment make their appearance. There is fever in the evening, and bimuriate of quinine, 16 grains, is given by hypodermic injection. During the following days the change for the better continues steadily; quinine, arsenic, and iron being administered.

On August 9th the crescent-shaped forms disappear from the blood.

On August 26th the hæmoglobin is 66 to 68 per cent.

The most prominent symptom in this case is the very severe and acute anæmia which rendered advisable the operation of transfusion according to Ziemssen's method. It is to be noticed that the cerebral symptoms ceased while the percentage of the hæmoglobin still remained extremely low. The blood manifested in an acute form those alterations which are found in serious states of anæmia (the macrocytes, the poichilocytes, &c.).[2]

5.

Tetanic Malignant Infection (Malignant Quotidian).

Case 17.—Marini F—, day-labourer, an able-bodied young man, [illegible] years old, suffered from malarial fever last year, but not this year till July 30th. On the 30th he had the first attack; on the morning of the 31st, probably before being again seized by the fever, he went on foot to his place of work (a furnace outside the Porta del Popolo). About noon he was found in a state of coma by his cousin, who had him taken to the hospital, which he entered towards 6 p.m. Hypodermic injections of quinine had been previously given by the local surgeon.

The patient is in a state of complete coma; there is trismus;

[1] Sodii Arseniatis gr. j (one grain),
Ferri Tartarati,
Quinæ Sulphatis,
Acidi Tartarici, āā gr. lvj,
Aquæ Destillatæ ℥xij.—Ed.

[2] This case and the three following were drawn up in association with [illegible]

after many attempts we failed to open his mouth; the arms are contracted, the forearm extended and prone, the hand and the fingers bent; the tetanic contraction ceases at intervals, and then suddenly reappears. An attack is not brought on by compressing the vessels and the nerves of the limbs during the periods of quiescence. There is no opisthotonos. The lower limbs are drawn together in extension; the soles of the feet are arched, and have a position tending to varus; the contraction increases at intervals, but never ceases entirely. The abdomen is sunken. The upper costal respiration is about 80 in the minute, and stertorous; the abdomen is tucked in in the act of inspiration. The pulse is 120, soft and rather full; the right side of the heart is dilated.

The eyes are turned upwards and outwards; the pupils are large, and react to the light. From time to time the patient has attacks, during which the rigidity of the trunk increases, and the pelvis is raised; there is also an incomplete erection of the penis. The reflexes of the knee-pan are exaggerated; the superficial ones are normal. 8.30 p.m., temperature 103·4°. Bimuriate of quinine, 48 grains, given by hypodermic injection. Temp., 9 p.m., 101° (after a cold pack). 12 p.m., 103·7°.

August 1st, 2 a.m., temp. 104°. 2·30 a.m., death.

The examination of the blood at 6 p.m. on July 31st revealed nothing abnormal but a few endoglobular forms with pigment at the centre, and some pigmented white blood-corpuscles.

August 1st, 9 a.m., autopsy.—The tension of the dura mater is increased; the meninges are intensely hyperæmic; the central grey matter is strongly melanotic; there is no hæmorrhage. Bilateral pulmonary serous infiltration; the heart healthy. The spleen is very soft and melanotic; the Malpighian corpuscles are not pigmented, and are very well marked. The liver is soft, and there is melanosis, but not very intense. The bile-ducts are full of bile. The intestines are normal, and loaded with bile. The kidneys are strongly hyperæmic. The bone marrow is not intensely melanotic.

Microscopic examination.—The cerebral capillaries are entirely filled with red blood-corpuscles, each one of which contains a parasite with pigment at the centre; there are also some similar parasites observed in a free condition. On the other hand, the blood taken from a cerebral vein and artery contains only a very few plasmodia. The spleen contains a very large number of parasites, with pigment at the centre, both endoglobular and free, and also in decolorized red blood-corpuscles, which last are rather

and a half pints of milk in the d[illegible] macrophagi), [illegible]
He takes Baccelli's mixture[1] of ir[illegible] the cells of the
the crescent-shaped forms are rar[illegible]
phagi with masses of pigment, s[illegible] found in the same
also macrocytes and red blood [illegible] some endoglobular
ances (poichilocytes).

6th.—The improvement g[illegible] part of the red blood-
in number; at the same [illegible] atic cells contain a con-
pigment make their app[illegible] rusty-coloured granules;
and bimuriate of quini[illegible] to have in them entire
injection. During th[illegible] gold.
continues steadily [illegible] malignant infection, proving
On August 9th [illegible] ned by a single generation
blood.
On August 26t[illegible] y the microscope showed
The most pr[illegible] n of the nervous centres,
and acute a[illegible] number of the amœbæ was
transfusion [illegible] that the malignant paroxysm
that the [illegible] the disease, after an initial
hæmoglob[illegible]
in an acu[illegible]
of anæm[illegible]

[illegible] with Cerebral and Bulbar [illegible]

[illegible] from outside the Porta
[illegible] ver two days ago. Three days
C[illegible] felt well and spoke well; he is
ma[illegible] serious condition. The house
th[illegible] quinine by hypodermic injection
m[illegible]

[illegible] the patient is very prostrate,
[illegible] speaks with an exceedingly slow
[illegible] syllables, and replies to questions
[illegible] lowing symptoms are observed:—
[illegible] well marked; the tongue turned
[illegible] the muscular force on the two
[illegible] disturbances of the sensibility; the
[illegible] erficial, are normal; the bladder is
[illegible] e are several plasmodia without pig-
[illegible] od-corpuscles; also many pigmented
[illegible] jections given of bimuriate of quinine,

[illegible] morning visit, the dysarthria is found

to be persisting, as well as the abnormal position of the tongue; the sensorium is a little dull; the bladder is full (it is found necessary to use the catheter regularly); the temperature is subfebrile. In the blood, at 10 a.m., there is a very small number of plasmodia, with granules of pigment, and white blood-corpuscles with masses of pigment. The urine contains traces of albumen.

On the 31st the paresis of the facial and of the hypoglossal nerve persists, as well as the dysarthria; the voice is nasal, owing to paresis of the velum pendulum. The patient walks with a staggering gait; in the night he has passed urine spontaneously. Nothing abnormal but pigmented white blood-corpuscles are found in the blood; there is now complete intermission.

September 1st.—The fever returns in the morning. Temp. 101·5°. Bimuriate of quinine, 16 grains, given by hypodermic injection. In the blood there are only a few pigmented leucocytes.

On September 2nd the bulbar symptoms become aggravated again, after another paroxysm of fever which supervened in the night. The patient passes urine unconsciously; the expression of the face is stupid, and he talks foolishly. There is nothing abnormal but a few pigmented phagocytes in the blood. After other injections of quinine a rapid improvement takes place, which becomes more pronounced on the following days, the patient continuing to take quinine, arsenic, and iron. Up to the fifth day pigmented leucocytes are still seen in the blood, but thenceforward none. The different nervous symptoms disappear successively, but the dysarthria persists, being limited to an imperfectly articulated pronunciation. On September 20th the patient is lost sight of.

This is one case among others observed by us where during the parasitic invasion cerebral symptoms (*e. g.* lethargy, dulness, &c.) are developed, as well as bulbar ones, such as dysarthria, paresis of certain bulbar nerves, &c., and it is noticeable that these latter have the greater persistence; they disappear slowly and by degrees, many days after the actual infection has ceased.

7.

Malignant Infection in an Old Man.

Case 19 (the Lancisi Division, No. 52).—The patient is an old man of 70 years, a watchman on the Tivoli Railway. He states that he has had intermittent fever for a long time, and insists on the fact that after the attacks he became drowsy and fell into a

abundant. There are no large phagocy... ...ist in a serious
are there any alterations visible in the nuc... ...estions, and has
pulp and of the follicles. ... the disease; he

In the bone marrow the parasites
condition as in the spleen; in add... ...d a serious arterial
spindle-shaped bodies are seen. ... hæmorrhages into

In the capillaries of the liver the g... ...ngue is diverted to
corpuscles contain no parasites. Th...
siderable number of hæmoglobinic ... in the blood; about
some of the hepatic cellules are ... ...graded, and in some of
red blood-corpuscles of the colour ... are observed. There

This is an instance of very sev... ...ment.—plasmodia without
rapidly fatal, and having been d... ...ference and at the centre,
of quotidian parasites. Exami... ...-shaped bodies; also an
an extremely serious parasitic ... blood-corpuscles, as many
while in the blood of the finger ...
very scanty. It is also notew... ...centre vary greatly in size;
developed on the second da... ... the red blood-corpuscle,
paroxysm of little importance ... between these extremes all
... of bimuriate of quinine
... the condition as regards

Malignant Infection ... described, but the number
... Towards 4 p.m. the
... of extreme prostration; he

CASE 18.—Biancini ... muscles are contracted and
S. Lorenzo, was attac... ... is small. Fresh injections
before entering the l... ...given.
now brought thithe... ... second day.
surgeon immediat... ...stance is of a dark red colour;
(August 29th, 18... ... membrane, and dilatation of

On the morni... ... of a recent softening in
almost in a leth... ...cerebral arteries. The heart is
articulation of t... ... atheromatous patches in the
with great diffic... ...cardium is coloured brown. The
paresis of the ... spleen is large and very black,
to the left; ... very clearly visible. The
sides equal; ... swollen; there is much bile in
reflexes, b... ... also contain a quantity of it.
very full. ... upper and lower thirds, is dark
ment, som... ... brown.
macroph... ...—All the red blood-corpuscles
24 grai... ... plasmodia without pigment, or

On A... ... are in the majority; the forms

with pigment at the centre are very scarce, and there are no forms in segmentation. Much of the endothelium in the cerebral vessels is pigmented. Also in the spleen the plasmodia without pigment prevail; the crescent-shaped forms are very rare. Almost all the white blood-corpuscles are pigmented; in addition there is a great deal of free pigment. In the bone marrow, besides those parasitic forms which the spleen contains, there is a large number of endo-globular bodies, round and ovoid, with pigment shaped like small rods, scattered about or collected together, in motion as well as motionless: the latter are the young forms of the crescent-shaped phase.

This case and other analogous cases demonstrate the deceptive course which the malarial infection may take in old people. Sometimes an enormous number of parasites is found in individuals, with regard to whom the clinical examination gives no warrant for suspecting the extreme gravity of the disease. Death can be foreseen by anyone who examines the blood, and it may take place only a few hours after the malignant symptoms have appeared.

8.

Malignant Infection attended with Coma.

CASE 20 (December 7th, 1891).—Corazza Antonio, 36 years old, working outside the Porta del Popolo, has had intermittent fever for eight days, but the type has not been recognised. On December 6th he was pretty well, so much so that he had passed the evening drinking with his friends. But towards midnight he was seized with intense shivering and very high fever, and soon after fell into a state of coma. In this condition he was brought to the hospital at 8 a.m. on December 7th; hypodermic injections of bimuriate of quinine, as well as different stimulants, were then immediately administered.

The patient is in profound coma, with complete relaxation of the muscles; the deep reflexes are effaced on the right side, and almost so on the left, while the superficial ones are also entirely wanting. The respiration is slow, noisy, short, irregular, and interrupted from time to time by long pauses.

The pulse is 110; it is regular and soft.

The patient's complexion is earthy, and the spleen is not much enlarged. His comrades assert that he has not had any other before the present attack of fever.

Temperature, 8 a.m., 98·8°. 12 noon, 99·4°. 3 p.m., 99·9° F. Blood: there is an immense number of plasmodia without pigment, and many bodies with pigment at the centre; also a moderate amount of crescent-shaped forms, both adult and young, as well as bodies of different sorts,—round, spindle-shaped, &c. Many pigmented white blood-corpuscles are seen, of large size, and abounding in shining granules.

Although at brief intervals during the day fresh injections of quinine, of camphor, &c., were given, death supervened at 4 p.m.

The autopsy.—The meninges are hyperæmic and dry; the cerebral convolutions are flattened, owing to increase of the subdural tension. The brain is melanotic; the capillaries are filled with red blood-corpuscles containing forms with a small mass, or with needles of pigment in a state of motion, at the centre. The spleen is twice the normal size; it is a little softened, and black in colour. The liver is melanotic, and at the same time of the colour of yellow ochre. The marrow of the ribs abounds in parasites, which are for the most part pigmented; it contains also many nucleated red blood-corpuscles, in one of which a parasite is found. There is nothing worthy of notice in the other organs.

9.

Malignant Infection with Cerebral Symptoms of Irritation. Appearances of Meningitis.

CASE 21.—A boy of twelve years of age is brought to the hospital, by people who know nothing of his history, in the night between the 11th and 12th of November. He has very high fever, and the house surgeon orders him to be wrapped in a cold pack (after which the temperature sinks to 101·8°) and administers a hypodermic injection of bimuriate of quinine, 32 grains.

Being visited on November 12th, at 8 a.m., the patient is found in the following condition:—he is very pale, and with an earthy complexion; there are some cutaneous hæmorrhages on the breast. The spleen is enlarged, but not overlapping the costal arch. The pulse is slow. There is a prompt response to stimuli, even to slight ones. The heart is dilated on the right side. Blood: there are many plasmodia without pigment, a few crescent-shaped forms, and several pigmented white blood-corpuscles. 4 p.m., blood: condition the same. The patient has fallen into a lethargic state. He mutters a few words in such a way that they cannot be understood. *Motus carpentes et ludentes.* The bladder is full. The teeth are pressed together; the mucous membranes are dry and covered with sordes. There is a remarkable hyperæsthesia, both superficial and deep. Vomiting now takes place. After 4 p.m. tonico-clonic convulsions set in, and continue for several hours. Then collapse follows. The pulse is small and arhythmic; there is also cyanosis; profound coma. Temperature, 4 a.m., 102·2°. 12 noon, 98·8°. 4 p.m., 98·6°. 8 p.m., 96·8°. 12 p.m., 98·5° F.

The patient dies at 4 a.m. on November 13th, notwithstanding that during the 12th several hypodermic injections were made of bimuriate of quinine amounting to 64 grains.

The autopsy.—There is well-marked anæmia of the skin and of the mucous membranes; also hæmorrhages into the skin of the breast, shoulders, abdomen, and thighs. The cranium is somewhat wanting in symmetry. The dura mater is tense; the pia mater is bloodless. The cerebral cortex is melanotic. The white substance contains but little blood; the grey matter of the bulb and of the medulla is hyperæmic.

The lungs are free, but in the posterior parts of the right one there is œdema. The heart is dilated on the right side, and empty; the myocardium is brown in colour. There is also anthracosis of the lungs and of the peribronchial glands.

Meteorism of the intestines is found; the liver is pushed up; the spleen does not extend beyond the costal arch, but is enlarged and melanotic, with thickened and tense capsule. The gall-bladder is full of bile. The kidneys are melanotic, with the glomeruli not very distinct. In the liver there is a melanosis which is chiefly perilobular. The marrow of the flat bones is of a dark red colour. Examination by the microscope reveals the existence of amœbæ, with and without pigment, as well as in the sporulation stage, in immense quantities, especially in the capillary vessels of the cerebral cortex.

10.

Malignant Infection attended with Coma. Protracted Course.

CASE 22.[1]—G. B—, a countryman 60 years old, enters the hospital on August 10th, 1886, and states that he has had several paroxysms on the preceding days. On the afternoon of the 10th he is without fever, but prostrated and pale; 32 grains of hydrochlorate of quinine are administered. During the night he is seized with fever, and he falls into a state of coma. On August 11th, at 9 a.m., profound coma continues, and hypodermic injections of quinine are given. The blood contains a considerable quantity of plasmodia without pigment, and some forms with a small mass of pigment at the centre. The coma continues during the whole day, and at 5 p.m. the parasites are found in the same condition as above.

[1] See Chart III, tracing 16.

On the 12th, at 8 a.m., there is a remarkable decrease in the number of plasmodia without pigment; but others are seen both pigmented and in process of fission. Again injections of quinine are given, but the profound coma lasts throughout the day. The respiration is frequent and superficial, the pulse small and frequent. At 4 p.m. there is sweating; the plasmodia without pigment have now become very rare, while many pigmented white blood-corpuscles are found.

On August 13th there is still profound coma; the pupils are contracted, and there are punctiform hæmorrhages into the skin of the eyelids, the forehead, and the ocular conjunctiva. At 8 a.m. the blood shows only a very few motionless plasmodia without pigment, and some pigmented white blood-corpuscles. During the afternoon the general state remains the same, as also does the condition as regards the parasites.

On August 14th, at 6 p.m., death takes place.

August 11th.—Temp., 4 a.m., 101·5°. 8 a.m., 103·3°. Noon, 104·4°. 4 p.m., 105·3°. 8 p.m., 105·1°. 12 p.m., 105·1°.

12th.—Temp., 4 a.m., 105·1°. 8 a.m., 104·4°. Noon, 102·4°. 4 p.m., 101·7°. 8 p.m., 102·4°. 12 p.m., 103·5°.

13th.—Temp., 4 a.m., 103·5°. 8 a.m., 103·1°. Noon, 102·6°. 4 p.m., 102·7°. 8 p.m., 103·3°. 12 p.m., 102°.

14th.—Temp., 4 a.m., 104·4°. 8 a.m., 104·6°. Noon, 104·6° F.

Throughout the whole course of the fever the patient was in a comatose condition, lying on his back and incapable of being roused by the strongest stimuli.

The autopsy revealed punctiform hæmorrhages in the cerebrum and in the retinæ; the cerebral capillaries contained a very small quantity of plasmodia, all without pigment; the spleen was enlarged and of a black colour, and there was pulmonary hypostasis.

This is an instance taken from a class of cases in which the high fever and the cerebral symptoms persist for several days, although the parasites, owing to the action of the specific remedy, continuously decrease in number. The anatomico-pathological examination sufficiently accounts for the aggravation of the cerebral symptoms, and for the fatal issue. The fever may take, as in the present case, a subcontinued course.

II.

Malignant Infection attended with Coma. Quotidian Fever.

Case 23.[1]—N. N—, an able-bodied countryman coming from Maccarese, has had fever for eight days. On the morning of

[1] See Chart III, tracing 17.

August 6th he was attacked by fever as he was walking to his work; after being carried to the hospital, he fell into a state of coma at 4 p.m. His complexion is slightly jaundiced, the spleen is enlarged, and there is high fever (temp. 104·9°). An immense quantity of plasmodia without pigment are found in the blood; some of the red blood-corpuscles are seen to have two, three, or four of them in different planes; there are also some forms with pigment at the centre, and several forms of fission, as well as many pigmented white blood-corpuscles; 56 grains of soluble hydrochlorate of quinine are administered, partly by hypodermic injection, partly by the mouth. The fever falls during the night; on the morning of the 7th the patient has recovered from the coma, and replies to questions, but his mind appears clouded. As regards the parasites, at 8 a.m. there is an extremely large number of plasmodia in motion and without pigment; only a very few being pigmented; some also are in process of fission. The temperature is 98·6°; 24 grains of quinine are given. The intermission lasts during the whole day; in the afternoon the temperature is 98·7°. At 4 p.m. the patient is awake, answers questions slowly, and complains of headache; the blood is found on examination to be in the same condition as in the morning. But towards 9 p.m. he again has fever (temp. 104·9°), and relapses into lethargy.

At 7 a.m. on the 8th the lethargy and the fever persist. Again injections of quinine are administered, as well as stimulants. At 9 a.m. the temperature has remarkably decreased (it is 99°); the parasites also have become less in number; a few plasmodia are seen without pigment, there are some forms with pigment at the centre, and many pigmented white blood-corpuscles. The lethargic condition lasts throughout the day; at 4 p.m. the blood is examined again, with results similar to those obtained in the morning.

The fever returns during the evening and night; the maximum temperature is 102·2°.

On the morning of the 9th the patient is very prostrate and has a jaundiced complexion, but is no longer in a state of lethargy; temperature 100·4°. A very small number of plasmodia are found in the blood, and pigmented white blood-corpuscles. The patient improves rapidly.

On the 10th plasmodia are still found in the blood, but they are very scanty; there are many pigmented white blood-corpuscles, and a very few crescent-shaped forms. The jaundice decreases, and the appetite returns. The maximum temperature during the day is 99·7° F.

On the 12th, at 8 a.m., there is a [illegible] from fever, the blood
number of plasmodia without pigm[illegible] of crescent-shaped
pigmented and in process of fissio[illegible] [illegible]rpuscles, and pigmented
are given, but the profound c[illegible]
The respiration is frequent and [illegible] malignant paroxysms,
frequent. At 4 p.m. there is [illegible] [illegible]died, and energetically
pigment have now become ver[illegible]
blood-corpuscles are found.

On August 13th there i[illegible]
contracted, and there are [illegible] *[illegible]a and Eclampsia. Third*
of the eyelids, the forehea[illegible] *[illegible]ever.*
a.m. the blood shows only [illegible]
out pigment, and some pi[illegible] [illegible] years old, coming from the
the afternoon the gener[illegible] [illegible] days in the month of July,
the condition as regard[illegible] [illegible] For three days he has had

On August 14th, at [illegible] [illegible]mber 22nd towards 8 a.m., and

August 11th.—Temp[illegible] [illegible]he fever appears to have been
104·4°. 4 p.m., 105[illegible]

12th.—Temp., 4[illegible] [illegible]ent was brought to the hospital,
4 p.m., 101·7°. 8 p[illegible] [illegible] Division. He is extremely pale;

13th.—Temp., [illegible] [illegible]es no answers. The pulse is very
4 p.m., 102·7°. 8[illegible] [illegible]een is large, and the abdomen

14th.—Temp., [illegible] [illegible] above 102·2°. 10 a.m., blood:

Throughout t[illegible] [illegible] plasmodia without pigment; a
a comatose cond[illegible] [illegible] with fine granules of pigment, and
roused by the [illegible] [illegible] pigment at the centre, and, in

The autops[illegible] [illegible] in size from a fourth to a fifth of
and in the re[illegible] [illegible] Also young crescent-shaped bodies,
quantity of p[illegible] [illegible]containing small masses of pigment.
and of a bl[illegible] [illegible] of quinine administered by hypo-

This is [illegible] [illegible] 102·2° : 10 grains of bimuriate of
high feve[illegible] [illegible]dermic injection. From this time the
although [illegible] [illegible] up to the time of death. 2 p.m.,
continu[illegible] [illegible], camphor, &c. 2.30 p.m., tonic and
examin[illegible] [illegible] and vertical nystagmus. The deep re-
cereb[illegible] [illegible] superficial ones are effaced. There is
take[illegible] [illegible] the parasites are as above, only
[illegible] plasmodia without pigment especially,
[illegible] they are discoid and annular in
[illegible] Also many pigmented white
[illegible]

[illegible] body is very pale in colour. The brain
[illegible] substance is somewhat anæmic.

[illegible] are congested, and a little œdematous. The heart healthy. There is a little serous fluid in the pleuræ and pericardium. The liver is melanotic, and the gall-bladder full of bile. The spleen is very large, with hyperplastic follicles; the pulp is plum-coloured and not very soft. There is a chronic enlargement together with an acute intercurrent one. In the kidneys the cortical substance is pale with yellowish striæ; the stellæ venosæ are very fully injected.

Examination by the microscope gives the following results:—in the brain there is an enormous number of sporulation forms, some about as large as a third of the size of the red blood-corpuscle and others still larger; many forms are also found with a small mass of pigment at the centre, as well as accumulations of free spores which block up certain of the capillaries (thromboses of spores). In the spleen the quantity of parasites is not so abundant as in the brain; in it forms with pigment at the centre, young plasmodia, and crescent-shaped forms both young and adult are found. In the bone marrow there is an immense amount of round, ovoid, and spindle-shaped forms, also of young amœbæ. In almost all the forms the pigment is disseminated irregularly. There are no forms of sporulation. In the liver the parasites are found in the same condition as in the spleen, only very few in number. The hepatic endothelium and Kupfer's stellated cells are pigmented.

In this case, as in the others described, the parasites are found in a condition denoting great malignancy, so much so that the severe infection can be diagnosed simply by examining the blood. The appearances of the amœbæ in the brain are noteworthy, and the distribution of them in the different viscera is characteristic.

13.

Malignant Infection accompanied by Delirium. Subcontinued Fever.

Case 25.[1]—Domenico de Rossi, 18 years old, able-bodied, works outside the Porta del Popolo. He was well up to August 21st, but towards 11 a.m. on that day he was seized with shivering and fever, which has been continuous up to the present. He enters the hospital on August 22nd, in the afternoon.

August 22nd.—Temp., 4.30 p.m., 103·1°. 8 p.m., 105·8°. 12 p.m., 105·4° F. At 4.30 p.m. there is sweating. Blood: there are many plasmodia with granules of pigment, and several in

[1] See Chart II, tracing 13.

brassy red blood-corpuscles: also a few forms with a small mass at the centre.

23rd.—Temp., 4 a.m., 103°. 8 a.m., 104·4°. 12 noon, 103°. 4 p.m., 104·9°. 8 p.m., 105·3°. 12 p.m., 106·2° F. During the night the patient is twice wrapped in a cold pack. There is frequent vomiting. 8 a.m., the patient is calm. Blood: there is a very small number of plasmodia without pigment, discoid, annular, and bacilliform; also an extremely scanty quantity of pigmented white blood-corpuscles. 9.30 a.m., there are plasmodia without pigment as above: also a minute quantity of discoid plasmodia with one or two very fine granules of pigment. One form is seen with a little mass of pigment at the centre, small in size, and another, larger—about one third of the size of a red blood-corpuscle—with signs of spore-formation; also a very small number of pigmented white blood-corpuscles. 3 p.m., there is severe headache and prostration. Blood: the parasites have remarkably increased, and consist of the following:—A moderate number of plasmodia without pigment, small, discoid and annular in shape, and in motion (the first and second forms being in the majority); discoid and annular plasmodia with very fine granules of pigment or with indefinite outline; one form with a small mass of pigment at the centre in a shrivelled blood-corpuscle—in size about one third of a normal red blood-corpuscle; one form of the same size with pigment at the centre and in motion, in a well-preserved red blood-corpuscle; and lastly, a very few white blood-corpuscles with small masses of pigment. 4.45 p.m., blood: the condition is as above. There is one form with granules of pigment at the centre, about as large as a third of the size of a normal red blood-corpuscle, enclosed in a brassy red blood-corpuscle. Also some white blood-corpuscles with small masses of pigment.

24th.—Temp., 4 a.m., 101·8°. 8 a.m., 101·6°. 10.30 a.m., 101·2°. 12 noon, 102·2°. 4 p.m., 100·6°. 8 p.m., 101·8°. 12 p.m., 100·8° F. 8 a.m., blood: a moderate number of plasmodia of medium size, annular and discoid in shape, all with clearly marked granules of pigment, some in brassy red blood-corpuscles or in those tending to become so; also a few pigmented white blood-corpuscles. 11 a.m., blood: the condition is as above, but the number of the parasites has a little decreased; there are several pigmented plasmodia in brassy red blood-corpuscles, also white ones with small masses of pigment. 2.45 p.m., blood: there are still plasmodia with fine granules of pigment, discoid and annular in shape, and in motion, enclosed in red blood-corpuscles both normal and brassy; but they are less numerous than in the morning. There is one form with a small mass at the centre; it is small in size, about one sixth of the red blood-corpuscle. 4.15 p.m., blood: condition is as above, and in addition there is one very young annular form.

25th.—Temp., 4 a.m., 104°. 8 a.m., 103·5°. 12 noon, 104·9°. 2 p.m., 103·5°. 4 p.m., 104°. 8 p.m., 101·1°. 12 p.m., 98·8° F. The patient has had an attack of shivering in the night. 8.30 a.m., the patient is agitated. Blood: there is a moderate number of plasmodia without pigment, discoid and annular in shape, and in motion; some also with indistinct outline, and none with clearly marked granules of pigment. The pigmented white blood-corpuscles are very scarce. 9.30 a.m., 24 grains of bimuriate of quinine injected hypodermically. 10 a.m., the patient is in a state of happy excitement. Blood: condition as above. 1 p.m., the patient is enveloped in a cold pack. 3.30 p.m., the happy excitement continues. Blood: there is a moderate number of plasmodia without pigment, as above; also one discoid form with small granules of pigment scarcely visible; and several pigmented white blood-corpuscles. 6 p.m., blood: the same. Thirty-two grains of bimuriate of quinine administered by hypodermic injection.

26th.—Temp., 4 a.m., 98·6°. 8 a.m., 98·1°. 12 noon, 97·7°. 4 p.m., 96·3°. 8 p.m., 98.° 12 noon, 99·9° F.

The patient is found in the morning in a state of astonishment; he appears occasionally to have alarming hallucinations; he speaks slowly, and frequently laughs. 8.30 a.m., blood: there is a moderate number of plasmodia without pigment, discoid and annular in shape and *in motion*, also plasmodia with fine granules of pigment, some of them in brassy blood-corpuscles. Thirty-two grains of sulphate of quinine given by the mouth. 11.15 a.m., the condition of the blood is as above; the parasites are perhaps less in number. There is a very small quantity of pigmented white blood-corpuscles. 2.45 p.m., temperature natural. The general condition is almost as above described; the patient speaks slowly and somewhat hesitatingly, as if scanning his words. Blood: there are a few plasmodia, with and without granules of pigment, in brassy blood-corpuscles; also a few leucocytes with small masses of pigment. 4.45 p.m., condition the same. The hesitation in articulation continues, the patient speaks with great difficulty, pronouncing many syllables imperfectly, so much so that some words cannot be understood. The coarse movements of the lips and tongue are normal. The deep reflexes are discernible. The tongue is coated and sticks to the mouth;

its margins are reddened. He recognises places and persons well. 6 p.m., 16 grains of sulphate of quinine administered by the mouth. During the night the patient mumbles constantly in a gay manner.

27th.—Temp., 4 a.m., 101·1°. 8.30 a.m., 99·4°. 12 noon, 99°. 4 p.m., 100·8°. 8 p.m., 100·4°. 12 p.m., 100·1° F.

The patient has almost a typhoid appearance; the tongue and lips are dry; he continues to talk senselessly and to articulate the words slowly and with hesitation. 8.30 a.m., 16 grains of sulphate of quinine given by the mouth. Blood: there are a very few plasmodia without pigment in normal red blood-corpuscles and in those tending to become brassy; also many leucocytes, several containing small masses of pigment. 11 a.m., blood: in one preparation there is a single plasmodium without pigment in a brassy blood-corpuscle. Towards midday the patient takes 32 grains of sulphonal. 5 p.m., he has become drowsy. Blood: examination gives a negative result. 6 p.m., 16 grains of sulphate of quinine administered by the mouth. Later on, in another preparation a single plasmodium without pigment is found.

28th.—The patient is apyretic, and has passed a quiet night. He is now calm, and there is no delirium; he speaks much more rapidly and clearly than yesterday. 8 a.m., 16 grains of sulphate of quinine given by the mouth. 4 p.m., the improvement becomes more pronounced. There are no parasites found in the blood.

31st.—The patient's condition is perfectly satisfactory, and he has appetite.

This is an instance of fever of tertian origin which has become subcontinued through the prolongation and overlapping of paroxysms.

As is evidenced by the examinations of August 22nd and 24th, the blood shows only the forms of a single generation of parasites, which, however, develop in groups at a certain interval of time, in such a way that, for a short period, the amœbæ are found in a complex condition. See the examinations of August 23rd.

The fever runs its course without serious symptoms until the 25th, when it becomes rapidly worse, but still without any signs of malignancy. The malignant symptoms—excitement, delirium, &c.—appear later, after quinine had been given, notwithstanding that the temperature had fallen and the parasites had diminished rapidly and progressively. The dangerous condition lasts a little more than two days.

What is remarkable in this case is the persistence of the malignant symptoms for two days, in spite of the progressive decrease in the number of the parasites. The different parasitic forms disappear successively under the action of the quinine; the last that remain are the plasmodia without pigment, and these vanish after the destruction of the blood-corpuscles which contain them. Here, too, we are enabled to foretell the aggravation of the infection by investigating the state of the blood.

14.

Subcontinued Fever, changed by the Action of Quinine into an Intermittent Tertian.

CASE 26.[1]—Puliti Bartolomeo, coming from Pratica di Mare, states that he had an attack of fever nine days ago, then two days of freedom from fever, after that a fresh attack, then one day he had a natural temperature, and lastly for four days a quotidian fever with shivering towards 10 a.m.; it appears, however, that the intermissions were never complete. He has taken quinine on several occasions. There is a marked enlargement of the spleen.

July 24th.—Temp., 11 a.m., 104°. Noon, 103·7°. 4 p.m., 103·3°. 8 p.m., 103·3°. 12 p.m., 101·7° F. 8 a.m., blood: there are large plasmodia, discoid and annular in shape, mobile, and almost all with small granules of pigment at the circumference; also several in brassy red blood-corpuscles; in addition, pigmented leucocytes. 10.30 a.m., blood: condition as above; the brassy corpuscles are more abundant. 4 p.m., blood: the parasites have much decreased in number; there are plasmodia in brassy corpuscles, and forms with a small mass of pigment at the centre; also very young plasmodia without pigment. 5.15 p.m., blood: the amœbæ are still extremely scanty; the brassy corpuscles have disappeared. There is a very small number of plasmodia without pigment; also a very few forms with a small mass at the centre.

25th.—Temp., 4 a.m., 102·7°. 8 a.m., 103·3°. Noon, 101·5°. 4.30 p.m., 104·6°. 8 p.m., 102·9°. 12 p.m., 101·7° F. 8 a.m., blood: there is only one form with a small mass at the centre; also a few young plasmodia in motion and without pigment, as well as pigmented white blood-corpuscles. 10 a.m., blood: the young plasmodia without pigment have increased in number; there are some plasmodia with granules of pigment at the circumference; also pigmented white blood-corpuscles. 3.30 p.m., blood: a moderate number of plasmodia without pigment; a very few with granules of pigment, and some pigmented white blood-corpuscles. 7.30 p.m., the patient is a little agitated, and has diarrhœa.

[1] See Chart II, tracing 12.

Blood: condition as above; in addition, one endoglobular, young, crescent-shaped form, also many pigmented white blood-corpuscles. [illegible] p.m., 32 grains of sulphate of quinine administered by the mouth.

[illegible]th.—Temp., [illegible] a.m., 101·7°. 8 a.m., 98·6°. Noon, 97·7°. [illegible] p.m., 101·3°. 12 p.m., 101·7° F. 8 a.m., the patient is quiet. Blood: there are a few large plasmodia with [illegible] granules of pigment, some in brassy blood-corpuscles; [illegible] with small masses of pigment. 10.45 a.m., [illegible]. Blood: condition as above; in addition there is [illegible] with a small mass of pigment at the centre. [illegible] a very small number of large plasmodia with [illegible] of pigment; also many pigmented white blood-corpuscles.

[illegible]th.—Temp., [illegible] a.m., [illegible]. [illegible] a.m., 103·3°. Noon, 104·2°; [illegible] in a cold pack. 1 p.m., 103·1°. 4 p.m., [illegible] p.m., [illegible]. 12 p.m., 101·8° F. 7.30 a.m., the [illegible] and the diarrhoea has ceased; the tongue [illegible]. Blood: a few plasmodia without pigment, some very small, [illegible]; also a few pigmented white blood-corpuscles. [illegible] p.m., blood: a few annular plasmodia without pigment. [illegible] p.m., the patient is somewhat lethargic. Blood: there are a few plasmodia without pigment; one form has a small mass at the centre; there is also one free form of sporulation, and a few pigmented white blood-corpuscles. 5 p.m., 32 grains of [illegible] of quinine given by hypodermic injection.

[illegible]th.—Temp., [illegible] a.m., 99·5°. 8 a.m., 98·6°. Noon, 96·8°. [illegible] p.m., [illegible]. 12 p.m., 101·2° F. 8.30 a.m., prostration. The mucous membranes are dry. Blood: there are a few pigmented white blood-corpuscles.

[illegible]th.—Temp., [illegible] a.m., 103·9°. 8 a.m., 101·3°. Noon, 102·2°. [illegible] p.m., [illegible]. 12 p.m., 100·4° F. 9 a.m., the patient is quiet. Blood: there are a very few plasmodia with granules of pigment enclosed in brassy corpuscles; also a few pigmented white ones. 3.15 p.m., blood: a very small number of pigmented white blood-corpuscles; one white corpuscle contains a form with a little mass of pigment at the centre; there is also one endoglobular, young, crescent-shaped form. No young amoeboid forms are visible.

On the morning of July 30th there is an intermission, the patient continues to take quinine, and the cure becomes complete.

In this case the fever is subcontinued at the outset. The forms of a single generation predominate in the blood, but, along with these, repeated examinations show the existence of certain parasitic forms more advanced in development. After quinine is administered a small number of parasites continue to develop, and they are all found in the same stage. In other words, a certain amount of amœbæ belonging to the generation which originally prevailed is all that now remains in the blood. Consequently the fever becomes an intermittent tertian.

The paroxysm following on the second administration of quinine is not attended with disturbances in the general condition, although the temperature is elevated.

15.

Malignant Infection accompanied by Coma, with Subcontinued Fever of Tertian Origin.

CASE 27.[1]—Balletti L—, 31 years old, has worked at Ostia; coming thence to Rome, he was seized with fever, from which he has now suffered for seven or eight days. He appears to have had intervals free from fever; occasionally there has been shivering. He was carried to the hospital on August 9th and put in bed No. 2, Lancisi Division. 10 a.m., the patient is prostrated, and seems rather dull; he recollects with difficulty and contradicts himself easily. The pulse is good. He complains of severe headache, and says that he cannot see well or distinctly. The fever is slight. The spleen is large; there are punctiform hæmorrhages on the trunk, and great pallor is observable. Blood: there is an immense quantity of plasmodia; forms are seen small in size, annular in shape, mobile, and without pigment; also larger discoid and annular forms with pigment at the circumference; and forms with a small mass of pigment at the centre, or with granules of pigment at the centre in a state of motion. The spore-producing forms are very few in number. There are several pigmented white blood-corpuscles with granular protoplasm, and having large shining granules; also many brassy blood-corpuscles. Forty-eight grains of bimuriate of quinine given by hypodermic injection. Noon, temp. 102·6°. 3.15 p.m., blood: the parasites appear to have decreased, the brassy blood-corpuscles especially so. For the rest, the same forms are observed: the small annular plasmodia without pigment predominate; next to these come the bodies with pigment at the centre; some of these are free, and there are others in which the process of fission seems to have commenced.

[1] See Chart III, tracing 15.

One form of fission is found enclosed in a decolourised red blood-corpuscle, about one third of it in size. The pigmented white blood-corpuscles have become fewer. The patient has fallen into a state of lethargy, and rouses himself with difficulty; there is incoherent delirium and agitation. The pulse is 124, and soft. The right side of the heart is dilated. 4 p.m., temp., 105·8°. A hypodermic injection is made of bimuriate of quinine, caffein, and camphor. The patient is swathed in a cold pack. He has now fallen into profound coma. After the application of the wet pack there is a considerable improvement, which, however, is only transient; he rouses himself on being called, and replies with great difficulty. The pulse is 95. 8 p.m., temp. 103·7°; 32 grains of bimuriate of quinine given by subcutaneous injection. 11 p.m., 16 grains of the same similarly injected. During the night stimulants continue to be injected. 12 p.m., temp. 102·6°.

August 10th.—Temp., 4 a.m., 100·8°. 8 a.m., 101·5°. The coma still persists. 16 grains of bimuriate of quinine injected subcutaneously. 8 a.m., blood; there are many discoid plasmodia without pigment and extremely mobile, also some very small annular ones, and forms with granules of pigment at the circumference. There are a very few forms with a small mass of pigment at the centre; no brassy corpuscles; many pigmented white ones, chiefly with small masses of pigment. 9.30 a.m., the profound coma continues. Blood: there are many plasmodia without pigment, some being in motion, and a very few with granules of pigment. The pigmented white blood-corpuscles are as above. The urine contains a moderate quantity of albumen, as well as granular cylinders. Noon, temp. 104·9°. Pulse 84, hard, cerebral. 3.15 p.m., coma: there is no reaction when the patient is pricked with a pin, not even when the face is thus tested; the collapse is complete. Blood: the parasites have greatly decreased; the plasmodia without pigment are in the majority; there are also a very few forms with granules at the circumference, or with a small mass of pigment at the centre. Many plasmodia without pigment are found enclosed in brassy red blood-corpuscles, or in those tending to become so. In addition, many melaniferous leucocytes. 4 p.m., temp. 103·8°. Pulse 104, and soft. The general condition is as above. The pupils still react to light and to mechanical stimuli. The patient is wrapped in a cold pack; 16 grains of bimuriate of quinine given by hypodermic injection; also caffein, &c. The profound coma continues through the whole night.

11th.—Temp., 4 a.m., 102·9°. 8 a.m., 104·9°. 8 a.m., râles

in the trachea. Pulse 140. Blood: there are a few plasmodia without pigment, some in brassy corpuscles; also an immense quantity of melaniferous leucocytes, some extremely large, and with black or rusty coloured pigment; in addition, white blood-corpuscles containing parasites. 10 a.m., the condition as to the amœbæ is the same. Noon, temp. 104·9°. 3.30 p.m., the profound coma and complete muscular relaxation persist. Blood: there is an enormous number of pigmented white blood-corpuscles, some of them of gigantic size. Temp., 4 p.m., 102·7°. 3 p.m., 105·8°. 11 p.m., 105·8° F. Death took place after midnight.

Autopsy.—The skin is remarkably pale. The dura mater is not tense. The veins of the pia mater are rather scantily filled with blood. The brain: the cortical substance is pale, neither hyperæmic nor melanotic; there are punctiform hæmorphages in the white substance of the hemispheres and subcortical structures, but none in the bulb. The heart: its volume is normal, and it weighs over 9½ oz. The right ventricle is full of fibrinous clots; the left contains a little fluid blood. The lungs: there are subpleural hæmorrhages; also hypostatic pneumonia, pulmonary congestion, and œdematous infiltration. Chronic perisplenitis and perihepatitis. The spleen is soft and black, measures 6½ × 4½ inches. The liver is congested, with extensive melanosis. The kidneys are normal in volume; the glomeruli can be clearly seen; the substance of the convoluted tubules is pale yellowish grey. There are punctiform hæmorrhages in the mucous membrane of the pelvis of the kidneys. The stomach and intestines contain a large quantity of bile.

Furthermore the microscopic examination reveals the following: —In the spleen there is an immense number of phagocytes loaded with pigment, with brassy red blood-corpuscles, and with free parasites; endoglobular parasites are very rare, and none are found except some endoglobular forms without pigment, some forms with a small mass at the centre, and a few forming spores; in addition some endoglobular ovoid forms (young crescent-shaped bodies?). In the brain a few capillaries are seen to contain amœbiferous red blood-corpuscles (also plasmodia without pigment in different shapes, with granules of pigment, as well as forms with spores). The endothelium is extensively degenerated and pigmented.

This is a case of comatose malignant infection, attended with subcontinued fever; there are several parasitic generations, but two are predominant, one consisting of adult forms ripe for segmentation, the other of young forms. It is noteworthy that the parasites gradually decrease in number until they entirely disappear in the blood of the finger (this is consequent on the administration of quinine), while otherwise the general state grows progressively worse. Another remarkable point is the influence which was strong enough from the very beginning to promote the development of the malignant form, in spite of the most energetic treatment,—a treatment which was unable to arrest the malignancy, although it was begun before the latter had really set in. The examination of the blood had, as a matter of fact, pointed to a prognosis of progressive aggravation.

16.

Malignant Infection attended with Coma.

CASE 28.[1]—(Of tertian origin.) Augusto B—, 33 years old, able-bodied, has been for about a month at Maccarese, where he never had fever; he then came to Rome, and remained without fever for a fortnight there or thereabouts, working near the Ara Cœli. He has now suffered for eight days from tertian fever, the paroxysms of which commence with shivering. He is carried to the hospital on September 6th in a state of coma, and put in bed No. 52, Lancisi Division.

September 6th.—3.30 p.m., coma, temp. 102·6° F. Blood: there is a considerable number of annular and discoid plasmodia without pigment, in a state of motion; a few with granules of pigment. Also a small number of forms with a little mass of pigment at the centre, or with pigment at the centre in motion (they are from a fourth to a fifth of the size of a red blood-corpuscle). In addition, a few adult crescent-shaped forms, and several pigmented white blood-corpuscles. Thirty-two grains of bimuriate of quinine given by subcutaneous injection. The patient does not rouse himself on being called, but pricking produces a sluggish reaction. The superficial reflexes are effaced; only the cremasteric ones are obtained very slightly in response to a strong stimulus. The deep reflexes are active and react readily. The pupils respond to light. The complexion is earthy; the spleen is very large and hard. 5 p.m., 16 grains of bimuriate of quinine administered by hypodermic injection; also caffein. 8 p.m., a similar injection given; temp. 102·2°. 11.30 p.m., another injection as above; temp. 101·3°.

7th.—There is now a ready reaction to pricking with a pin.

[1] See Chart 3, tracing 18.

The patient appears to understand, but he opens his mouth and puts his tongue out with difficulty; he does not seem able to see, and does not speak. The pulse is frequent, small, and soft. 8 a.m., temp. 100·4°; 16 grains of bimuriate of quinine injected subcutaneously; also caffein. Blood: the plasmodia without pigment predominate, and they are for the most part annular. There are a few adult crescent-shaped forms, and also several pigmented white blood-corpuscles. Noon, temp. 100·8°. 2.30 p.m., the general condition is unchanged. Blood: the parasites have greatly decreased in number: there are a few plasmodia without pigment, some of them in brassy blood-corpuscles; also many pigmented white ones, some with small masses of pigment, and a few crescent-shaped forms. 4 p.m., temp. 100·4°. 12 p.m., temp. 100·2°; 16 grains of bimuriate of quinine given by hypodermic injection.

8th.—The patient is agitated and delirious, he speaks with difficulty, and with exaggerated movements of the lips, pronouncing the consonants—especially the labials—indistinctly, and articulating the syllables with a little hesitation. Temp. 4 a.m., 99°. 8 a.m., 99·2°. 9.30 a.m., intermission. Blood: there are many crescent-shaped forms and round bodies; also a very few forms with pigment at the centre, and many pigmented white blood-corpuscles. Noon, temp. 97·2°. 3.30 p.m., the patient complains of severe headache, but the general condition has much improved. Blood: there are many crescent-shaped bodies, ovoid and spindle-shaped, some in process of disintegration; also several pigmented white blood-corpuscles. The apyrexia continues.

9th.—The patient feels much better. The trouble over his words, however, still remains; he speaks slowly, hurrying over some of the syllables, and pronouncing certain consonants, especially the labials, with difficulty. (There is slowness of speech, scanning and insufficient movement of the lips and tongue.) 9 a.m., blood: there are several adult crescent-shaped forms, and some pigmented white blood-corpuscles.

The patient rapidly improves during the following days; he takes daily 32 grains of sulphate of quinine by the mouth.

On September 12th a slight difficulty in talking still persists, and in the blood there are still several adult crescent-shaped forms and pigmented white blood-corpuscles.

The skin kept cool till September 21st, and the patient made a good and complete recovery.

The examination of the blood always yields the same results: there are crescent-shaped forms, round and flagellated bodies,

tation, the other of young forms. It is notewor[illegible] parasites gradually decrease in number until they [illegible] appear in the blood of the finger (this is consequent on [illegible] tration of quinine), while otherwise the general state [illegible] gressively worse. Another remarkable point is the in[illegible] was strong enough from the very beginning to prom[illegible] lopment of the malignant form, in spite of the m[illegible] treatment,—a treatment which was unable to arrest th[illegible] although it was begun before the latter had really [illegible] examination of the blood had, as a matter of fac[illegible] prognosis of progressive aggravation.

16.

Malignant Infection attended with Co[illegible]

CASE 28.[1]—(Of tertian origin.) Augusto B—, 33 [illegible] bodied, has been for about a month at Maccarese, [illegible] had fever; he then came to Rome, and remain[illegible] for a fortnight there or thereabouts, working n[illegible] He has now suffered for eight days from te[illegible] paroxysms of which commence with shivering [illegible] to the hospital on September 6th in a state [illegible] in bed No. 52, Lancisi Division.

September 6th.—3.30 p.m., coma, temp. [illegible] there is a considerable number of annular and [illegible] without pigment, in a state of motion; a fe[illegible] pigment. Also a small number of forms wi[illegible] pigment at the centre, or with pigment at the ce[illegible] are from a fourth to a fifth of the size of a r[illegible] In addition, a few adult crescent-shaped form[illegible] mented white blood-corpuscles. Thirty-two g[illegible] quinine given by subcutaneous injection. The p[illegible] himself on being called, but pricking produce[illegible] The superficial reflexes are effaced; only the [illegible] obtained very slightly in response to a strong [illegible] reflexes are active and react readily. The pu[illegible] The complexion is earthy; the spleen is [illegible] 5 p.m., 16 grains of bimuriate of quinine a[illegible] dermic injection; also caffein. 8 p.m., a si[illegible] temp. 102·2°. 11.30 p.m., another inject[illegible] 101·3°.

7th.—There is now a ready reaction to [illegible]

[1] See Chart 3, tracing 12.

In this case the maximum temperature in the rectum was 100·2° during the period of acute infection, in the night between the 25th and 26th of September. Recovery was extremely rapid owing to the disappearance of the cerebral symptoms, which left no trace behind them. With regard to the red blood-corpuscles, the ratio sank on September 26th to 1,950,000.

18.

Hæmorrhagic Malignant Infection.

CASE 30.—A lady had been staying for a few months at a place in the Roman Campagna, and after having suffered for two days from headache, which became more severe in the evening, she grew seriously unwell on February 5th, 1888; she was seized with bleeding at the nose, which, beginning as a slight oozing, constantly increased in quantity. On the following morning she was brought to Rome, and was so prostrated that she was obliged at once to take to her bed.

When first visited the patient was found in an exceedingly weak state; she moaned and spoke with difficulty; the bleeding at the nose was still going on; the skin, especially that of the neck, breast, and abdomen, was covered with hæmorrhages; the oozing of blood from the gums was continuous. The temperature was 104°, the pulse small and frequent, the respiration hurried, the skin earthy in colour, and the spleen a little enlarged. The nostrils were plugged, and 32 grains of bisulphate of quinine were ordered, hydrochloric lemonade, &c.

During the night there were agitation, slight delirium, flux from the intestines, and vomiting of blood.

In the morning the temperature was 103·8°, the loss of strength alarming, and the sensorium dull. The blood, on being examined, showed *an enormous number of endoglobular plasmodia without pigment and in motion, a few with a small mass of pigment at the centre and in different stages of the process of fission.* Sixty-four grains of bihydrochlorate of quinine were accordingly administered in the course of the day by hypodermic injection: towards midnight abundant sweating came on, the fever ceased, and the hæmorrhage stopped.

On the following day the patient had somewhat recovered; there was a slight attack of fever, and the treatment with quinine was continued.

On the third day without fever, being extremely anæmic and weak, she had a miscarriage of a three months' embryo. The

and frequently pigmented white blood-corpuscles, bu
become progressively less.

On September 21st, towards 11 a.m., the patient
and shows a tendency to vomiting, headache, &c., a
rature rises to above 100·4°. From this day a rem
mittent quotidian fever begins, which does not en
October 5th, and this notwithstanding that th
completely disappeared; indeed, so soon as the
September, examination failed to detect any.

During the whole of this period of fever (
no amœbæ were found in the blood; but the
be totally ineffective.

In this case it is to be noticed that after th
during which the condition of the parasit
characteristic, a period of freedom from fe
for about ten days; throughout this period
of quinine were daily administered by t
being found to contain parasitic forms belo
crescent-shaped bodies. When these dis
tent fever set in which was clearly not of
no parasites whatever were discovered in
the salts of quinine of any avail against
objective examination showed no lesio
this fever. The patient left the hosp
re-established in health.

17.

Hemiplegic Maligna

Case 29.—A middle-aged man, p
into the hospital of S. Spirito (Bagl
1889. He complains of pain in
indeed, the temperature is subno
ment of the spleen. A few h
loses consciousness, and become
on the left side; there is also
the deep reflexes,—symptoms
normal temperature. A car
of this state of things is made.
shows the presence of immens
the majority of them withou
with intra-venous injections
days, remaining, however, ve

n at
first
patient
sleep at
. He thinks
headache and
He comes to
ion, showing a
pression. Puncti-
trunk: the mucous

m., 99·2°. 6 p.m.,
Bimuriate of quinine
mic injection. Blood:
s without pigment in
ount of pigmented white

m., 100·8°. 9 a.m., 100·2°.
m., 99°. 11 p.m., 99·2° F.
erable number of plasmodia
brassy blood-corpuscles;
The pigmented white blood-
; they have a single
a.m., blood: the para-

decreased in quantity. The
quinine and camphor

kably improved,
blood there are
blood-corpuscles;
ed forms, and many

the blood contains pig-

gative result. During the
from the anæmic condition

20.

Malignant Infection.

. 54 years old, coming from Porta S.
cook, was brought to the hospital in a
September 5th, 1890, being accompanied
He has been ill since the 2nd instant.
now very difficult, and when left to himself
ous; he has a frightened look, the pupils are
n is cold all over the body and covered with
: there is cyanosis of the lips and the extremities;
hread-like and extremely frequent. In the morning
a diarrhœa and vomiting, which occurred also on his
hospital, where he continues to suffer from retching,
discharges at stool are as those of choleraic diarrhœa.
een is slightly enlarged. The examination of the blood
the presence of a considerable number of amœboid para-
but nothing else abnormal. Thirty-two grains of quinine are
en by injection, and thirty-two more by the mouth; friction
also employed, and stimulants administered (ether, camphor,
&c.). At 8 p.m. there is a profuse sweating, the skin remaining
cold; the delirium has ceased, and a continuous moaning has
taken its place; the pulse keeps all the time small and frequent,
and the diarrhœa persists. During the night the diarrhœa decreases, the skin becomes warm again, and the patient has rest
for some hours.

On the morning of the 6th of September the improvement is
remarkable; the pulse is 90 and strong; the coldness has passed
away, the temperature is 97·9°, and the cyanosis has disappeared,

but there are still some diarrhœa-like evacuations. Thirty-two grains of quinine were administered, as well as some stimulants and wine. The blood contained a few plasmodia without pigment, and in a state of motion. At 6 p.m. in the evening there is no fever and the pulse is good, but prostration and pallor to a remarkable degree still remain. The diarrhœa has ceased. Sixteen grains of quinine are given.

On the following days the improvement is maintained; strength is slowly recovered, and the appetite returns; the parasites disappear, and there is no more fever.

CHAPTER VIII.

THE ACTION OF THE SALTS OF QUININE ON THE PARASITES OF MALARIA.

Researches by various authors with regard to the action of quinine on the amœbæ of the quartan and tertian, and on the amœbæ of the summer-autumn fevers—Modifications of the thermic curve produced in the summer tertian by the action of quinine—Effect of the salts of quinine on the parasites of the summer fevers at different periods in their life-cycle—How the action of the salts of quinine on the malarial parasites may be interpreted—Considerations as to the best way of administering the remedy in the summer-autumn fevers.

§ 42. The researches which have been made with reference to the action of quinine on the malarial parasites have chiefly to do with the amœba of the quartan and the amœba of the tertian. According to Antolisei,[1] the adult forms belonging to the quartan are not hindered in their development by quinine (see p. 11 and following of the reprint); the sporulation takes place all the same, and so also does the paroxysm of fever, which, at the most, is delayed one or two hours, while the subsequent paroxysm does not occur. Antolisei has noticed, moreover, that in the paroxysm following after the administration of quinine only an extremely small number of young forms were found within the red blood-corpuscles. The forms of fission disappeared from the blood, as in the other paroxysms, but—contrary to what was seen in these latter—they were not succeeded by the usual quantity of amœboid forms without pigment; indeed, the number was much less. It is clear that in the present paroxysm they experienced the deleterious action of the quinine, and only a certain portion of them succeeded in escaping from it.

Romanowski[2] has devoted his attention to the changes which

[1] Antolisei, "L' ematozoo della quartana," 'Rif. Medica,' Gen., 1890.

[2] Romanowski, 'Zur Frage der Parasitologie und Therapie der Malaria,' St. Petersburg, 1891.

quinine produces in the intimate structure of the amœba (tertian). In studying it he has employed a certain method of staining of his own, which enables the nucleus of the parasite to be clearly distinguished. The stain of which this author makes use, is made by mixing one part of concentrated aqueous solution of methylene blue with two parts of 1 per cent. aqueous solution of eosin. It appears that the action of quinine is specially manifest in the adult endoglobular forms, where the nucleus undergoes change until it entirely disappears, the parasite takes the round shape of rest, the protoplasm assumes a homogeneous colouring, the pigment is evenly distributed, or, in some cases, collected at the circumference, while in place of the nucleus, and resulting from its actual destruction, fine granular appearances may be observed. Romanowski has also found alterations in the forms of segmentation after the employment of quinine. In these the protoplasm is seen to be uniformly coloured; the nucleus has no intense colouring, and is not surrounded with the normal pale halo. It is in this destructive action of quinine on the parasites that the specific activity of the remedy for malaria lies.

But the most complete researches on this subject are due to Golgi. This author has chiefly studied the action of quinine on the quartan parasites, and has arrived at the following conclusions:

The administration of quinine, given in ordinary therapeutic doses, does not stop the development of the parasites when the transformations characterising the process of segmentation have already commenced. The attack of fever is not thereby prevented, but the young generation of parasites resulting from the segmentations which have taken place is killed, whence a lasting cure is obtained by a single exhibition of the remedy. (The quinine is given four, five, or six hours before the attack.)

The same effect is produced when very strong doses of quinine are given, whether by the mouth or by hypodermic injection.

The young amœbæ, which are found on the first day of the intermission in the quartan, offer a remarkable resistance to the action of quinine; in some cases they may arrive at maturity and the stage of segmentation, in spite of the administration of the remedy; in others the development becomes irregular, causing thereby the first paroxysm to be wanting or to be delayed. But the recurrences are frequent, because the infection has not been destroyed. On the second day of apyrexia, when the changes which should lead to segmentation are commencing, the amœbæ are more sensitive to the action of the remedy.

The effect of quinine on the tertian amœba is not exactly the same as that which it has on the parasites of the quartan. The difference would appear to consist in this, that the tertian amœbæ, in any stage they may have reached in their endoglobular growth, are much more easily affected by quinine than the quartan parasites are during the corresponding period.[1]

As regards the summer-autumn fevers, we remind our readers that, from the time of their first notes on the subject, Marchiafava and Celli have drawn attention to the specific action of the salts of quinine on the plasmodia (on the young endoglobular forms of the parasites), noticing how they have been found to disappear in a fairly short time after the remedy was given.[2] Baccelli[3] has investigated the effect on the malarial parasites of the direct injection of quinine into the veins, studying the blood from half-hour to half-hour. He has observed that for the first six hours after the injection no sensible alterations can be noticed either in the number or in the form or in the amœboid movement of the parasites, except that during the first two or three hours he thinks that he remarked an increased activity of motion. "It is certain, however, that after twenty-four hours almost all the parasites could be said to have disappeared, while it was impossible before this to trace any phase of destruction or of death. Laveran's pigmented sickle-shaped forms remain visible in the blood even several days after the introduction of quinine into the veins, and the cessation of the fever."[4]

[1] Golgi, "Azione della chinina sui parassiti malarica e sui corrispondenti accessi febbrili," 'Rendiconti del R. Istituto Lombardo di Scienze e Lettere,' 1892.

[2] Marchiafava and Celli, "Weitere Untersuchungen über die Malaria-Infection," 'Fort. der Medicin,' N. 24, 1885.

[3] G. Baccelli, "Le injezione intravenose dei sali di chinina nell' infezione malarica," 'Riforma Medica,' Gennaio, 1890.

[4] Laveran's and Dock's observations have but little value with reference to this subject, as Golgi also has observed. Laveran ('Du Paludisme e de son Hématozoaire,' Paris, 1891, p. 185) treats in a general way of the disappearance of the parasites from the blood of patients placed under quinine. As regards the action of quinine on the different parasitic forms, he simply says, "The effect of quinine on the hæmatozoa may be directly studied by mixing a drop of the solution of sulphate or hydrochlorate of quinine with a drop of malarial blood: these conditions suffice to prove that the movements of the flagella are no longer observable, and that the hæmatozoa assume the form which means their death."

Dock (see 'Centralblatt für klin. Med.,' 1891, p. 643) writes that "under the influence of quinine the plasmodia become motionless, and no flagella are protruded." In his recent work, 'Sull' azione della chinina,' &c. (above-

quinine produces in the intimate structure [illegible] investigations as to
In studying it he has employed a certain [illegible] us types of fever,
his own, which enables the nucleus of th[illegible] ical study shows
distinguished. The stain of which th[illegible] fevers offer to the
made by mixing one part of concentr[illegible] sorts of malarial
methylene blue with two parts of 1 per [illegible]—for instance, in
eosin. It appears that the action of [illegible]
in the adult endoglobular forms, wh[illegible] state that the resist-
change until it entirely disappears, th[illegible]y in the infections
shape of rest, the protoplasm assum[illegible] the common quartan
the pigment is evenly distributed. [illegible] the details which
the circumference, while in place [illegible] summer-autumn tertian
from its actual destruction, fine [illegible] are investigated, first,
observed. Romanowski has also [illegible]ermic curve through
of segmentation after the employ[illegible]ministered in different
protoplasm is seen to be uniform [illegible]y the remedy on the
intense colouring, and is not [illegible]
halo. It is in this destructive [illegible] paroxysms and on their
that the specific activity of the [illegible]nfluence on the recur-

But the most complete rese[illegible] method of adminis-
Golgi. This author has chief[illegible]
the quartan parasites, and [illegible] *produced in the summer*
clusions: [illegible] modifications vary accord-

The administration of qu[illegible] administered. But even if
doses, does not stop the dev[illegible] the same time with refer-
transformations characte[illegible]s of fever, the results
already commenced. [illegible]nd tertian, so that they
vented, but the young [illegible] laws, as they can be in
the segmentations wh[illegible] mind the remarkable
lasting cure is obtain[illegible]asitic resistance in the
(The quinine is given [illegible]

The same effect is [illegible] the salts of quinine are
are given, whether b[illegible]tical elevation (that is

The young amoeb[illegible]n a single dose, in the
intermission in the [illegible]y in several doses while
action of quinine ; in [illegible]day ; (*b*) during the six
the stage of segmen[illegible] at the beginning of
remedy ; in others [illegible]begins to rise ; (*d*) during
thereby the first par[illegible]
the recurrences a[illegible]our conclusions without
destroyed. On th[illegible]
which should lead [illegible] in a manner obvious enough
are more sensi[illegible] the biology of the malarial

ducing the clinical details of cases; as the greater number facts set forth is demonstrated by the instances detailed and the rmographic charts given by us in another connection. We have ed the same doses of the remedy as are usually employed in our hospitals for summer infections. The first prescription is seldom less than 32 grains of sulphate or bimuriate of quinine, taken, as a rule, in two doses from two to four hours apart; after this, other doses are generally given every twelve hours, the amount varying from less than 16 grains to 24 grains. This is for infections of ordinary gravity; when the fever is serious, even though it be not attended with malignant symptoms, the first dose of the remedy is usually given by hypodermic injection, and the quantity is generally from 16 to 32 grains.

In the malignant infections subcutaneous injection is always adopted; it is administered every four or six hours, beginning with large doses of from 32 to 48 grains; these are followed by smaller ones, usually of 16 grains. We have seldom found it necessary to alter the quantity to suit the condition of individual patients, because the sphere of our observations is almost entirely limited to able-bodied young men coming from the country, with no disease except the malarial infection.

Having detailed these premises, we proceed to state our conclusions:—(*a*) If the salt of quinine be administered a little after the pre-critical elevation, and the doses continued during the twelve hours of intermission immediately following the crisis, then the expected paroxysm may be entirely absent; in this case on the day after the crisis there are only slight elevations of temperature, somewhat above 98·6°. Judging from our experience of the last malarial season, this is what most frequently happens in the mild infections, and we have met with a great number of instances.

More rare are the cases in which, although the quinine be given in the same way, and even in doses larger than usual (*e. g.* 48 grains during the crisis of a paroxysm and 32 grains by the mouth during the succeeding apyrexia), the following attack is not prevented, but *it is delayed* for several hours (the limit being about six). This delayed paroxysm may be considered as abortive, as it consists of a simple elevation of temperature, which in the instances to which we refer is a little above 102·2° F. The retardation may sometimes be very remarkable, even for almost twenty-four hours, as we happen to have seen in one patient. But it is also possible that the expected paroxysm may assume an abortive form, and take place without any considerable delay.

§ 43. It follows from the facts described that investigation the action of quinine must be made in all the various types of and on the different varieties of parasite. Clinical study the varying amount of resistance which the fevers offer action of the remedy, not only in different sorts of infection, but even in one and the same group—for in that of the summer-autumn fevers.

Our own researches, indeed, enable us to state that ance to quinine varies much more considerably in the belonging to this latter class than it does in the comm and tertian; this will become manifest from the we shall now give. We have made the summer- the chief object of our studies, and we have in the changes which are produced in the thermic the agency of the salts of quinine, administe ways; and secondly, the action effected by the life and development of the amœbæ.

Lastly, the influence of quinine on the paroxy succession must be distinguished from its influ rences of fever, in accordance with the m tration.

1. *Modifications of the thermic curve pro tertian by the action of quinine.*—These modific ing to the time that the remedy is admini it be given, in the different cases, at the ence to the development of the paroxysm are not so constant as in the quartan an cannot be formulated in simple and fixed these latter. We must always bear in variability of the thermic and the par group of fevers now under consideration

The results, then, vary according as ... im- administered (*a*) a little after the pre- ... sub- to say, during the crisis of an attack ... y, or space of several hours, or else success ... re the crisis lasts and on the following ... hours preceding the expected attack ... the paroxysm just as the temperatu ... the paroxysm.

For brevity's sake, we shall

mentioned), Golgi has criticised these conc to anyone familiar with the latest resear parasites.

in other cases a slight retardation is noticeable, and the paroxysm may also be less severe than the preceding; yet even in these cases the curve resembles the typical one of the summer-tertian.

(*c*) The result may be the same if the remedy be administered at the beginning of the paroxysm, just as the temperature is beginning to rise, or a little before; that is to say, the paroxysm may delay its commencement somewhat, or it may also become abortive without any retardation. However, in the majority of cases the paroxysm develops normally, but not without exhibiting certain modifications in the curve which must be attributed to the effect of the quinine. The alteration in the curve may be due to an exaggeration of the pseudo-crisis to such an extent that the attack tends to lose its own individuality, and becomes, as it were, divided into two; or else the initial elevation of the temperature may be followed by a brief crisis, whereby the paroxysm is considerably shortened. These changes in the curve are generally to be noticed when the remedy has been administered in large doses (*e. g.* 32 grains and even more), and by hypodermic injection.

(*d*) If the salts of quinine be given during the paroxysm of fever, the first dose a little after the beginning, followed by others during its course, then in one series of cases we have found no appreciable modification of the tertian typical curve; in another series the curve has shown various alterations; (i) the pre-critical elevation either disappears altogether, or is diminished; or (ii) the pseudo-crisis is exaggerated, the length of the paroxysm remaining unchanged; or (iii, and lastly) the paroxysm is protracted despite the quinine, and lasts, it may be, even many hours longer than the preceding one. We shall have occasion to return to this fact of the prolongation of paroxysms during the course of which quinine is administered even in large doses. When the remedy is given liberally during a paroxysm there is a whole series of cases in which the succeeding paroxysm entirely disappears, or only slight and tardy elevations of the temperature occur on the day or days following the suppressed paroxysm.

§ 44. In the malignant tertians, or in the malignant infections with irregular fever of tertian origin, it is impossible to analyse the facts presented as accurately as can be done in the mild fevers and in those of medium gravity, because in the former our observations naturally only commence at the moment when we begin to use the remedy by hypodermic injections repeated at short intervals of time. In one series of cases the temperature falls promptly (as it may do in the fevers of medium gravity), even when the malignant symptoms still persist for two or three days.

It is only in a few cases that we have been unable to any appreciable influence exerted by the quinine on paroxysm; it was given in the same way, and also in doses (for instance, 96 grains in a little more than hours). Nevertheless even here it has usually return of a later paroxysm. But if the quantity during and after the crisis be insufficient, *e.g.* which is also too small when injected subcutaneously, only is the following attack not checked, as far observed, but it may even be succeeded by a second attack, which is developed in spite of the remedy thus insufficiently administered, can be met various forms; thus in some of the cases we have abortive; in others, on the contrary, it shows the the summer tertian, while in others it may even as prolonged. In several instances we have found paroxysms that are subsequent to the administration display certain oscillations of temperature which pronounced than usual, while the intermission between two attacks are more clearly defined length than generally happens in the common facts are in themselves sufficient to give clusion we have already expressed with regard thermic resistance observed in these fevers. the proposition becomes still more manifest when that the same thing may occur—that is to say, second and of a third paroxysm—notwithstanding remedy, and this not only if it be given in as we have explained, but also when really doses are administered—for instance, 32 grains every twenty-four hours.

In the fevers in which the intermissions perfect and disappear, *i. e.* where there is an continuity, if the quinine be administered in the end of an attack, and subsequent doses intervals of about twelve hours, then it may is succeeded by a complete intermission unlike of things; but other attacks which are to follow although they may be modified in one of ways [11].

(*b*) If the quinine be given during the the expected paroxysm, in the ordinary effect may be manifested on the curve of the

experience goes, the recurrence is a very frequent event, whatever be the method in which the quinine is given, nor can it be avoided, as a rule, even when the remedy is continued for several days following, as all physicians know. But this is not all; despite repeated and liberal doses of quinine, a relapse, even in a serious form, may possibly occur, although very rarely, after a short interval without fever lasting for four or five days.

§ 46. Summing up the preceding in a few propositions, we formulate the following conclusions:

In the summer tertian, if the quinine be administered during the crisis of a paroxysm and during the subsequent intermission, in the majority of cases the following paroxysm is prevented; it may happen, however, that the paroxysm is not completely suppressed, but takes an abortive form, or is delayed (even for a considerable period of time,—from six to twenty-four hours). Only exceptionally do we find no discernible influence exerted on the next paroxysm. In cases which offer much resistance to the remedy, if the quantity given be insufficient, or even if ordinary doses be administered, then a second, and perhaps also a third paroxysm may occur. This third paroxysm is generally abortive, but there are instances where it shows the normal curve of the tertian, or it can even be prolonged. When the quinine is continued in the same way—that is to say, during the period of apyrexia intervening between two attacks,—we have never observed the recurrence of other paroxysms beyond the third, counting from the one after which the remedy was first prescribed. If the fever be a complex one owing to the presence of several generations of parasites, the quinine having been given at the end of an attack, and repeated on an average every six or twelve hours, does not usually prevent at least one fresh paroxysm, which may be more than ordinarily protracted and even malignant.

When the quinine is administered during the period of about six hours before the impending attack, then this paroxysm may be delayed, or it may become abortive, or, lastly, it may show an alteration in the curve, either on account of the initial elevation being followed by a rapid fall of the fever, or because of the exaggeration of the pseudo-crisis.

Finally, a paroxysm is not shortened by the administration of quinine during its course, but generally its curve is modified. The change may either be caused by the lengthening of the pseudo-crisis to such an extent that it appears to be a real crisis, or else it may be due to the fact that the pre-critical elevation is

In anoth... ...times it happens that,
the remedy ... is even more than
high, ... facts are observed in
days be...

Betw... ...i phenomena is found—
althoug... ...ction which the salts of
succe... ...parasites. Let us now
the ... ...bæ of the summer tertian

If, ... times, with respect to the
fever ... and in the same doses as
the... r the sake of brevity we do
fre... ...ails in support of the facts
lib... which we must separately
si... ...he quinine influences the life
m... ...globular stage, *i. e.* the plas-
m... ...e of motion; (2) the way in
... felt by the forms in course of
... the process of fission has already
... ...wards completion, *i.e.* plasmodia
... ...ence, those with pigment at the
... and (3) we must investigate the
... the amœbæ a little after they
... ...gmenting forms, and before they
... ...ed-corpuscles. Hence, in order to
... be necessary to inquire how the
... ...dified, according as the quinine is
... ...ter an attack of fever, (*b*) during
... ...ding paroxysm, and (*c*) at the
... ...elopment of the hot stage.

... ...nistered in close proximity to the
... the blood except young plasmodia
... ...of motion, and if the doses be con-
... ...urs, then the amœbæ still remain
... ...nger for almost twenty-four hours,
... ...e blood-corpuscles; after that, they
... further, while the red blood-cor-
... undergo alteration by shrivelling up
... ...ss or old gold. In some few cases the
... rapidly, and they may even do so in
... ...er hand, the pigmented white blood-
... ...nd in the blood for two days after the
... remedy, and in the dangerous fevers
... we shall see. These are the pheno-

mena belonging to one series of cases. In others, if the quinine be given in the same way, but soon (after a few hours) suspended, then it may happen that the young amœbæ persist for more than twenty-four hours (thirty-six and even forty-eight); during this time they go on developing; and, becoming slowly pigmented, they produce a delayed attack, as we have already explained.

Lastly, in other cases, if the quantity given be insufficient or even if the dose be a large one, for instance, 32 grains of bimuriate of quinine taken by the mouth or injected subcutaneously, it is possible that there will be no apparent effect of the remedy on the development of the parasites, which are succeeded by a fresh generation, and consequently a new paroxysm ensues. In instances of this sort we must assume a certain resistance in the infection above the usual average.

(*b*) If the quinine be given at the time when the blood only contains pigmented plasmodia in process of development, that is to say during the last twelve hours, roughly speaking, which precede the expected attack, then the evolution of the amœbæ proceeds till the fission stage is reached; it is, however, not unreasonable to suppose that the parasitic forms do not all attain to completely maturity, because the following paroxysm is usually abortive. During this attack no amœbæ belonging to the young generation are, as a rule, found within the red blood-corpuscles, so that, as far as the parasites are concerned, the examination of the blood may yield an entirely negative result, saving the presence of pigmented white blood-corpuscles. The effect is the same whether the remedy be administered by the mouth or by hypodermic injection.

In other instances the attack is found to be not only abortive, but also delayed.

Another series of cases shows the following phenomenon. If the quinine be given while the parasites are in this phase of their development, then the bodies belonging to the group of the crescent-shaped forms make their appearance. It would appear that here the adult forms, instead of arriving at sporulation, take the other course of development, which leads to the formation of bodies in the semilunar phase, the significance of which is, as we have already stated, still obscure.

If it be remembered that, as regards the parasites of th summer tertian, the changes preceding fission are carried out in a short space of time, it will be understood how impossible it i to study the effect of quinine exclusively on this particular lif stage of the amœba; these forms are always found in com pan with others less advanced in development, as well as with forms of fission already completed, on all of which the action of the remedy is simultaneously exerted.

(*c*) If the quinine be administered at the beginning of a paroxysm, when the blood only contains forms in which either the fission is accomplished or is still in progress (although these are but rarely seen in the blood of the finger), then the amœbæ of the new generation are found to be affected in a marked manner. During the course of the paroxysm they become extremely scanty in number, and disappear within twenty-four hours, especially if the remedy be continued when the attack has become advanced; at the same time the red blood-corpuscles containing them shrivel up, and assume the appearance of the so-called brassy blood-corpuscles, while the young amœbæ show not the least signs of development.

In spite of the remarkable paucity of parasites during its course, *the paroxysm may nevertheless be severe*, owing to the duration and height of the fever, as well as on account of the accompanying symptoms. There are, indeed, cases in which, when the quinine is given as above stated—that is to say, at the beginning of the paroxysm—and continued during its course, the fever is protracted beyond the length of an ordinary paroxysm. Now in these instances an accurate examination of the blood will show that the new generation of amœbæ appears a long time (even twenty-four hours) after the fever has begun, and for the most part in very moderate numbers. It is probable that this fact—that is, the slow invasion by the young amœbæ of the red blood-corpuscles consequent on the action of the quinine—stands in a causal connection with the prolongation of the paroxysm beyond the usual duration. For just as the paroxysm arises from the diffusion in the blood of the materials derived from the fission, so it would seem that the cessation of the paroxysm results from the entrance into the red blood-corpuscles of the young amœbæ derived from the spores. It is as if every cause for fever was removed simultaneously with the disappearance of the free foreign elements scattered about in the blood-plasma. We have, indeed, already observed that the number of young endoglobular amœbæ progressively increases during the course of a paroxysm, and attains its maximum at the close.

This being so, it may be supposed that the process, whereby the plasma is relieved of the free parasites diffused in it, is retarded through the action of the quinine given at the beginning of the paroxysm, and that consequently there is a corresponding delay before those of the amœbæ which succeed in escaping, or resisting the effect of the remedy, begin their endoglobular life, whence results the prolongation of the paroxysm.

We ought to add that, at least according to our experience, exceptional cases are to be found in which the quinine, when administered as described at the beginning of this paragraph, has but a minimum effect on the life of the plasmodia; this especially happens if an insufficient quantity has been employed (*e. g.* 16 grains of sulphate or bimuriate of quinine), and if it has been given by the mouth.

The facts which we have set forth in the three preceding sections receive additional confirmation from a study of those cases where parasites in different stages of development are found in the blood at the time of administering the remedy. In these instances it is possible to trace in the blood itself the action of the quinine on the various phases of the life of the plasmodia. The results of our observations are as follows:

If the parasites consist of young forms together with adult ones ripe for multiplication, as is usually the case in the dangerous fevers (malignant subcontinued, &c.), the first to disappear are the adult forms, which are not succeeded by a fresh generation, while the young amœbæ (the plasmodia without pigment) remain till the last,—for more than twenty-four hours, and in some cases for a still longer period, as from thirty-six to forty-eight hours. The red blood-corpuscles also which contain them undergo alteration, and present the characteristics of the "brassy" condition; furthermore, along with the parasites, the pigmented white blood-corpuscles persist in the circulating blood. This is the result which ensues when the administration of the remedy is continued in three or four doses at intervals of from six to twelve hours.

Even in the most dangerous fevers, and in the fatal malignant infections, there may be observed the same progressive decrease and successive disappearance of the parasites up to the time of death, in consequence of the effect of strong and repeated doses of quinine. But it is easy to foresee, from what has been said above, that also in this latter group cases may be found in which the sequence of phenomena is somewhat different from that described, causing us to suppose that there is a peculiar resistance offered to the action of the remedy. Thus it sometimes happens that, although the quinine is repeatedly given, a portion of the young parasitic generation goes on developing until a fresh paroxysm is produced, *which may even be prolonged.* It is remarkable that the generation of parasites in course of development may be so limited as to numbers that it escapes notice, even for a long time, *e. g.* twelve hours; but the endoglobular amœboid forms increase in number during the paroxysm, corresponding in a certain ratio with the gravity of the latter. We have already remarked that it is no rare occurrence to see the crescent-shaped bodies appear, or (if they were already in the blood) increase in number, at the same time that the endoglobular amœbæ become fewer under the influence of the quinine. In cases belonging to this last series the same fact is more frequently and more clearly observed. Generally speaking, it is a question that has to do with dangerous fevers which have already lasted for a certain time, and where the parasites are very numerous; which, in our opinion, is the explanation of the phenomenon.

It is well known that, during the periods of freedom from fever subsequent to a series of paroxysms, the forms of the crescent-shaped phase frequently persist in the blood from one to two weeks.

On this (the crescent-shaped) phase in the life of the amœba, the salts of quinine even when liberally employed (*e. g.* from 16 to 32 grains per diem) exert no appreciable influence; Laveran was the first to notice this, and it has been confirmed by Chenzinski, Councilman, Marchiafava, Celli, Guarnieri, &c.

§ 48. We now proceed to sum up the facts we have described in the following propositions:—When the quinine is administered at the end of a paroxysm, there being none but non-pigmented plasmodia in the blood, then as a rule the development of these plasmodia is checked, and they disappear between from twelve to twenty-four hours, less frequently from thirty-six to forty-eight hours; or else they develop partially, and become slowly pigmented, thus giving rise to a delayed paroxysm; or, lastly, in exceptional cases, where we must assume a great resistance on the part of the amœbæ to the influence of the alkaloid, they develop normally both in time and manner. This is especially the case when the whole quantity of quinine prescribed is taken in one dose.

If the remedy be given during the apyrexia preceding a paroxysm, there being in the blood only adult forms, which are just beginning or have already commenced to display the changes which end in fission, then, although, as is well known, the impending paroxysm is not prevented, the new generation fails to make its appearance within the red blood-corpuscles. If, however, the temperature is already beginning to rise at the time that the quinine is administered, a different result generally obtains; for in this case we find that the new generation is either visible during the paroxysm in a very small and feeble form, and then rapidly disappears, or else that it appears a long time—even twenty-four hours—after the fever has begun.

Finally, if the condition of the parasites be complex at the time when the remedy is first employed, then the different forms usually vanish one by one, the longest to remain in the blood being the plasmodia without pigment, the pigmented white blood-corpuscles alone survive these. The last-named parasitic forms are either arrested in their growth, while the red blood-corpuscles become "brassy," or else their development is only partial.

§ 49. Essentially the same facts are observed in the quotidian. Thus, when the quinine is administered after the crisis of a paroxysm, the young forms persist in the blood for rather a long time, it may be even for more than twenty-four hours; after which they disappear, without showing previously any sign of development.

If an insufficient amount of the remedy has been employed, or even where large quantities are used (*e. g.* 32 grains injected subcutaneously), provided they are administered in a single dose, it may happen that the development of the young amœbæ proceeds, and that no appreciable effect of the quinine can be detected. If the remedy be administered a little before the commencement of a paroxysm, or exactly at the beginning, the paroxysm is not thereby averted, but the new generation of young amœbæ are prevented from invading fresh red blood-corpuscles.

§ 50. The conclusions above established sufficiently determine the modifications consequent on the action of quinine which the parasites in the summer fevers undergo, as well as the length of time during which the various forms still persist in the blood after the use of the alkaloid, &c. We have now to inquire more closely into the morphological and biological changes which the alkaloid produces on the different phases of the amœba's life.

The young endoglobular amœbæ, endowed as they are with extremely rapid movement, do not seem to be affected in the least for some hours after the administration of the remedy; the movements continue, indeed in many cases they appear to be actually increased, as Baccelli also has remarked. But after the lapse of several hours the amœbæ assume the discoid or annular form, their movement first becomes sluggish and then entirely ceases, while the red blood-corpuscle shrivels up, and its colour changes and grows darker than usual. What is more interesting to observe is that the nutritive processes of the amœba become feeble and then cease altogether; in fact the non-pigmented parasite does not proceed to develop and acquire pigment; and in cases where very fine granules of pigment, arranged at the circumference of the amœba, have already appeared, the pigmentation goes no farther. This may be taken as the general rule.

On the other hand, there is a certain characteristic belonging to this group of summer-autumn fevers, which is analogous to what Golgi has observed in the quartans; we refer to the fact that those intimate modifications which accompany the act of fission are carried out despite the action of the remedy, until the entire process is completed, as may be arrived at not so much from examining the blood of the finger, as from noting the presence of numerous fissional forms in the cerebral capillaries, even when death has occurred after several hours from the time that liberal doses of quinine were given [12]. But the new generation resulting from this production of spores, which is accomplished under the influence of the alkaloid, does not invade any other red blood-corpuscles.

Other changes, manifested, for instance, in the appearance of the parasites, in their shape, in the characteristics of the pigment, &c., cannot be seen in this class of fevers.

While the other phenomena we have described may be satisfactorily interpreted without difficulty, the last-mentioned fact cannot be itself directly observed, and hence it is possible to frame various hypotheses with a view to its explanation. The question is, what becomes of the spores formed during the period in which the quinine is active, and are they or are they not the source from which the new generation springs? We know that not only the free spores, but also the amœbæ, previous to their invasion of the red blood-corpuscles, pass, as a rule, undetected. Now, with regard to this matter, one may suppose (i) either that the quinine has a fatal effect on the spores, or on the young amœbæ which are evolved from them; (ii) or else that it does not destroy the spores, but prevents their transformation into young plasmodia. Of these two hypotheses, the first is opposed by the fact that all the malarial infections belonging to this group are nearly invariably followed by the recurrence of the fever; hence, supposing we assume that the quinine has the power to kill the spores and the young amœbæ which spring from them, it must nevertheless be admitted that not all the forms are subject to this lethal action, which, consequently, cannot be said to be general, or without exception. Otherwise we should be obliged logically to maintain that no fever ought to be succeeded by a recurrence, provided it be energetically treated before the onset of a paroxysm, so that the maximum influence of the remedy is exerted on the spores and on the free amœbæ in the blood-plasma. But experience shows that, as a matter of fact, in the majority of cases recurrences do occur, notwithstanding the most active measures; they are observed, indeed, in patients who have been kept for a long time in the hospital, where it would be out of the question to suppose that a fresh infection had arisen. Therefore the inference to be drawn is that, granting the quinine destroys the spores or the young amœbæ resulting therefrom, there is always, or almost always, a certain number of parasites which escape, and that it is these which, after a period of incubation, determine the recurrence.

In support of the second hypothesis we have the fact of the tardy appearance of the plasmodia within the red blood-corpuscles in the case of those prolonged paroxysms which succeed (as we have pointed out) the administration of quinine. The phenomenon may be interpreted as follows:—If the remedy be given at the beginning of a paroxysm, or a little before, at the time when there is nothing but adult forms or those in process of segmentation in the blood, the development of the spores is arrested; but when, after some hours, the quantity of quinine in circulation, owing to its rapid elimination, has become too little to continue to induce this effect, then the amœbæ are evolved from the spores, and penetrate into fresh red blood-corpuscles, but more slowly than they usually do. Whatever be the true explanation one fact remains certain, and this is, that both in the summer and in the quartan and tertian fevers *the maximum and most rapid action of the remedy is exerted on that phase of the parasite's extra-globular life which is subsequent to the completion of the spore formation.* With regard to the other phases of the amœba's life, it may be said that the quinine operates so far as to hinder nutrition and development, but it is powerless to prevent the process of fission, even when it has hardly commenced.

From these facts we can deduce a law, which may be formulated thus:—*Quinine acts on the amœba of malaria in those phases of its life which are occupied in nutrition and development; when, however, the transformation of hæmoglobin into black pigment is arrested, and in consequence the nutritive activity ceases and the reproductive phase begins, then against this latter process quinine is of no avail.*

This resistance of the adult forms, which in spite of the action of the remedy complete the phase of fission or sporulation, explains the powerlessness of the drug in so many cases of fatal malignancy. *The fission of the adult forms takes place, whatever be the quantity of quinine employed, and however it be administered.* Now if, as is more than probable, poisonous materials are formed during the fission, it is clear that the treatment is incapable of counteracting the injurious effects which these produce, and (what is more important) that it is still less able to prevent the accumulation of parasite-laden red blood-corpuscles in the vessels of the different organs, especially in those of the brain. In the cases of fatal malignancy which we have observed, the autopsy revealed a great predominance of adult forms (*i. e.* plasmodia with a small mass of pigment at the centre) and of fissional forms, especially when we came to examine the internal organs. We have already indicated that this also is one of the reasons why the presence in a malignant infection of a large number of adult forms leads one to make a very serious prognosis.

But if all these facts place it beyond doubt that the quinine actively hinders and changes the nutritive processes which are carried out in the amœba, so, on the other hand, it cannot be denied that the remedy may also possess a more complex power of action, and may exert an indirect influence on the life of the parasite. Certain experiments carried out by Binz and his *collaborateurs* have demonstrated that quinine has a directly preventive effect on oxidation and some other processes which are due to the presence of hæmoglobin. If a neutral salt of quinine be added to blood, no spectroscopic modification of the hæmoglobin takes place, but the conduction of oxygen from ozonised turpentine to guaiacum—which is induced by a certain property of hæmoglobin—is either stopped or distinctly retarded. Rossbach attributes this action of quinine to the following cause:—"Quinine does not modify the property of hæmoglobin whereby it is a conductor of oxygen; it only makes the latter (the oxygen) combine more closely with the colouring matter, and does not allow it to pass so readily into other substances."

If now we take due account of these ascertained facts, we cannot but admit that the action of the remedy not only extends directly to the parasite, but that it also alters the red blood-corpuscle in such a way as to render it less fit, or unfit, for the amœba to live in.

Hence it seems to us that in our investigations as to the mode in which quinine influences the malarial parasites, it is of importance to bear in mind the possibility that this action partly consists in modifying the fluid in which the amœba lives, whose normal nutrition is thereby hindered.

After this statement of facts, we feel bound to record here that all recent researches afford the fullest confirmation of the theory which Binz has upheld for many years, and which both he and his school have defended in a series of works—a theory which maintains that the cause of the remarkable efficacy of quinine against malaria lies in the specific action of the drug on the malarial parasites, and not in a hypothetical and unproved effect on the nervous system.

§ 51. After all the experience gained and accumulated by physicians of every country with regard to the effect of quinine on the malarial fevers, the method of administration, the most suitable time of employing it in connection with the succession of the paroxysms, &c., it was not reasonably to be expected that the above studies could do more than confirm and rationally interpret certain rules or laws which have been already adopted by everybody, and the usefulness of which is generally recognised. The only result that we could hope these researches might yield, was that such confirmation might be of real use in practice.

Many practitioners, owing to lack of other means of investigation, are compelled, in many cases where the diagnosis is doubtful, to form their judgment of the malarial nature of a fever through the action of quinine. Now it is clear that the only sure guide in diagnosing is the exact knowledge of the modifications produced by the drug on the thermic curve in the different groups of fevers; and this is the reason why we have devoted so much time to the consideration of this series of facts.

With regard to the course to be followed as to the administration of the remedy in this group of fevers, the foregoing conclusions indicate that the method usually employed in our hospitals is the most advisable. At the close of his inquiries into the effect of quinine on the quartan amœba, Golgi expresses a strong belief that the most rational mode of treatment is to employ the remedy some hours before the paroxysm, so that its maximum action may be spent on the young forms resulting from the fission while they are still free in the blood-plasma; for this is the period of their life on which the influence of the drug has the greatest effect. In the summer-autumn group of fevers we have proved that quinine operates with great efficacy on all the amœba's life-phases, that alone excepted wherein the process of reproduction is completed. But even if the remedy be given at the time when the blood contains nothing but parasites which are ripe for or actually in course of fission, a beneficial influence is nevertheless brought to bear on the amœbæ produced from the spores. We have also seen that the administration of a single dose, and even of a large one, is less efficacious than a number of doses repeated every five or six hours, even though they be collectively smaller in quantity. Now, seeing that these fevers in the vast majority of cases are dangerous, and moreover that the drug is not without a useful effect at whatever time it be employed, it is clear that recourse to it ought not to be put off until some hours before a paroxysm begins (which in the quartan and tertian is the best course); it will be well to administer it *as soon as possible, and repeat the dose at intervals of from four to six hours, no matter what may be the particular point in the course of the fever at which the remedy is first commenced.* This is exactly how nearly all the cases in our hospitals are treated, and it is a plan which is strictly and completely rational.[1]

It may be asked whether it is possible to escape the recurrence if the quinine be continued for several days after the cessation of the fever. As far as our own experience goes, we cannot give an affirmative answer to this question. In several cases we have administered the remedy for four or five days, and even for a longer time, after complete absence of fever had been secured,

[1] In obstinate quartan infections Puccinotti advises that the quinine should be given one or two hours before the attack. By following this method "prompter and more certain results are obtained" than from the other plan, which is to employ the remedy at a time as far removed as possible from the paroxysm. But in the malignant infections (he says) the quinine must be administered without delay during the paroxysm itself, in as large a quantity as can be given, and in the most effective way possible; so that the rules which Puccinotti succeeded in forming from clinical observation evidently agree in the most perfect way with recent researches. He closes the discussion of this subject as follows:—"In all the intermittent malarial infections, both benign and malignant, excepting where it is necessary to make use of some preparation of quinine during the paroxysm itself, it may be maintained, as a general therapeutic rule, that the strongest dose of quinine ought to be given immediately before the onset of a paroxysm, and that in the intermittent quartans and tertians which are of benign nature, we may and ought to defer the administration of the remedy until this favorable time arrives. The longer the fever has persisted, and the more it has shown resistance to the system of small and divided doses, the greater is the need for employing this method; whereas in the malignant infections the safest and most efficacious course to pursue is to give the quinine during the whole period of the apyrexia, the doses being gradually increased in strength up to the last moment before the new paroxysm begins." ('Opere Mediche di Francesco Puccinotti,' p. 326, Milano, 1856.)

and yet, though we also made use of rather large doses (*e.g.* 32 grains per diem), the recurrence was not prevented; for the rest, this is an event with which physicians are very familiar. It would seem, therefore, that quinine has no appreciable effect on those parasitic forms which keep up the infection in a latent condition, and which, after a certain period of incubation, determine the recurrences. By far the greatest number of these infections are put an end to gradually, through a progressive weakening of the recurrences. Each time one of these occurs, a large number of parasites develop in such forms, as are then destroyed by the action of the remedy; in this way the inherent energy of the infection tends little by little to become exhausted. Hence it is our opinion that the complete cure of a malarial infection may be looked upon as a sort of *fractional sterilisation*, which we produce on the advent of each recurrence through the agency of quinine, until the strength of the disease is at last completely spent.

CHAPTER IX.

PHAGOCYTISM IN THE SUMMER-AUTUMN FEVERS.

Phagocytosis in the circulatory blood in the spleen and in the bone marrow—Cyclic development of the phenomena of phagocytosis in the summer-autumn fevers—Cyclic development of the same phenomena in the quartan and tertian—Differences which are noticeable in these two groups of fever, from the point of view of phagocytosis—Importance of phagocytosis in relation to spontaneous cure, and in relation to recovery brought about by quinine.

§ 52. OUR study of the cure effected in these fevers by quinine leads us now to inquire how far the processes of phagocytosis are of importance in connection with the resistance shown to the infection. The principal facts known with regard to the phagocyte action of the leucocytes in malaria are to be found in various published works on the etiology and pathological anatomy of this disease. Marchiafava, Celli, and Guarnieri have studied the phenomena of phagocytosis directly, under the microscope, in the blood as it circulates. Guarnieri and Bignami have observed the same processes in the organs of persons who have succumbed to a malignant attack. Their investigations have enabled them to describe the characteristics of the leucocytes which perform this function. For the most part they present the form of large mononucleated cells with finely granular protoplasm. Sometimes these phagocytes attain gigantic proportions, and are provided with large shining granules of varying size, which are only to be seen in fresh preparations; in the Ehrlich-Koch preparations they remain unstained. It has been remarked that the largest elements belonging to this species are found in great quantities, especially in the malignant infections. But the phagocyte function has been recognised not only in these large elements of spleno-medullary origin, but also in the endothelial cells; the latter, equally with the former, contain adult parasitic forms, and bodies of which the fission is already completed or still in progress, as well as amœbiferous red blood-corpuscles which have undergone alteration, either through becoming shrivelled up (brassy blood-corpuscles) or through loss of the hæmoglobin (decolourised red blood-corpuscles); in addition to these may be seen amœbæ-laden red blood-corpuscles, to all appearance normal in condition; the bodies also which belong to the group of crescent-shaped forms are found enclosed in the white cells. But of all the elements thus met with, it is the black or rusty-coloured pigment which constitutes by far the greatest part; it may be either collected together in large groups, or in small spherical blocks, or else divided into fine granules or needles. In preparations it can be seen not infrequently that the enclosed bodies are contained in a large cavity formed in the protoplasm of the white cell, as described and figured by Bignami. The polynucleated cells (elements with neutrophil granules) are not so often pigmented as the large mononucleated leucocytes, while the lymphocytes and eosinophil white blood-corpuscles never contain pigment or other *debris*. It has further been observed that the development of the phagocyte function is accompanied by profound alterations not only in the bodies included in the white cells, but also in the white blood-corpuscles themselves which enclose them; these changes can be better studied in the phagocytes collected in the spleen, in the liver, and in the bone marrow, than in those which are seen circulating in the blood during and after the paroxysms of fever. The pigment, comprised in small blocks or in granules, gathers together in large shapeless masses; at the same time the hæmoglobin of the amœbiferous red blood-corpuscles passes through its well-known modifications until it is turned into rusty-coloured pigment. The parasites then become disintegrated and disappear in a short time, but the enclosed spores remain longer visible. The leucocytes which contain them have been observed to undergo a series of degenerative changes, shown in the structure of the nucleus—changes which allow us to state with certainty that, as a general rule, these elements degenerate and perish after the completion of their phagocyte function, and when they have been deposited in the spleen, liver, and bone marrow.

In the meantime leucocytes are found in the spleen and bone marrow with their nuclei in process of fragmentation or in karyokinesis; these are never pigmented, and bear witness to the existence of an active reparative process. The phagocyte function is therefore generally carried out by a species of spleno-medullary leucocytes (large mononucleated leucocytes) which degenerate and die in large numbers (as Guarnieri and Bignami have noticed) in consequence of their performing it; they are then succeeded by young elements of the same species, which rapidly multiply in the spleen and bone marrow.[1]

Notwithstanding these phenomena of cellular reproduction in the spleen and bone marrow, in the majority of cases the white blood-corpuscles decrease in number, both relatively and absolutely, during the malarial infection, as the researches carried out by Kelsch and Dionisi have proved. According to Kelsch, it is only during the malignant paroxysms that the white blood-corpuscles increase, but even then not with any steadiness, and in any case merely for a short time. In the opinion of Dionisi, the white blood-corpuscles share the fortunes of the red ones; but sometimes they take an opposite course, that is to say, they become enormously reduced in quantity, while the red blood-corpuscles tend to recover their normal proportion. All these facts lead us to the conclusion that in malaria there does not exist any leucocytosis in the proper sense of the word. The ordinary leucocytosis, which occurs in many diseases and especially in infections of pyogenic nature, is marked by a transitory numerical increase of the white blood-corpuscles in the blood, chiefly of the variety that has a polymorphous nucleus and a finely granular protoplasm, endowed with great power of motion (Ehrlich's cells with neutrophil granules, or Max Schultze's cells with granular protoplasm).[2] It may be well to repeat here that malaria, by itself, does not determine this sort of leucocytosis, which is found to a very pronounced degree in inflammatory diseases for instance. So that when the blood of persons suffering from malaria happens to show a considerable increase of polynucleated neutrophil white blood-corpuscles, we must assume the existence of another infection, which, being associated with the malarial fever, is the cause of this change in the blood. Thus on several occasions both Dr. G. Bastianelli and ourselves have been led to suspect the presence of a complication, *e. g.* pneumonia, or suppuration, or erysipelas, simply from examining the blood; because, in addition to the alterations that properly belong to malaria, we

[1] A complete study on the pathology of the white blood-corpuscles in malaria was recently read by Dr. G. Bastianelli before the Medical Academy of Rome (sitting held May 22nd, 1892). Our own conclusions agree with those which Dr. Bastianelli has arrived at.

[2] Dr. H. Rieder, 'Beiträge zur Kenntniss der Leukocytose,' pp. 29 and following, Leipzig, F. C. W. Vogel, 1892.

succeeded in discovering this leucocytosis. The clinical examination was found to confirm the opinion we had formed [13].

§ 53. Golgi[1] has studied the method whereby the phenomena of phagocytosis in the quartan and tertian are evolved in cycles, and has expressed his results in a comprehensive article, which we shall again have occasion to quote. The law which he has formulated is as follows :—"Phagocytism is a process which is periodically evolved as a regular function of the white blood-corpuscles—which develops in precise correspondence with fixed phases in the malarial parasites' evolutionary cycle, and during a determinate period in each paroxysm of fever."

It now remains to inquire how the process of phagocytosis is characterised in the summer malarial fevers during the course of the paroxysm, and whether the sequence of facts is as regular as in the quartan and tertian.

If we take into consideration the results obtained from autopsies on malarial subjects, we must conclude that phagocytosis takes place in the entire vascular system, but preferably in that of certain of the viscera (the spleen and bone marrow), so that what we find in the blood taken from the finger must be looked upon as an episode in a process which is carried out by preference in the vessels of the internal viscera; and hence it follows that, should no instances of phagocytosis be met with in the blood of the finger, we cannot infer with certainty that there are none elsewhere at the same time.

When we examine the blood taken from the finger at different stages in the attack, and in the interval it is found that phagocyte forms begin to make their appearance at the commencement of the paroxysm, they chiefly consist of white blood-corpuscles, enclosing the same small round masses of pigment that are seen at the centre of the forms of fission. During the course of the paroxysm they go on increasing, until towards its close they sometimes become extremely numerous. In typical cases of summer tertian the maximum quantity of pigment-laden white blood-corpuscles is usually to be met with about the time of the pre-critical elevation.

In the short period of apyrexia they decrease considerably, or else disappear (though this a rare occurrence) only to reappear in

[1] C. Golgi, 'Il fagocitismo nell' infezione Malarica, Riforma Medica,' May, 1888. In this article the author has set forth the history of the questions that have gathered round the subject, and has given the observations of Laveran, Metschnikoff, Marchiafava, Celli, Guarnieri, and others; and to it we refer our readers for further information.

large numbers when the fever returns. The presence of phagocyte forms during the paroxysm may be almost always verified; indeed, there are cases of mild summer tertian where sometimes it is impossible to find parasites in the blood of the finger during short intervals of time, but the pigmented white blood-corpuscles enable the physician to diagnose the infection as malarial.

This cyclical function of the white blood-corpuscles, which is carried out in correspondence with the paroxysms of fever, may be easily traced in cases where the infection is recent; but its course cannot be followed if the disease has lasted for a fairly long time. In instances of this sort, pigmented white blood-corpuscles are found every time the blood is examined, and it may be impossible to say when they are increasing or diminishing; moreover the shortness of the periods of apyrexia is another difficulty in the way of forming a judgment. That in these cases phagocytes are met with not only during and a little after the paroxysm, but also throughout the whole apyrexia, is no hard matter to explain. As a matter of fact it is well known that large numbers of pigmented white blood-corpuscles, and generally phagocyte forms as well, are found in the organs of those who have died from a malignant infection. After the acute stage of the fever has passed away these bodies slowly leave the vascular system of the lungs, kidneys, intestines, &c., and gather together in the spleen, liver, and bone marrow. Now experience shows that this process of purifying the vascular system takes many hours, and in some cases several days to complete; hence, when, owing to the succession of different paroxysms, the capillary system of the various viscera has been polluted by a great quantity of phagocytes, it is obvious that these forms must still be seen circulating in the blood during an apyrexia intervening between two paroxysms; and the difficulty of following the cycle of the phagocyte function will be found to vary directly as the gravity and extension of this pollution. For the same reasons it will be understood how it is that in the apyrexia which is interposed between a series of paroxysms and the relapse, a small quantity of pigmented white blood-corpuscles may still be seen in the blood, even for several days (for instance, four or five), at a time when the parasites have completely disappeared. It will also be perceived why the severe and malignant infections show the same state of things; in these cases, even after a cure has been effected by the extinction of the acute infection, one may still see pigmented leucocytes in the blood for [illegible] or eight days; they consist for the most part of the large pigmented or blood-corpuscle-laden macrophagi, showing signs of degeneration or of necrosis.

It may be frequently noticed that just in proportion as the endoglobular parasitic forms go on decreasing under the action of the specific remedy, so the number of the phagocytes increases—in fatal cases till death supervenes, and this even when the parasites have almost entirely disappeared.

When the fever is cured by treatment with quinine the pigmented leucocytes continue to be seen in the blood for one, two, or three days, and it may be for a longer time in instances where the parasites and also the phagocyte forms were found in very large quantities previous to the employment of the remedy. Sometimes, indeed, after the administration of quinine the pigmented and blood-corpuscle-laden leucocytes become exceedingly numerous,—in fact, so much so that it may be possible to judge of the increase on examining the ordinary preparations of blood, without making use of one of the well-known methods of estimation. As we have already remarked, this phenomenon is usually more frequently to be seen in the malignant fevers, and not only in those which end in recovery, but also in those which do not—a point which is worthy of notice.

Finally, in cases where, despite the action of the remedy, the life-cycle of a portion of the parasites is continued, and the fever, in consequence, persists, the pigmented white blood-corpuscles still remain visible even for several days (four, five, six, and it may be more), and diminish progressively and proportionately with the parallel decrease in the amœbæ. In instances of spontaneous recovery we have carefully examined the blood from this point of view, but have not succeeded in obtaining any constant results. In some cases, as the attacks were becoming less and less until they entirely vanished, we have thought we could detect an increase in the phagocyte forms when compared with the amount observed on the days preceding the time when the infection showed a tendency to pass away; in other cases, on the contrary, the pigment-laden white blood-corpuscles appear to diminish in correspondence with the gradual disappearance of the parasites.

When the fever has ceased, and bodies of the crescent-shaped phase persist in the blood, then so long as these forms remain (about twelve or thirteen days) pigmented white blood-corpuscles continue to be seen at intervals.

§ 54. The evolution of the phagocyte function in the quartan and tertian has been followed by Golgi, and we can confirm his observations.

We will give the summary of his investigations in his own words:[1]—"It would be useless to look for signs of phagocytism in the blood as it circulates at the time when the parasites of malaria are in their endoglobular stage, or when they are passing through the phases preceding complete maturity; on the other hand, when the amœbæ are full-grown and are ripe for segmentation, or when the segmentation has just taken place, then the activity of the phagocytes may be seen easily enough. This begins simultaneously with the onset of the paroxysm, becomes more marked in the course of three or four hours, and terminates some hours after its close, although even later than this certain facts pointing to the continuance of the process may be verified. The phenomena, in their entirety, run their course in a period of six, eight, or twelve hours." The author then proceeds to describe how, during the period when the paroxysm is being prepared, the blood contains white blood-corpuscles enclosing forms which are either still in process of segmentation or have already separated, or, it may be, they comprise isolated masses of pigment. Later on, the same malarial forms are found included in white blood-corpuscles, but in a state of disintegration, which constantly increases until nothing is left but extremely fine granules of pigment. After ten or twelve hours, *when the destruction of the materials contained in the leucocytes has been completed,* the phagocyte forms disappear, only to reappear with the subsequent attack, and pass through a similar evolution.

§ 55. If now we compare these facts with those observed in the dangerous fevers, certain important differences will become evident. First and foremost, we must draw attention to what we have already noticed, namely, the fact that in the dangerous infections one frequently meets with blood-corpuscle-laden cells, and especially with large leucocytes containing brassy red blood-corpuscles laden with plasmodia, while the enclosed red blood-corpuscles may be either entirely decolourised, or may retain an almost normal aspect; and they may comprise young plasmodia without pigment and discoid in shape, or pigmented forms, or corpuscles with pigment at the centre in process of fission; or, lastly, bodies belonging to the group of crescent-shaped forms. *Therefore in*

[1] C. Golgi, "Azione della chinina sui parassiti malarici," 'Atti Istituto Lombardo,' vol. xxv, No. 5, p. 357.

the dangerous fevers the process of phagocytosis is developed even "when the parasites are in their endoglobular stage, and when they are passing through the phases preceding maturity." In speaking of the malignant infections we have had occasion to point out that the parasites of the summer-autumn group are not only more virulent—that is to say, capable of greater reproductive energy —than those of the spring fevers, but that they are also more poisonous. This higher degree of virulence is shown in part by the swiftness of the change which the amœba, as it grows, works in the red blood-corpuscle; its chemical and physical properties, its appearance, its colouring, its elasticity, &c., are all modified. It is more than probable that in these profound alterations lies the reason why amœbæ-laden red blood-corpuscles are found enclosed in the white cells even long before the fission, and, moreover, at a time when a large portion of the substance of the invaded blood-corpuscle still remains intact. This process, whereby amœbiferous red blood-corpuscles, to all appearance in a normal condition, are included in white cells, would lead one to suppose that the poisonous change in the blood-corpuscle is already far advanced even before it is manifested through visible modifications in regard to colouring, form, &c. As we have said, these phenomena are not to be seen during the corresponding stage in the development of the tertian and quartan amœba.

If now the whole series of facts as set forth be borne in mind, it is believed that they may be summed up and formulated in the following law:—"*The phagocyte function of the white blood-corpuscles in the summer-autumn fevers is carried out on the parasites, and the small masses or granules of pigment, which have become extra-globular, and are shed abroad in the plasma in a free state, is also carried out on those red blood-corpuscles in which profound degenerative alterations have been determined by the amœba.*" As a matter of fact, the process of sporulation towards the beginning of the attack is coincident with the liberation of a large number of blocks of pigment, and, on the other hand, with the death of a great many adult forms, which are enclosed in brassy red blood-corpuscles, and do not reach the stage of reproduction. At this point the phagocytosis begins in full activity (leucocytes pigmented or containing either red blood-corpuscles or plasmodia); as the paroxysm proceeds it continues, and attains its maximum during the pre-critical elevation,—that is to say, when the adult forms, whether free or contained in brassy red blood-corpuscles, the sporulation, and all the other bodies entirely disappear from the blood.

We have mentioned at the beginning of this chapter that the phagocyte function is also performed by the endothelial cells; this is known not only from examining organs like the liver or brain in cases of fatal malignancy, but also because, in severe infections, the blood of the finger is found to contain endothelial cells enclosing pigment, parasites, and plasmodia-laden red blood-corpuscles, as Marchiafava and Celli have already noted.[1]

We have now to inquire what is the importance of this process with reference to the resistance offered by the organism to the infection. It is clear that the possession of exact conceptions, with regard to the way in which spontaneous recovery is effected, would be a very important factor towards the solution of this question. But as yet we have nothing of the kind. It is impossible to affirm that the phagocytosis is more active when recovery from the fever is spontaneous, because on this point the observations made are contradictory, as we have before remarked. In the second place, it is not certain that the phagocytes destroy the enclosed spores, and these probably represent the only forms capable of development that are included by the white blood-corpuscles. If the enclosed spores are all destroyed, how is the relapse to be accounted for, which is almost always consequent on the summer fevers? On the other hand, we have no means at present of objectively determining what becomes of these included spores.

For the production of spontaneous cure we must not forget the importance which may attach to the death of the malarial parasites, and especially of the adult forms which have become free in the plasma. Various observers (Celli, Antolisei, &c.) have described certain processes of degeneration which are carried out in the large pigmented forms, as well in the quartan and tertian as in the summer fevers. In the latter, degenerative changes of this sort are seen not only in the bodies belonging to the group of crescent-shaped forms, but also in the forms with pigment at the centre, which in their normal state divide into spores: we have traced in these forms, as in the large pigmented forms of tertian fever, a process whereby they become vacuolated and disintegrated into hyaline spherules, which undergo rapid changes. It is only the bodies which have divided into spores and have become free in the plasma that

[1] It is well established that the phagocyte property of the endothelial cells is manifested in other infectious diseases, and Metschnikoff considers it of great importance in relation to the question of phlogosis (Metschnikoff, 'Leçons sur la Pathologie comparée de l'Inflammation,' 1892, 9me leçon).

show no alterations visible by the microscope, while we have reasons for maintaining that all the forms in other phases of life, when once the protecting envelope of the red blood-corpuscle has disappeared, die more or less quickly, owing to a certain deleterious influence which the constituent parts of the plasma exert on them. This hypothesis is also sustained by Faggioli's recent experiments.[1]

The importance of these facts in spontaneous recovery cannot be denied; but here, too, the objective solution of the question is not as yet possible.

It remains to consider the importance of phagocytosis in cases of cure effected by quinine. We have often observed a remarkable development in the phagocyte phenomena after the administration of the salts of quinine; but, in our opinion, this is not due to an increase in the phagocyte energy brought about by the drug, but to the greater quantity of necrotic forms, and of free pigment, which is diffused in the blood in consequence of the direct action of the remedy on the parasites; the phagocytes remove the dead forms which render the blood impure. All that objective observation allows us to say with certainty is, that the salts of quinine do not hinder the phagocyte activity of the white blood-corpuscles, nor is their mobility modified, so far as can be judged from microscopic examination. For the rest, Disselhorst[2] and others have proved by experiments on the frog that the motility of the leucocytes in the vascular system of the living animal remains unimpaired by the action of quinine. The phagocyte function continues to be performed owing to the fact that the leucocytes are unchanged both in power of motion and in other biological properties; but all the researches which we have described unite in confirming the truth, that the cure of malarial fevers by the salts of quinine is effected by the action of the drug on the nutritive processes of the amœbæ.

If the facts actually are as we have set them forth,—if, that is

[1] Dr. F. Faggioli ('Arch. Italiens de Biologie,' vol. xvi, Nos. 2, 3, 1891) in his Laboratory of Experimental Pharmacology at Genoa has studied the poisonous action of the blood on the protozoa, and has arrived at the following conclusions:—The blood in the whole animal series is endowed with a property which is deleterious to inferior unicellular organisms; this property is due to the presence of salts, especially of chloride of sodium, and may be looked upon as a means of protection of the species; the representatives of any given species show no absolute constancy with regard to this poisonous quality; variations may be observed, which pass gradually even into negative values.

[2] 'Virchow's Arch.,' vol. cxiii, p. 108, 1888.

to say, phagocytosis is only carried out on forms contained in red blood-corpuscles which are profoundly modified, or else on the free forms which probably die through a poisonous property in the plasma, if this be not strong enough to destroy the spores—we cannot but conclude that the most important result of the phagocyte process is the cleansing of the vascular system by the removal of the dead forms, and of the refuse entering it during the acute stage of the infection. This phenomenon is, without doubt, nothing else than a part of the functions of resistance to the disease, whereby recovery is worked out. If this theory be true, the white blood-corpuscles are pre-eminently *carriers and consumers of débris.*

According to Golgi, phagocytosis has a very important bearing on the course of the infection in the quartan and tertian fevers; indeed, he says it seems certain that the white blood-corpuscles, in correspondence with each paroxysm, destroy not only the products of parasitic disintegration, but even certain numbers of the amœbæ themselves. If this were not so, and if all the parasites were to invariably complete their cycle, then, in the opinion of the author above mentioned, "every malarial intermittent fever would necessarily and by fixed rule become aggravated, so as finally to pass into malignancy." But this is not the case, as everyone knows. We, however, guided by our observations, cannot attach such importance as this to phagocytosis; thus we are unable to admit that the aggravation of every fever, including the advent of malignant symptoms in our spring infections, is prevented solely by the action of phagocytes.

Since the time when the parasites of the tertian and quartan were first known, *there is no instance on record of a malignant infection caused by them; and no autopsy has ever been made in connection with a malignant spring tertian or quartan.*

Hence we are led to seek the cause of this constant feature, not in the functions of resistance and of individual reaction, which confessedly show the greatest variability, but in the biological properties of this group of parasites. *The malignant infections* (as we have shown in detail) *are due to another special class of parasites; and malignancy, in spite of the evolution of the phagocyte functions, developing as it does in a much more active way than in the spring fevers, is chiefly produced by the particularly virulent and poisonous attributes of this parasitic group.*

NOTES.

[1]

Page 41. So as not to enter into a question which at present would be difficult to solve, we have intentionally abstained from treating of the nomenclature of the parasites of malaria in the text. It may not be superfluous, however, to explain why we still continue to use the term "*plasmodium*" in treating of the younger forms of parasites, although its adoption has aroused so much criticism that we are compelled to admit is in great part justified. Marchiafava and Celli in their first publication proposed the term "plasmodium," wishing thus to designate the parasite in its early period as being composed simply of an amœboid mass of protoplasm. Several zoologists and botanists have adopted the term in this sense, as will be seen by referring to the publications quoted by Celli and Guarnieri in their article "On the Etiology of the Malarial Infection," 'Transactions of the Royal Academy of Medicine in Rome, 1888–89,' p. 399,[1] as also to the dissertation on *Protochytrium spirogyræ* by Borzi. Later on it was justly observed that this term "plasmodium," in its restricted sense as used by zoologists, signified those bodies formed by the aggregation or fusion of many amœbæ, each retaining its own nucleus. Thus, in scientific language, a "plasmodium" is a polynuclear mass of protoplasm. For this reason various names have been proposed by different observers, of which, however, none has been universally accepted. Grassi proposed the term "amœba," which both Golgi and ourselves subsequently adopted. Later on, however, he abandoned it, as he thought it best, from the standpoint of our present knowledge, to differentiate between the term "amœba" of the zoologists and the parasite of malaria. Mannaberg, holding that it is

[1] "Sulla etiologia delle infezione malariæ," 'Atti della R. Accademia Medica di Roma, 1888–89,' p. 399.

to say, phagocytosis is on[illegible]ure until the zoological red blood-corpuscles which [illegible]een better defined, makes the free forms which probab[illegible] expression "parasites of in the plasma, if this be not [illegible] "plasmodium malariæ," —we cannot but conclude [illegible] Hæmogregarinidæ," which the phagocyte process is t[illegible] blood-corpuscles of the the removal of the dead for[illegible] the term "plasmodium," as the acute stage of the in[illegible] state of the parasites of doubt, nothing else than [illegible]derstood; and further, of all the disease, whereby re[illegible] generally used. true, the white blood-[illegible] [illegible]menclature as proposed by *consumers of débris*.

According to Golgi [illegible] a term which, later on, was on the course of the [illegible] indeed, he says it [illegible] correspondence with [illegible]veran). ducts of parasitic [illegible] Metschnikoff). amœbæ themselves [illegible] Marchiafava and Celli). were to invariably [illegible] Osler). the author ab[illegible] (quartan). would necess[illegible] tertian). finally to pass [illegible] quotidian). everyone k[illegible] *[illegible]ulata.* cannot attac[illegible] semilunar), Grassi and Feletti. are unable [illegible] cluding th[illegible] is preven[illegible]

Since [illegible] times insisted upon the fact that were fir[illegible] finger for amœbæ in the stage of *infecti[illegible]* their initial period may often be *connec[illegible]* taken from the spleen forms of [illegible] However, we are compelled to add

Her[illegible] cases of medium gravity, it may at in the [illegible]dies are absent even in the blood confe[illegible] the onset of fever or during the prop[illegible]rimarily, however, those endoglobular (as w[illegible] in their centre, which precede the *para[illegible]* visible, and when properly stained easily *cyt[illegible]* sporulation. This fact leads us to *th[illegible]* has the segmentation of the body con-*vir[illegible]* and the formation of sporules taken place [illegible] scattered, and for this reason it is so rare to [illegible] rosette shape (see Plate I, figs. 52—66). [illegible] may also apply to the parasite of malignant

[3]

Page 52. During the summer and autumn of 1891 we observed many cases of this form of tertian, several following a completely regular course. The greater number of the cases of pernicious fever that came under observation during that malarial period also appeared to belong to the same clinical type.

On the contrary, cases of quotidian and of pernicious quotidian were less frequent. However, the proportion between the two forms of summer-autumn fevers is not always the same in all seasons. Marchiafava and Celli have already alluded to this fact in former communications. During the present year (1893), moreover, Dr. Bastianelli, who has observed many cases of malarial fever with us at the Santo Spirito Hospital, has found more cases of quotidian than tertian fever, whilst the condition was exactly the reverse during the preceding season (1892). We have merely wished to call attention to this fact in order that the importance we attach to the tertian type may not appear exaggerated. It is necessary to remember that not only do the different clinical forms vary in frequency in various malarial districts, but also during successive seasons in the same one. We hold that this fact can be easily explained by admitting that the different types of parasite correspond to the varied fundamental clinical forms. For those who wish to test our observations by personal research, it is necessary to note these facts, and to remember that in order to present a more or less complete description of these fevers several years of observation are requisite. It is more difficult to offer a reason for other variations in observations made by us during successive years.

Thus, for example, during the period 1888 and 1889, Marchiafava and Celli had opportunities for studying many cases of malarial infection with scarcely any melanæmia. In one case of comatose pernicious fever the capillaries of the brain were found by them to contain numerous unpigmented plasmodia, the greater number of which were in the stage of segmentation or had already split up. We were never again able to find this condition till 1893.

In a case studied towards the end of October in this year we were able to observe at the post-mortem examination several instances of precocious segmentation without pigment in the capillaries of the brain. These were found in a boy coming from the Campagna, who died in the Santo Spirito Hospital after about three days' illness in spite of repeated hypodermic injections of full doses of quinine. In this case an enormous number of parasites had invaded the vascular system of all the organs, and the young forms without pigment were chiefly met with.

We have preserved in the Pathologico-anatomical Institute specimens of malarial brains, in which the capillaries are filled with parasites without any trace of melanosis.

[4]

Page 56. In several cases of pernicious fever observed during the present year (1893) conjointly by Dr. Bastianelli and ourselves in the Santo Spirito Hospital, forms of segmentation with a great number of spores up to twenty, thirty, or even more, were noticeable. Indeed, in one case the capillaries of the brain presented various types of sporulation with many spores, whilst the spleen and the bone marrow demonstrated, in prevailing numbers, forms of endoglobular division with ten to twelve spores.

[5]

Page 57. In this description of the amœba of the summer tertian, as well as in the preceding ones, regarding the other varieties of malarial parasites we have always treated of the endoglobular development of the parasites, without discussing whether or not they are really endoglobular, or simply attached to the red blood-corpuscles. As is well known, Laveran thought the parasites were either free in the plasma or simply attached to the red corpuscles. Marchiafava and Celli, in calling special attention to the younger forms (unpigmented amœbæ), maintained that they were found within the blood-corpuscle. To sustain their view they affirmed that the pseudopodia of the amœba never extended beyond the limits of the red corpuscle, which must have occurred were the parasite merely attached to it. Furthermore they noted that in slowly moving the fine adjustment they were never able to observe the parasite either above or under the corpuscle, but that it always appeared within its substance. Later observers, in studying the parasites of malaria, have never doubted their endoglobular position. It is only recently that Mannaberg has again brought up this question. He believes he is able to demonstrate that the adult forms, the spherical variety belonging to the semilunar, and the larger forms of the tertian type, are endoglobular. In fact, the best proof of this is obtained by watching under the microscope that on the exit of the parasite from the corpuscle the latter becomes decolourised and splits up.

However, he does not look upon the younger forms (unpigmented amœbæ) as endoglobular. According to him, even if their pseudopodia do not extend beyond the border of the blood-corpuscles, this may be due to the viscidity of the parasite, and not to its being endoglobular. Again, he observes that the transparency of the blood-corpuscle will not permit us to establish with exactness whether so hyaline a body as a young parasite be above, within, or under the corpuscle itself. In examining the blood Mannaberg recommends oblique light, keeping the diaphragm of the microscope entirely open. In this manner the high lights and shadows appear more marked, and the observer can often convince himself that the young parasites are situated in a sort of niche or concavity on the surface of the blood-corpuscle. However, this question, after all, is of but little importance. Admitting the endoglobular position of the adult forms, it merely remains to be settled at what period of the development of the younger forms they *enter* into the substance of the blood-corpuscle. We still maintain that the greater number of the young forms are endoglobular. In some cases we have been able to observe the unpigmented amœba change its position *in toto*—a complete movement of transposition—within the corpuscle, whilst in others we have seen the parasite immerse itself, as it were, in its substance, and then again coming into view, appear close to the surface of the corpuscle—a series of movements impossible were the parasite not within the substance of the corpuscle. Again, we have been able to study the red blood-corpuscle containing the young plasmodia, as seen in their vertical aspect. During their change of position we have almost convinced ourselves that the parasite appeared surrounded on all sides by a stratum of globular substance.

Besides these undoubtedly endoglobular forms, there are those in indentations upon the surface of the blood-corpuscle alluded to by Mannaberg. Marchiafava and Celli, who at the beginning of their first studies described and illustrated them exactly as described by Mannaberg, based upon them their view that the hyaline bodies were extraneous elements having penetrated into the corpuscle, and not products of degeneration of the corpuscle itself. Up to within recent years this fundamental question was still doubted by many. Only Marchiafava and Celli interpret this appearance as the form in process of escaping from the red blood-corpuscle. These particulars, which in themselves are of but little importance, may indicate to us how the youngest plasmodia penetrate into the corpuscle. This process may be conceived as follows. The youngest amœbæ, the offspring of sporulation, by virtue of the viscidity of their protoplasm adhere to the surface of, and by their movements bury themselves in, the contour of the red corpuscle. In this position the parasite attacks the external strata of the corpuscle as a means of nourishment, and after altering these layers is able to penetrate within, and thus becomes entirely endoglobular.

[6]

Page 58. Besides those alterations already alluded to (shrinking, decoloration), the red corpuscles containing the adult parasitic forms may be subject to another change, *i. e.* fragmentation. Under the microscope it is at times possible to observe the red corpuscle divide by constriction into two parts, one containing the parasite, the other being tenantless. Thus the microcytes or schistocytes, according to the nomenclature of Ehrlich, are formed.

This fact, however, is of little importance in malaria, as microcytes are but seldom found, and if found at all they occur only in small number, in the blood of malarial subjects. We have also observed a red corpuscle containing two parasites divide in such a way that each part presented a parasite surrounded, as it were, by a zone of hæmoglobin.

[7*[1]]

Page 95 [line 7, after "parasites"]. The facts alluded to in the above-mentioned paragraph, treating of the relation between the course of the fever and the development of the parasites in the blood, must be accepted with certain limitations. In the fevers pursuing a regular course, such as in most of the mild fevers, and often in cases of considerable gravity as well, it may be accepted as a general rule that "the paroxysm corresponds to the development of a generation of parasites," and that "the phase or period of multiplication of the parasites determines the initial stage of the access." In the dangerous fevers, and above all in those of pernicious type, a series of disturbing elements intervene, whose influence often renders the intimate relation between the course of the temperature and the period of life of the parasites unrecognisable. This view has been already alluded to in discussing the facts treated of in the text, as also in several of the clinical cases cited as examples. Thus there are cases of pernicious infection without

[1] An apology is due for the numbers marked by an asterisk not having appeared in the text, as they were brought to notice too late for insertion.—Ed.

' out any characteristic type, in
..lood reveals the presence of
. All practitioners are familiar
forms of pernicious malaria. On
s in which the temperature remains
successive diminution, even total dis-
'es in the blood. Thus in Case 27, an
nicious fever of the tertian type, in which
.ned high for several days, and in which
sed by a marked increase of fever, the para-
beginning of the disease were most numerous,
ished in number and disappeared in the blood
e finger, whilst but few were found at the autopsy
of the organs. Neither is it possible to find any
tween the course of the temperature and the life of
ites. We could cite many similar cases, and these facts
prove that there can be a great increase in number of
ites without an access of fever; and, on the other hand, that
eat rise of temperature may be independent of the state of the
arasites. These facts furthermore attest to the great complexity of the phenomena. Being entirely ignorant of the precise methods by which the multiplication of the parasites produce the fever, we naturally cannot enter into the discussion analytically why in some cases this effect is wanting. We can only surmise that in cases of the grave type disturbing elements come into operation, which change the regular succession of phenomena. In those instances, great elevation of temperature, noticeable in certain cases of cerebral pernicious fever, to all appearance, independent of the biological state of the parasite, one may suppose that they can be due to, or are in relation with, the secondary functional or organic changes produced by the parasites in the nervous centres. According to this view, these fevers would bear a certain resemblance to those occurring in cerebral hæmorrhage, in cases of traumatism of the brain, &c.

[8*]

Page 101 [line 16, after "regular"]. Our statement that cases of pernicious fever do not exist in which the diagnosis cannot be established by the microscopic examination of the blood has been contradicted by some observers, and probably will be by others yet to come. This must naturally be the consequence, as long as the result of observation of one or only a few ca
entitles any observer to formulate a law on a general b

We maintain our point, based as it is on numerous observations extending over several years of study. Two facts, however, must not be overlooked; the first, that in some cases of pernicious fever the parasites may disappear from the blood after full doses of quinine, and notwithstanding this the disease may tend to become aggravated, and may even have a fatal issue. We have treated of this fact in a preceding chapter. In the second place, it must be remembered that some of the grave morbid symptoms may develop in individuals in whom the malarial infection has recently spent itself. At the end of this chapter we have called attention to these types, and have termed them "post-malarial," an expression which, while it indicates the course of facts, does not include a fixed conception of their pathogenesis.

[9*]

Page 103 [line 21, after "autopsy"]. We shall briefly treat of those rare cases of severe general infection, at times even fatal, in which there are but few parasites, in the second Appendix.

[10*]

Page 112 [line 10 from below, after "predominant"]. The observations made referring to the distribution of the parasites in the vascular areas of the organs of those who have died of pernicious fever, allude almost exclusively to that group of pernicious fevers with cerebral symptoms (coma, delirium, convulsions, &c.), a group which could be called "pernicious cerebral fever." These cases, as we have already remarked, are the predominating ones occurring among us, and form the greater number of the cases studied by Bignami in his publication. Bignami has already observed that in the forms of pernicious fever the accumulation of parasites may, by preference, take place in other organs than in the brain, *e. g.* in the intestines in choleraic pernicious fever. From this point of view one may distinguish various groups of cases in pernicious fever.

1st. Cases in which the entire organism is invaded by the parasites to such an extent that a comparative examination of the brain, of the spleen, and of the bone-marrow will render it impossible to establish in which organ the accumulation is greatest.

2nd. Cases in which the greatest number of parasites are found in the capillaries of the brain, the adult forms or those in the process of sporulation predominating.

3rd. Cases in which the greatest accumulations are observed in the spleen, in the bone-marrow, and occasionally in the capillaries of the intestines.

To the second group belong the greater number of cases of cerebral pernicious fever, which we have stated to be so common with us. This will explain why almost all of our descriptions, and the conclusions we have arrived at while treating of the distribution of parasites, and of the changes in various organs, in cases of anatomico-pathological examination of cases of pernicious fever, almost exclusively refer to this group. We further wish to add that it is possible to find the parasites accumulated exclusively in the brain; thus in a case of comatose pernicious fever studied during this year (1893) in the Santo Spirito Hospital by Dr. Bastianelli, and by us, post-mortem examination revealed the capillaries of the brain filled with parasites in various stages of development, whilst no trace of them could be found in either the spleen or the bone marrow. However, in another case of algid pernicious fever the spleen and the bone marrow were full of parasites, whilst but few were found in the brain. To the third group belongs the following case studied by Marchiafava in the summer of this year (1893), and in which the parasites were found almost exclusively in the intestine; the case was one of algid pernicious fever with hæmorrhagic diarrhœa, and the post-mortem examination revealed an acute enteritis, with superficial sloughing of the mucous membrane as the main feature. The accumulation of parasites was almost exclusively limited to the superficial capillaries of the mucous membrane corresponding to the necrotic portion. This observation tends to strengthen our view, already expressed at other times, that in some way local causes enter into action, and modify the general laws relating to the distribution of parasites in the vascular areas of the organism.

[11]

Page 158. The cases which we allude to at the end of paragraph (*a*) demonstrate that the thermal resistance, and also the resistance of the parasites to the action of quinine, vary within rather large limits. We have mentioned cases in which, notwithstanding the most proper administration of this remedy, the fever has persisted for two, three, or even more days. In some cases it seems that the resistance to the influence of quinine is greater in recent infections, and gradually diminishes in the later progressive paroxysms. In fever patients coming from the country, presenting themselves at the hospital on the third or fourth day of the fever, and who either have not been treated or the treatment has been carried out in a most imperfect manner, we seldom see more than one attack after the administration of several grammes of quinine. However, in some cases it appears that the action of the remedy is not as prompt if administered earlier. Subcontinued fevers, as we have already mentioned, present the same variations in the resistance to quinine; this is probably most marked in the so-called subcontinued "d'emblée." In one case of this type, notwithstanding the administration of quinine at the very onset, and its being continued regularly, the fever kept its course, uninfluenced by the remedy, for about five days. We do not know of any cases in which the resistance to the influence of quinine was greater.

[12]

Page 168. The facts alluded to in the text, relating to the action of quinine on the parasites of summer-autumn fevers, refer merely to what is observed in studying fresh preparations without fixing or staining. We must add, however, that staining brings out the more minute alterations produced by quinine. Besides the observations already cited of Romanowski, there are those of Mannaberg, which treat specially of the parasites of the quartan and of the common tertian type. In examining the blood of a quartan or of a tertian, a few hours after the administration of the first dose of quinine, the greater number of the small and medium-sized parasites will be observed to have their nucleoli no longer stained, whilst the small vesicle which represents the nucleus continues to be stained as before. According to Mannaberg, this disappearance of the nucleolus demonstrates the necrosis of the minute parasite. Furthermore, he observes that many sporulating forms undergo special alterations, after the administration of quinine a few hours previous to the attack; whilst to all appearances the fresh specimens seem normal, when stained with hæmatoxylin, the nucleoli of the greater part of the spores remain uncoloured. Mannaberg considers these thus altered forms as stillborn spores. These observations lead him to conclude that the spores of all the various forms of parasites of malaria are the most susceptible to the action of quinine. He also holds that these facts contradict the hypothesis of Bignami, *i. e.* that the relapses are due to the development of spores which have remained latent in the spleen, and have escaped the destructive action of quinine, of the phagocytes, &c.

We have been very reserved in our judgment regarding the action of quinine on the spores of the summer-autumn parasites. In the face of Mannaberg's objections to the possibility of the latent vitality of the spores, we can adduce the fact that in individuals who have succumbed to pernicious fever, and to whom quinine had been administered in the largest doses, we have often been able to find in different organs very numerous forms of sporulation. These specimens stained most perfectly with hæmatoxylin and the aniline dyes, and presented no recognisable changes whatever; so evident was this that we had no cause to consider them as necrotic forms. Furthermore, we wish to note that in cases of pernicious fever the spores, normal in structure, and when stained by hæmatoxylin to all appearances perfectly preserved, are often seen enclosed in white blood-corpuscles. Dr. Bastianelli and ourselves have often been able to make this observation. It does not seem to us as likely, therefore, that the spores of the parasite of summer-autumn fevers are the forms most susceptible to the influence of quinine, nor do we believe that Bignami's hypothesis regarding the latent vitality of the spores should be so easily abandoned.

[13]

Page 177. As we have stated in the text that the number of leucocytes diminishes absolutely and relatively during an attack of malarial infection, we must add that this diminution, which may be very marked, involves the polynuclear, neutrophil leucocytes. As Dr. Bastianelli has observed, the proportion in number between the various kinds of leucocytes is noticeably altered, while there is a diminution of the polynuclear neutrophil white blood-corpuscles, there exists instead a relative increase of *large mononuclear leucocytes* and of the so-called *transitional* forms (according to the nomenclature of Ehrlich and Einhorn). This is especially noticeable in cases of advanced malarial infection and in cases of the pernicious type, and is less evident in the initial period and during the first paroxysms.

At times the number of lymphogenic leucocytes is diminished, at others not. At this point it is interesting to remember that the large mononuclear leucocytes pre-eminently fulfil the function of phagocytes; in regard to this all observers are in accord.

As we have observed that to replace the loss of leucocytes many elements are found in a karyokinetic state in the spleen and in the bone marrow, we further wish to add that the increase of leucocytes also takes place in the circulating blood, in which also, as both Bastianelli and the authors have observed, leucocytes in a karyokinetic state may be found.

One may also find in the blood of malarial subjects, especially in the pernicious type, structures which bear all the characteristics of splenic and osseo-medullary cells. Thus leucocytes somewhat smaller than the ordinary large mononuclear cells, whose protoplasm and nuclei are more deeply stained by hæmatoxylin, may be observed. Leucocytes bearing these characteristics are very frequently found in some cases of spleno-medullary leuchæmia, and have recently been considered as young immature forms of mononucleated leucocytes (Bastianelli).

In two cases of pernicious fever we also found a few mononucleated eosinophil elements identical with those found in the bone marrow. According to some observers, these cells are only found in cases of spleno-medullary leucocythæmia. However, it appears that they occur in other diseases of the bone marrow, *e. g.* Bastianelli observed them in the blood of an anæmic patient in a case with fatal termination of multiple lympho-sarcoma of the osseous medulla.

The presence of a true leucocytosis—that is, a marked increase of the polynuclear leucocytes in malarial blood—may justify one in suspecting complications of an inflammatory process. We must, however, add that other pathological conditions may also determine a similar increase in malarial patients, in the same manner as they do in other diseases. Thus we have observed marked leucocytosis in malarial subjects who suffered from profuse diarrhœa or were collapsed, and the same condition may exist during the failure of vital power immediately preceding death, &c. In consequence of the most recent observations, we have grounds for believing that leucocytosis may also be met with in malarial hæmoglobinuria.

APPENDIX I.

ON THE CLASSIFICATION OF THE MALARIAL FEVERS.

The classification adopted by us has, if we mistake not, this advantage over the others which have been suggested: it rests on carefully ascertained matters of fact, while the standpoint employed as its criterion is a practical one.

Golgi admits the existence of the following fundamental types of fever:

(1) Intermittent fevers depending on parasites whose cycle of evolution is completed in two days. This group corresponds to the clinical types of the tertian, and of certain quotidians which are due to the daily alternate maturation of two generations of tertian parasites.

(2) Intermittent fevers depending on parasites whose cycle of evolution is completed in three days. This class includes the clinical types of the quartan, the double quartan, and the triple quartan.

(3) Intermittent fevers depending on the presence in the blood of those forms which are as yet not well understood, and which are generally called "crescent-shaped," the period of their development being variable. Under this division may be included many intermittent fevers of irregular type; the intermittent infections with long intervals, as well as many others with short ones, belong to this division; also some quotidians, and certain subcontinued fevers and subintrant quotidians.[1]

This last class corresponds to what we have named the *summer-autumn* group; and inasmuch as these infections, both in their clinical types and in their parasitic characteristics, differ in the clearest manner from the other two groups, we have placed

[1] C. Golgi, "On the Intermittent Malarial Fevers with Long Intervals: Fundamental Criteria for grouping the Malarial Fevers," 'Archivio delle Scienze Mediche,' 1890.

them in contrast to the latter; for, in our opinion, it is of great practical utility to draw a sharp line of division between the group of mild fevers, and the group composed of those fevers which may become malignant.

It is surprising to find that Golgi, in his theory of this latter class of infections, ranks the fevers with long intervals in the same category with those which have very short ones, such as the quotidians. Later on we shall give our reasons for being unable to believe that a group of the so-called long-interval fevers ought to be formed by itself. Only we cannot help here noticing how Golgi's indefiniteness of conception disappears before the clinical and parasitological study of these fevers, as carried out by us. Furthermore, all the facts and arguments set forth in this work go to show the impossibility of our accepting the view maintained by Golgi with regard to the parasitic variety which produces these infections.

The classification proposed by Grassi and Feletti[1] is drawn up from the zoological point of view. They distinguish two genera of malarial parasites:

I. The Hæmamœba.

II. The Laverania.

In the genus Hæmamœba they include the following species:

(1) The *Hæmamœba malariæ* (found in man, and producing the quartan fevers).

(2) The *Hæmamœba vivax* (found in man, and producing the tertian).

(3) The *Hæmamœba præcox* (found in man, and producing the malignant infections).

(4) The *Hæmamœba immaculata* (found in man, and also producing the malignant fevers).

In addition to these pathogenic species observed in the human subject, the above-named authors mention the following, found in birds:

(5) The *Hæmamœba relicta.*

(6) The *Hæmamœba subpræcox.*

(7) The *Hæmamœba immaculata.*

Under the genus Laverania they group three species:

(1) The *Laverania malariæ* (found in man, and producing the quotidian fevers, the subcontinued infections, and the "long interval" fevers).

(2) The *Laverania Danilewsky* (in birds).

(3) The *Laverania ranarum* (in frogs).

[1] 'Contributions to the Study of the Malarial Parasites.'

Without entering at length into the merits of this classification, we may observe that the fundamental grouping of the malarial parasites into two genera (the Hæmamœba and the Laverania) is based on the interpretation which assumes that the crescent-shaped forms (Laverania) represent a separate species of parasite entirely different from the species which give rise to the dangerous fevers (the *Hæmamœba præcox* of Grassi and Feletti). But this theory is not accepted by any of the other observers who have devoted themselves to these questions; on the contrary, they all maintain, as we do, that the crescent-shaped forms are in reality a certain phase in the life of the parasites of the summer-autumn infections. Whatever be the final solution of this matter, it is sufficient to remark here that Grassi and Feletti's classification is constructed on one of the most contested of all the facts connected with the biology of the malarial parasites. Moreover, as far as our knowledge at present goes, we cannot allow that a distinction should be drawn between the *Hæmamœba præcox* and the *Hæmamœba immaculata* as two separate species. The latter is said to be characterised by premature sporulation, which takes place before the pigmentation of the parasite.

This occurrence has been observed by Marchiafava and Celli, but only in very rare cases; and where these forms of fission did occur, sporulating forms *with* pigment were also present; so that in these instances we should have to admit a double infection produced both by the *Hæmamœba præcox* and the *Hæmamœba immaculata*—a hypothesis which at present is destitute of all foundation. We shall feel unable to change our opinion until we meet with cases of malarial infection which may show no trace of melanæmia, and which would consequently mean a *pure culture* of this presumed species of parasite, the *Hæmamœba immaculata*. There are, however, instances of malignant malarial fever where the melanosis of the organs, consequent on the melanæmia, is so slight that it may escape detection without a microscopic examination of the organs in which it is usually most intense.

Mannaberg[1] does not accept Grassi and Feletti's classification, especially refusing to admit the division into the two genera of Hæmamœba and Laverania. He agrees with the Roman school in maintaining *that it is one and the same amœboid parasite which either arrives at sporulation in the well-known way, or else changes into the crescent-shaped body.* His theory as to the structure and biological signification of the semilunar forms is that they are

[1] 'Die Malaria Parasiten,' Wien, 1893.

then[illegible] conjunction of the smallest
prac[illegible] starting from this position,
gro[illegible] two groups,—those which
whi[illegible] Thus:

It [illegible] segmentation, but without the forma-
clas[illegible], without crescent-shaped bodies.
same [illegible] quartan parasites; (*b*) the tertian
the [illegible]
una[illegible] segmentation and with the formation
fev[illegible] with crescent-shaped bodies. This
noti[illegible] pigmented parasite of the quotidian;
the [illegible] of the quotidian; (*c*) the
out [illegible]
in th[illegible] is almost identical with the
view [illegible] fact that the author draws a
whi[illegible] pigmented and non-pigmented parasite of

Th[illegible] we cannot endorse for the reasons
from [illegible] the fundamental grouping
of m[illegible] biological signification of the

I [illegible] is not shared by other observers,

II. [illegible] Whatever be the result which

In [illegible]annaberg's classification, to say the

(1 [illegible] is open to doubt.
the q[illegible] in the biology of the malarial

(2[illegible] has induced us rather to take
terti[illegible] phenomena as the fundamental

(3[illegible] malarial fevers. This method is
mali[illegible] for the physician than one which

(4[illegible] seem that we are fully justified in
duci[illegible] "to the group of fevers

In [illegible] and autumn. As a matter of fact
subj[illegible] special clinical aspect, which
in bi[illegible] only familiar with the milder

(5) [illegible] The parasites present such special
[illegible] diagnosis may be made *on the*
[illegible] Then, again, near Rome they usually
[illegible] at the end of June and the
[illegible] have been taught by an experience of
[illegible] during the whole autumn, the
[illegible] their appearance in the winter, while in
[illegible] primary infection is never observed.
[illegible] common quartan and tertian) by
[illegible] may appear less justifiable; for in

reality these fevers are found in all seasons of the year, and in the districts of mild malaria they even prevail during the summer and autumn. It is, however, necessary to bear in mind what we have already pointed out—the fact that it is *solely* at the close of the winter and during the spring that these infections predominate, to the exclusion of the other types of fever; while in the cases met with in the summer and autumn they occupy a subordinate position with regard to the endemic fevers peculiar to these seasons. Nor should it be forgotten that the nomenclature here adopted is "*a potiori.*" In order to understand the exactness and the practical usefulness of this classification, one must take the point of view of an observer who, in those countries where malaria is intense, watches the clinical phenomena of the infection, as they develop and as they succeed each other. And because all the clinical forms of the disease cannot be seen except in districts of this sort, it is only logical to start from researches which have been carried out on such a field.

To group these fevers solely from the standpoint of the parasitological criteria—that is, to employ a purely zoological method —is, in our opinion, premature at present. We have already remarked that several points connected with the biology of the malarial parasites are still *sub judice,* and some of these are such as would necessarily be of great moment in a zoological classification. The most important of these contested questions concerns the biology of the so-called crescent-shaped forms. In the present treatise we have assumed our attitude towards this subject, without any minute discussion of the facts on which we rest our view, and without examining opposite opinions; the essentially clinical nature of our work prevented us from doing so. But we willingly recognise that researches are still needed to test the facts upon which Grassi and Feletti and also Mannaberg have built their theories, and it is with such investigations that we are now engaged.

In our classification the so-called *long-interval* fevers as well as the so-called *irregular* infections have no place. The reasons which have led us not to form a group of the fevers with long intervals have been stated by Bignami in a short monograph,[1] the conclusions of which we will here briefly give. In studying the cases which have been classed together under this name it is necessary to distinguish the regular from the irregular "long-interval" fevers. The regular infections with long intervals were

[1] "Sulle Febbri Intermittenti Malariche cosi dette a Lunghi Intervalli," 'Riforma Medica,' 1891, No. 165.

meant by the old writers (from Hippocrates and Galen down to our own Borsieri) when they spoke of fevers recurring every six, seven, eight, &c., days. With regard to these, considering what we now know, there is really nothing to say, because, since the discovery of the malarial parasites, no one has had the opportunity of observing a single case. As to the irregular infections with long intervals, all the physicians who practise in malarial districts agree in admitting their existence, and in regarding the irregular return of the paroxysms as a series of recurrences. Somewhat similar to this type of fever are certain cases which we have studied, as well as one investigated by Golgi,[1] in which latter there were groups of paroxysms separated by intervals of apyrexia from five to ten days in length. As a general rule we find two, three, or four paroxysms coming together in groups which succeed each other at various intervals in different cases, varying from ten or fifteen days to a month. With respect to the parasites in some of these cases we find that the variety which characterises the summer-autumn fevers (as in the instance observed by Golgi),—that is to say, the small amœboid parasites are seen during the paroxysms, and the crescent-shaped bodies during the apyrexiæ; other cases show the parasites of the mild tertian, as in some instances which have come under our own notice. Of these two series the explanation of the first, produced as it is by the summer-autumn parasites, may be debatable, owing to the fact that our knowledge of the crescent-shaped bodies is still incomplete; on the other hand, the second series, which is due to the parasites of the mild tertian, can be interpreted without difficulty. We certainly cannot suppose that the tertian parasite undergoes such changes in its biological properties that it produces forms which slowly develop during the course of the long apyrexia until at last they give rise to fresh attacks of fever; in point of fact, such forms do not occur in the blood of the patient. Consequently a period of apyrexia which lasts for ten, fourteen, or sixteen days can bear no resemblance to one which intervenes between two tertian or quartan paroxysms, during which a parasitic generation is matured. It is therefore right to regard the fresh attack as a recurrence, which occurs after an interval manifestly equal to the time required for the parasite's incubation; so that these "loug-interval" fevers are presumably the product of a series of recurrences, which succeed each other at a nearly equal distance of time. According to this theory the

[1] "Sulle Febbri Intermittenti Malariche a Lunghi Intervalli," 'Arch. delle Scienze Mediche,' vol. xiv, f. 3.

intervals of apyrexia must be considered not as *intermissions* in the proper sense of the term, but as periods in which the malarial infection is *latent*. The recurrence connected with the summer-autumn fevers are frequently to be seen in the winter.

As regards the so-called *irregular* fevers our view may be deduced from all the facts set forth in this work, and may be thus summed up. There is no group of fevers which are naturally and *per se* irregular, but fevers of every class may *become* irregular, and in different ways: some types are less liable to this change, while in others, like the summer-autumn group, it takes place very frequently. If we bear in mind the law that "a fever with regular periods is caused by the maturation of a single parasitic generation"—a law which is valid for all kinds of malarial infection, a conception may be formed even *a priori* of the various ways in which a given type of fever can become complex and irregular. But there exists no variety of parasite characterised by uncertainty and irregularity in development; hence it follows that the conception of a group of essentially irregular fevers has no foundation on fact.

APPENDIX II.

ON THE MALIGNANT INFECTIONS.

The additional experience we have gained in regard to this subject during the last two malarial seasons, since our treatise was published, enables us to confirm our previous statements in all essential points.

In the first place, we can still further establish the fact on which we have insisted in the text, that *the malignant infections are always produced by the summer-autumn varieties of the malarial parasites.* The practical importance of this law has induced us to devote careful study to every additional case of malignant fever that has come under our notice, and there have been several such; the result has been that each new instance has only supplied additional confirmation of the principle we have laid down.

We return here to this subject because the law as enunciated by us has been called in question. Thus it has been alleged that we deny the possibility of malignant infections making their appearance in the winter. It is almost needless to add that we have never made this statement. As a matter of fact, malignant infections during the winter may be found, although not frequently, in districts where malaria is intense; and we have reported an instance in Case 30. But these cases, rare as they may be, are nevertheless determined by the parasitic varieties which we have called *a potiori* the summer-autumn.

With regard to the factors of malignancy in these malarial infections, we have brought into prominence the following facts:

(*a*) The vast quantity of parasites in the majority of cases;

(*b*) The frequent presence of two, and sometimes of more than two generations or colonies of amœbæ;

(*c*) The high reproductive activity; and

(*d*) The specially poisonous nature of the summer-autumn group of parasites.

With respect to the first of these points: after ascertaining that the quantity of parasites in fatal cases is usually much more abundant in the blood of the viscera than in that of the finger, we wrote as follows:—"The contradiction frequently met with in life between the number of parasitic forms and the severity of the disease, and also the degree of anæmia, *disappears in most cases when at the autopsy an examination of all the organs is possible.*" This assertion contains a reservation which requires explanation and justification. There are, in fact, certain cases of malignant malarial infection in which, on examining the blood during life, one is surprised at the relative scarcity of the parasites; their numbers are not proportioned to the gravity of the clinical symptoms. And when, in spite of energetic treatment with quinine, death ensues, even then the microscopic examination of the viscera reveals no such accumulation of amœbæ in the vascular areas of the brain, the spleen, the bone marrow, &c., as is usually met with in the majority of instances. Some fevers of this sort have come under our notice during the past year; and Dr. G. Bastianelli has observed two similar cases at the beginning of the present season. But these instances are rare in comparison with the others in which the quantity of parasites is extremely large; the latter constitute the rule, the former the exception. We have generally noticed them at the beginning of the malarial season, in the month of July, never in the autumn. The victims for the most part are peasants from the country at the time of thrashing the corn, when they are weakened by toil, by the burning sun, and by their miserable food. The nervous symptoms are those which predominate, such as coma, convulsions, &c. The anatomical examination shows the signs of a malarial infection at work, of recent date; in fact, not only are the parasites relatively few, but the melanosis of the viscera is also slight—a circumstance which makes it very improbable that the final paroxysms were preceded by any other serious ones.

Cases of this sort easily rouse the astonishment of anyone who is observing an endemic of severe malaria for the first time. He sees that invasions of parasites in relatively small numbers are followed by severe, and sometimes by exceedingly grave paroxysms of fever; and as he finds this phenomenon difficult to understand, his attention is more arrested by it than when he observes severe paroxysms to be consequent on the presence of large quantities of amœbæ—a matter easily enough explained. Hence it comes about that the rule is forgotten in the exception, and on the exception it is attempted to construct theories.

If we desire to look for the explanation of these phenomena, we should remember first of all that analogies capable of verification occur in all the infections. In the experimental infections, where we can approximately measure the quantity of the material inoculated, it is admitted, and, indeed, well known, that if the amount of the material of a culture of bacteria, which is injected into the animal be varied within certain limits, then, *cæteris paribus*, different effects will be produced with regard to the [illegible] the [illegible], and the issue of the infection thus artificially developed. Nevertheless it is common knowledge that exceptions to this rule are not infrequent, and these may be explained by the fact that different subjects show different degrees of sensitiveness to the same dose of infective material. And it would certainly be remarkable if malaria were to give [illegible] analogous phenomena. Indeed, if we look at the matter closely it will be seen that the question is not so much one of finding the cause of occurrences like these, as of [illegible] the reasons why they happen only exceptionally. This consideration leads us to regard it as probable that the [illegible] of the degree of the parasite's virulence have [illegible] importance as one might *a priori* suppose; because, if [illegible] cases to which we have drawn attention would [illegible]. The severe symptoms observed in these [illegible] relative paucity of the parasites, might [illegible] quantity of poisonous products which they [illegible] greater virulence of the products them[illegible] hypothesis: but we cannot conceal [illegible] arbitrary to ascribe, as some have [illegible] substances whatever in the sympto[illegible] has hitherto escaped a better [illegible] On the other hand, when we take [illegible] it does not seem improbable that [illegible] addition to the infection, go to make [illegible] the severe symptoms: these are the [illegible] &c.

[illegible] discover the reason why these cases [illegible] number of parasites is relatively [illegible] by preference (as we have before [illegible] the malarial season. We have [illegible] when work in the country [illegible] But speaking generally, we must mention that, with regard to the way in which the disease behaves, certain remarkable differences exist between persons who are subjects of the fever for the first time, and those who are suffering from recurrences. Many writers have called attention to these differences; but there is one difference, less known than the others, which is at present being studied by us, and which has to do with the relation between the intensity of the symptoms of the fever and the amount of the parasites. It is, indeed, known that when in two cases, one of primitive infection and the other of the recurring fever, the quantity of the amœbæ is apparently equal (we say *apparently* because in the living subject, from a single examination of the blood of the finger, it is very difficult to form an exact idea as to the extent of the parasitic invasion), then the symptoms in the former are severer than in the latter case; in the former the fever is more intense, and sometimes continued, the nervous symptoms are more pronounced and frequent, and there is a greater fall in the proportion of the hæmoglobin, and in the number of the red blood-corpuscles, than in the latter, where the patient is already depressed and anæmic in consequence of the preceding infection. This general fact, which probably finds its explanation in certain phenomena of adaptation and compensation, may also supply materials for the interpretation of the infections of which we have here been speaking, and which are characterised by severe symptoms combined with a relatively small number of parasites.

The second point connected with the factors of malignancy, to which we drew attention, relates to "*the frequent presence of two, and sometimes of more than two generations of amœbæ.*" We ought, however, to say that there are certain malignant infections which show the presence only of a single generation of parasites, both during life when the blood is examined, when the cases terminate fatally, and at the autopsy. As we have only made a passing allusion to this phenomenon in the text, it seems desirable to confirm it here; indeed, since our treatise was published, in the course of studying additional cases of malignancy, we have found ourselves able to establish the fact, apparently in a greater number of instances than before.

There is one fact among others which specially deserves notice and discussion, while we are investigating the fevers belonging to this group; we refer to the tendency of the adult parasites and of the forms of fission to accumulate in the vascular system of certain organs, in such a way that when, during life, the blood taken from the pulpy point of the finger is studied, one is very rarely successful in tracing the whole of the parasite's life-cycle up to the point of fission: *as a matter of fact, the fission of the amœbæ is effected for the most part in the capillary system of certain of the viscera.* On the other hand, in the mild tertian and quartan it is well known that this is not the case—a circumstance which renders the study of the parasites of these fevers much easier. We have mentioned in the text the principal facts concerning the distribution of the parasitic forms in the different viscera, making use of Bignami's work for this purpose; but we did not stop to discuss the possible causes of such distribution.

According to Bignami,[1] the chief reason lies in the grave changes induced by the parasites in the red blood-corpuscle—changes which have the effect of gradually destroying the blood-corpuscle's capacity for free circulation; so that it finally behaves as a foreign body does, and, like the latter, accumulates either in the capillary system of the purifying organs (*e.g.* the spleen, &c.), where the circulation is relatively slow, or else in the very fine capillaries of other organs (*e. g.* the brain), where the resistance is great. In consequence of this accumulation of amœbiferous red blood-corpuscles, which contain chiefly adult parasites and forms of fission, alterations occur in the endothelium of the capillary vessels (*e. g.* pigmentation, swelling, fatty degeneration, and detachment): these changes, which are especially frequent and noticeable in the brain, become in their turn the cause of a fresh accumulation of amœbæ, principally in the adult phase and in forms of fission. This interpretation, if accepted, explains how it is that the internal organs tend to become loaded with the last-named rather than with the young forms; for, generally speaking, the younger amœbæ are contained in red blood-corpuscles which have undergone less alteration than those in which the advanced phases abound. Furthermore it may be supposed that the parasite's development is fostered by the slowness of the circulation, which is physiological in some organs (*e. g.* the spleen), and pathological in others (*e. g.* the brain), owing to the lesions in the vascular endothelium. Whence it follows that the parasitic forms which reach sporulation are, for the most part, those which are found in certain well-defined vascular areas. To this may be added the probability that the fission and separation of the spores in this variety of parasite require but a very short time for their completion; and the spores being quickly set free from the red blood-corpuscle, which con-

[1] "Ricerche sull' Anatomia Patologica delle Perniciose," 'Atti Accademia Medica di Roma,' see 5th series, ii, p. 32, *et seq.*

stitutes their envelope, are at once lost in the blood-plasma, where they can no longer be recognised with any certainty.

It cannot be denied that the red blood-corpuscles are more rapidly affected by the parasites of this species than by those of the mild tertian and quartan, and that as they lose their capacity for circulating, they tend to behave like foreign bodies introduced into the blood; hence a certain value undoubtedly attaches to the considerations above set forth. Nevertheless the difficulty remains of understanding how it is that at the beginning of the paroxysm the forms of fission are to be found accumulated in the capillaries of certain organs (*e. g.* the spleen and the brain, and also in *great quantities*, as has been recently observed, in the small vessels of the pia mater), but are yet not to be seen in the capillaries of the skin, although in the latter parasites are present (frequently, too, in large numbers), enclosed in red blood-corpuscles already profoundly changed. The most typical instance of this phenomenon is furnished by the summer tertian. The difficulties here described incline us to look for a possible explanation in processes more intimate and complex than the mechanical factors we have alluded to. We know that there is a certain order of frequency in which the malarial parasites are found enclosed in the white blood-corpuscles. Of these intraglobular amœbæ the most common are the free adult forms; then come the forms of fission, and lastly those which have produced premature changes in the red blood-corpuscles. We also know that these phenomena of phagocytosis occur to some extent in all the vascular areas of the body, but especially in certain of the viscera, *e. g.* the spleen, liver, and bone marrow,—organs which abound in elements adapted for this function. In view of recent researches on the *chimiotaxis* of the leucocytes, we must suppose that the fact of the inclusion of certain parasitic forms, while certain others are excluded, is due to *chimiotaxic* action, and further, that this *chimiotaxic* action is exerted in an *elective* way. This theory of *elective chimiotaxis* is, moreover, strengthened by the knowledge of the two following facts:—(*a*) The endothelium of *all* the organs does not act as a phagocyte, but rather those belonging to particular viscera,—for instance, the liver and the brain (at least, in the malignant infections). (*b*) Neither does *all* the endothelium of these organs perform this function; just as not *all* the varieties of the white blood-corpuscles, but only some of them,—that is to say, the ordinary polynucleated and the large mononucleated leucocytes (spleno-medullary elements); the quantity of these in the blood of malarial patients is in excess of the normal,[1] and they multiply rapidly in the spleen and bone marrow. Now it has been demonstrated by observation that the adult amœbæ and forms of fission in this group of fevers tend to accumulate exactly in those vascular areas in which the phenomena of phagocytosis take place. Hence it appears probable that the same elective chimiotaxic action which determines the retention and enclosure of many of these forms is also the cause of delay in the case of those others which, after escaping from confinement, succeed in developing later on. This hypothesis explains satisfactorily the distribution, which is elective up to a certain point, of the parasitic forms in the capillaries of the different viscera, and may perhaps explain as well why the quartan sporulations always occur also in the capillaries of the skin. In the quartan and mild tertian the chimiotaxic action between leucocytes (probably also endothelial cells) and parasites is probably less vigorous than in the summer-autumn fevers; moreover the phenomena of phagocytosis do not, as a matter of fact, take place in the two groups of fever exactly in accordance with the same law. The phagocytosis in the quartan and mild tertian is not seen till after the sporulation is completed, or while it is in process of completion; in the summer-autumn infections it is visible even while the parasites are still in the phases preceding maturity.

Such considerations of course do not diminish the importance of the mechanical factors above mentioned. These must especially be taken into account in dealing with the worst forms of malignancy, when the blood is invaded by enormous quantities of parasites.

As we have already stated, this group of summer-autumn fevers is marked not only by the amœbæ which complete their life-cycle in all its details as described; there are the crescent-shaped forms as well. This class of bodies comprises both those that have, properly speaking, the semilunar form, and the other shapes which approximate to, or are derived from it, including the flagellated forms,—in a word, all which do not belong, at any rate apparently, to the amœba's life-cycle, and which differ so far from the latter that, according to some (Grassi and Feletti), they constitute an entirely separate parasitic species (Laverania). The biology and the significance of these forms are not well understood; what is known about them, especially in connection with the clinical course of the malarial infection, has been

[1] See G. Bastianelli, "I Leucociti nella Infezione Malarica," 'Bollettino della R. Accademia Medica di Roma,' 1892.

described partly in the text, and partly in the first Appendix, in which we have also brought forward the different theories suggested with reference to their significance. It is, however, worth mentioning that there are cases of summer-autumn malarial fever in which these forms do not occur, provided the infection be promptly checked by a resort to the specific remedy; neither in certain cases are they found at any rate during the first recurrence, nor when death speedily ensues. In some of these cases no crescent-shaped forms are visible even when the different organs are examined, while the amœboid parasites are present in immense numbers. On the other hand, there are certain instances of fatal malignant infection, in which, although during life but few crescent-shaped forms show themselves in the blood, the autopsy reveals an extremely large number of them. But they are not uniformly distributed in the vessels of each of the viscera; *a very large preponderance* is found in the bone marrow, where they may be seen in all stages; the spleen contains them in smaller numbers; while in the other organs they are very scanty, or else wanting altogether, as in the brain and the meninges, the capillaries of which are filled with red blood-corpuscles enclosing small amœbæ. This prevalence of the crescent-shaped forms in the bone marrow, which Bastianelli and we have already verified, inclines us to suppose that this organ forms, if not the only, at least the most suitable site for the growth of these bodies. From this point it would seem that they make their way into the stream of the circulation (where they are sometimes met with in great quantities), in the same way as the nucleated red blood-corpuscles in certain states of the organism pass into the circulatory system from the part where they are usually generated,—that is to say, the same bone marrow.

APPENDIX III.

A CRITICAL REVIEW OF PROF. C. GOLGI'S RECENT PUBLICATION ON SUMMER-AUTUMN FEVERS.

The greater part of this translation had already been in the press when Golgi's publication,[1] treating of the biology of the parasites of summer-autumn fevers, in which he arrives at conclusions partly at variance with ours, came under our notice.

Although the review of this publication compels us frequently to reiterate facts already alluded to, in order to better convey to the reader our most careful examination of Golgi's conclusions, of the methods by which these have been arrived at, of the tendencies which they lead to, and above all, that we are in no way compelled to change the facts or views treated of in this work, we deem it best to deal briefly with these. At this very point we hasten to state that Golgi's publication presents no new facts satisfactorily established; nor are there, according to our judgment, any original views that will bear criticism.

Golgi had already treated of the same subject in two former notes, arriving at conclusions which we at the time combated.

In the first[2] of these, Golgi tried to establish the relation between the so-called semilunar bodies of Laveran and that type of malarial fever characterised by recurrences which take place at intervals of five, six, eight, ten, twelve, even fourteen or fifteen days. The cycle of development of these semilunar bodies which cause these

[1] 'Summer-autumn Malarial Roman Fevers.' Communication of C. Golgi to G. Bacelli. Pavia, 1893.

[2] 'Gazzetta degli Ospedali,' No. 65, 1889.

fevers does not take place in a constant or well-determined period of time, but varies in different individuals, and even at various periods in the same case, according to circumstances as yet not well defined; this should afford the explanation of accesses of fever at long and irregular intervals.

Golgi, treating of the same subject in his second article,[1] gives an explanation and description of the cycle of development of the semilunar bodies, which had merely been alluded to in his previous publication. He adds that the presence of Laveran's semilunar bodies in the blood not only produces intermittent fevers at long intervals, but also "many fevers with accesses at short intervals, some of the quotidian type, and even those with subcontinued and subintrant quotidian characteristics." He further states "that, within the sphere of his own observations, these forms occurred in very limited proportions."

The most salient points of Golgi's description are as follows. Corresponding to each attack of fever of this variety, the blood is found invaded by young unpigmented bodies, endowed with amœboid movements, and in part immobile, arranged in annular shape. These bodies, instead of developing progressively, as is the rule in the endoglobular forms of the tertian and quartan variety, within twelve, twenty-four, and thirty-six hours, and after exhibiting few and very minute grains of melanin, disappear, probably after having undergone granular degeneration. *The author, however, does not exclude the possibility that these young parasites may exceptionally develop into forms similar to those of the tertian and quartan.*

Besides these bodies, Golgi, during the period of fever, further observed a few of the flagellated type, which seemed to disappear within a few hours. The examination of the red blood-corpuscles during the apyretic period gave only negative results. Instead of endoglobular forms, he observed a greater or smaller number of free semilunar bodies, which presented "in slow and regular gradation the change of the round into oval and then into spindle shape, with and without the curve, and finally into the characteristic semilunar, the curve gradually becoming more pronounced." The semilunar bodies, after having reached their full development, present internal structural changes which lead to the formation and throwing off of young corpuscles; the latter attack other red blood-corpuscles, and thus are the factors of renewed periods of fever. Accordingly, the facts dwelt upon in this publication are as follows:—1st, that the semilunar bodies

[1] 'Arch. per le Scienze Mediche,' 1890, No. 3.

multiply by "a process of internal structural changes;" 2nd, that the young amœbæ found in the red blood-corpuscles during the febrile attacks do not ultimately develop, but, probably owing to granular degeneration, disappear.

We have already given our reasons in the first Appendix for discountenancing the custom of treating of long-interval fevers as a separate class.

Again, in this and in preceding publications we have described the development of the young amœbæ, circulating in the blood, into bodies with a central accumulation of pigment and the segmentation of the latter. Furthermore we have expressed our serious doubts regarding the development of the semilunar bodies; although we have had abundant and suitable material at our disposal, we have never been able to trace them up to the stage of multiplication. These discrepancies in opinion, however, may in part be ascribed to the facility in variously judging the significance of certain forms of the parasites, above all of the forms of segmentation. This may occur especially if one unhesitatingly considers all bodies in the shape of small corpuscles that are divided or segmented, studied in fresh specimens, as types of segmentation. In our more recent researches we have established it as a rule, never to accept any forms of parasitic segmentation as types of multiplication unless thay have been studied in coloured preparations, and present the structure of spores.[1] It seems almost superfluous to add that Golgi's hypothesis of the possible development of the young amœbæ of summer-autumn fevers into those of the tertian and quartan type is not only not borne out by facts, but the latter, in reality, oppose it. Again, it is an error to look upon the semilunar bodies as generally free; Marchiafava and Celli, a long time ago, demonstrated their endoglobular origin, and showed that they retain this state during the greater part of their existence. In face of these and the other divergences stated, Golgi has felt the necessity in the publication, of which we will now treat, of re-arguing the questions. His monograph is divided into two parts, one of which is critical; the other treats of original observations.

In the first we shall merely touch upon the principal points. Golgi commences with a criticism of our division of malarial fevers into two great groups. While he accepts the term of "summer-autumn" for one of them, he does not approve of the

[1] Golgi, in his work, treats of various forms of segmentation different from those described by us. His descriptions, however, are by no means convincing, nor does it appear that they have been thoroughly studied.

nomination of "spring" or "winter-spring" fevers for the other group. We have already treated of the arguments he adduces, a part in the first chapter, and again in the first Appendix of this work; accordingly, we deem it superfluous to repeat. We now immediately approach one of the most important facts in the biology of the parasites of summer-autumn fevers, namely, a feature studied and insisted upon by us in all our reports as one of the most important characteristics of this group of fevers, that *the segmenting forms are almost never found in the circulating blood.* Were we to refer to our reasons for attempting to explain this fact, we should be compelled to repeat what has already been treated of in other parts of this work. Some of our considerations referring to the questions in argument are dwelt upon in the second Appendix. We merely wish to recall that we regard the presence in the blood of endoglobular amœbæ, presenting finely granular pigment, which gradually disappear from the circulating fluid as the new febrile attack approaches, as the sign of impending multiplication; these accumulate in the internal organs, where the process of reproduction by means of division takes place. Now Golgi does not hesitate to affirm that this fact—*i. e.* the accumulation of the parasitic forms in the internal organs, and their consequent multiplication in connection with the febrile paroxysm—if not entirely, in the main, still awaits confirmation, and that our observation is merely an induction based on collateral knowledge. As he expresses himself (l. c., p. 19 of the reprint), "I must note that it is neither the act of sporulation, nor of segmentation in progress, that is here considered as a symptom of the approaching attack of fever, but another sign that is interpreted as an indication of approaching sporulation. Now as the latter has as yet not been directly verified, being more of a supposition based on collateral knowledge, one may assert, and not without grounds, that the sporulation of the summer-autumn amœbæ *circulating in the blood* is more an hypothesis than a recognised fact."

Certainly several passages in our treatise must have escaped Golgi's attention. Thus on page 41 we note, "Although in the blood taken from the finger we but very seldom found structures in fission, still the presence of adult forms (plasmodia containing granules of pigment and forms enclosing masses of pigment) may lead one to infer with certainty that multiplication is about to take place in the internal organs. This is, in fact, demonstrated *by examination of the blood extracted from the spleen* during life, and by examination of the parasitic contents of the various organs in cases of fatal pernicious fever." The monograph of Bignami and Bastianelli[1] published several years ago, describing the methodical study of these fevers by means of frequent puncture of the spleen, seems also to have escaped Golgi's attention.

These observers, treating of this subject, state, "On studying these patients in the initial paroxysms of the fever, and in carefully observing the development of the parasites, *above all, availing oneself of frequent punctures of the spleen,* only the various forms of the amœba of Marchiafava and Celli in various phases of its development, from the unpigmented amœboid protoplasmic body to that containing pigment, or in a state of segmentation, will be found to be in relation with the paroxysms. In the greatest number of cases, in order to determine in the patient the forms of multiplication of the parasite, it is necessary to resort to puncture of the spleen. The blood extracted from the finger in the primary paroxysms generally only demonstrates unpigmented plasmodia or those containing only very minute granules of pigment. Marchiafava and Celli, in their preliminary publication, had already called attention to this fact; and evidently not bearing this in mind, it would be easy to think, as Golgi has affirmed, that the plasmodia of this group of fevers do not, as a rule, mature." It is also stated in previous portions of this publication that one may follow the development of the parasite, making use of puncture of the spleen, in *all the fevers of this group*.

Therefore, that multiplication of the parasites does take place in correspondence with the febrile paroxysm is not *an hypothesis*, but a *fact, confirmed* by numerous observations and studies, carried out with the same methods of investigation that Golgi has deemed fit to adopt in his own researches. Accordingly, it will appear as natural if we, in our latest researches into other points, have no longer practised repeated punctures of the spleen—an operation, although devoid of all danger in malarial patients, always unpleasant. Insisting upon its being a hard fact, confirmed by numerous experiments, we may pass over other observations made by Golgi in treating of this question, these no longer pertaining to the fact itself, but rather to his interpretation thereof. As it is, it would not be difficult for us to demonstrate also that these latter are not well founded.

We first of all felt the difficulty of satisfactorily explaining the reason why in this group of fevers, whilst the younger

[1] "Observations on Summer-autumn Malarial Fevers," 'Rif. Med.,' Ottobre, 1890.

; the more developed ones and
mulated in some of the internal
. The discussion of this question
fully prove it. Golgi, however,
fission of the tertian and quartan
even after the red blood-corpuscles
destroyed, it should be more easy
of the parasites of summer fevers,
lar and occupy only a part of the red
answer to this, first of all we wish to
usual not to observe products of fission
ven in classical tertian, whilst they are
internal organs. In fact, this tendency
rasites in the internal viscera is not only
vers, but, as Antolisei,[1] Bastianelli, and
also takes place in the classical tertian.
w, the difference between these two groups
most noticeable, is but one of degree.
bear in mind the peculiar alteration which
ce in the red corpuscles, an alteration which
nvolves the properties of the corpuscle, it
ting in the circulation as a foreign body.
taking into account other considerations treated
econd Appendix, we may assume that the adult
forms of the parasites are retained in the spleen
us through chimiotaxic action, this taking place
constituent elements and the hæmatozoa. Finally,
that a method of criticism by denying or doubting
shed fact, merely because it is, and ever must be,
satisfactory explanation, is hardly a fair one.

ng the mechanical reasons adduced by us to explain
ulation of the segmenting form in the organs, Golgi
But if the process of sporulation is always endoglo-
d if, as is a well-known characteristic, the size of the
of summer-autumn fevers is smaller than that of the
tertian; if, moreover, the size of the blood-corpuscles
by the small parasites at a period corresponding to the
attack be always smaller than the normal ones, we do
ee how the mechanical hypothesis can have a plausible
tion."

ording to Golgi, the diminished size of the red corpuscles

n the Hæmatozoa of Tertian Fevers," 'Riforma Med.,' Gennaio, 1890.
alarial Infection of Spring Fevers," 'Riforma Medica,' June, 1890.

must favour their normal circulation. However, the great and special alterations which they, due to the endoglobular parasite, have undergone, does not seem to have been considered. Now arises the question whether the circulating quality of the red corpuscles depends alone on their size, or not rather and mainly on their inherent elasticity, the state of their superficies, &c. That these qualities of the corpuscles do undergo profound alterations in summer fevers may be proved by direct observation. On examining microscopically fresh blood in which there are many corpuscles containing parasites, especially of the adult type, and making pressure on the covering glass, thus producing a change of position, the normal red corpuscles will usually be observed to rapidly move in all directions, rolling and gliding over each other, whilst those altered by the presence of the parasites barely move or change their places. This alteration in elasticity is not noticeable, adopting the same mode of procedure, in the red corpuscles invaded by the parasites of the classical tertian.

But, whatever be the reasons that the parasites prefer the internal organs to complete their cycle of development, we have certainly demonstrated this fact by repeated punctures of the spleen during life. It is in this sense that we must deny Golgi's charge, that the well-known state of segmentation of parasites found in the organs in fatal cases of pernicious fever "constitutes the principal basis of the doctrine that attributes the so-called summer-autumn fevers to the cycle of development within twenty-four to forty-eight hours of the small summer-autumn amœbæ" (l. c., p. 21). This assertion is entirely arbitrary on Golgi's part.

The conditions found in the above-mentioned autopsies contribute to our general knowledge of parasitic accumulations in internal organs, and permit us to have a clearer conception of the laws governing the distribution of parasites in the vascular areas of the viscera. There are cases in which, on microscopic examination, one may find within the narrow confines of one cerebral capillary, side by side, types of the various phases of development of the parasite, from the unpigmented amœba up to the period of segmentation. But what relation have these facts with the theory of the cycle of development in one or two days? This last is based upon an entirely different series of observations, made during life. Accordingly, Golgi's strictures can have but little weight, in face of the fact that he has not kept an important part of our researches in view.

Another point of divergency is the duration of the cycle of development of the amœbæ of this group. Golgi does not commit himself on this point, but he does not admit of its being as rapid as we describe. One argument which he adduces against our view of the rapid cycle of development is the great resistance which these fevers not unusually offer to the action of quinine. Even admitting that this intractability is as general an occurrence as Golgi is inclined to believe, we think that many physicians would not agree with him regarding its frequency. In any case, it is interesting to follow Golgi's train of reasoning in treating of this point. "It is well known that the action of the drug in cases of quartan and classical tertian fevers is, as a rule, energetic and prompt. Furthermore we know that in these fevers the young forms are most susceptible to the influence of the drug. Now, if the development of the amœbæ of these summer fevers does take place within twenty-four to forty-eight hours, we should have the certainty that quinine, administered at whatever period, due to its persistent action on the organism, should always act upon the young forms in their earliest stage and destroy them." Because this does not take place, Golgi's doubts regarding the cycle of development of these parasites as described are strengthened.

This mode of reasoning has the grave defect, that facts which are entirely different are treated of as similar or identical. It is implicitly taken for granted that the younger amœbæ of the tertian and of the quartan varieties share the same qualities as regards the action of quinine as do those of the summer group. However, this remains to be demonstrated, and, indeed, facts would indicate a contrary state of things.

The differences in the biology of these two groups of the parasites of malaria being so great, why not seek in these factors an explanation of their differing resistance to the action of quinine?

It is by no means arbitrary to assume a special hypothetical anatomical condition, by which the parasites are protected against the action of the drug, rather than an inherent degree of resistance of the parasites to it. Elsewhere we have laid stress upon the necessity of studying the action of quinine on each variety of the parasites, and accordingly cannot think it proper to apply to one variety, peculiarities belonging to another, without thorough corroboration of the facts.

We shall not treat of other points of controversy, of minor importance, such as the significance of the "brassy red corpuscles," the more so as Golgi agrees with us, "that of the various hæmatological appearances that point to an approaching development of fever, the one in question (the presence in the blood of red blood-corpuscles containing parasites) is indisputably of notable importance" (l. c., p. 14).

As we have amply illustrated our observations by examples and thermometric tracings annexed to our publication, we similarly prefer not entering into argument upon points referring to the clinical course and the variety of these fevers. Furthermore, we shall not dwell upon some inexact criticisms which Golgi's work offers; as example, on p. 14, in treating of the greater virulence of the parasites of summer-autumn fever, he states that this co-efficient "has, up to the present, never been taken into consideration in malaria," whilst we in our publication have paid special attention to it in the chapter "On Pernicious Fevers." Were we to combat, point by point, the criticisms levelled against us even in the most trifling details, we should of necessity be compelled to repeat continuously facts already treated of in this work. To avoid this, we shall pass on to the second part of Golgi's work, that based on original researches. The principal and fundamental propositions that result from Golgi's observations are essentially two in number; we shall present them as nearly as possible in the author's language, namely—

1st. In contradistinction to what occurs in the classical intermittent fevers—of the tertian and quartan types—in summer-autumn fevers the pathological state of the circulating blood (essentially due to the presence of the small summer-autumn parasite) does not represent *a necessary, however almost constant*, "index" of this special group of malarial fevers.

2nd. "The entire process (*i. e.* the cycle of development of the parasite) *does not take place in the circulating blood, but in the internal organs.*"

According to Golgi, all the changes found in the circulating blood represent "merely an accidental, not necessary, index of this special group of malarial fevers" (l. c., p. 33). Let us now look into the facts upon which he bases this proposition, and the consequences to which it leads. It is essentially based upon the circumstance that the examination of the blood in certain cases, notwithstanding the existence of malarial infection, may give negative results. We need not remind the reader that these negative results are entirely exceptional; we cannot recall a single case of malarial infection in which repeated and properly conducted examination of the blood did not reveal the presence of parasites.

Mannaberg, in 130 cases, records only three in which examination gave negative results. Besides, we have called attention to the variations in the number of the parasites during the varying phases of the course of the infection, indicating the periods most opportune for diagnostic examination (see chapter on "Summer Tertian").

Examination in cases of classical tertian, at times, also may result negatively, and even when yielding positive information, in certain cases, will not demonstrate the various phases of parasitic development up to fission. Based upon this, Golgi assuredly would not assert that also in cases of common tertian the alterations found in the circulating blood are purely accidental.

However, in treating of summer-autumn fevers, this mode of reasoning seems to him valid. For example, Golgi, "under the influence of observations made on the common type of intermittent fevers" (l. c., p. 34), at first accepted the possibility of negative results in examining the blood during the initial period of malarial fevers with a certain amount of diffidence. On the contrary, in the summer-autumn fevers he immediately accepts it, and considers it of great importance.

The fact, however, that this was *observed for the first time in two cases of common tertian by* Gualdi and Antolisei *in our Medical Clinic* seems to have escaped Golgi's notice.

The truth is that Golgi's assertion seems manifestly based on a preconceived doctrinal idea. Taking it for granted, as is stated in the second proposition, that the parasites of summer-autumn fevers only develop in the internal organs, one can easily understand "that, in any case, the presence or the absence, or the number of the young amœbæ in smaller or greater quantity in the circulating blood, will always constitute an accidental factor." However, all of our researches, the fact especially of the successive development of the parasitic elements in the blood, up to a given phase in their cycle of life, when they slowly disappear, and again, the regular repetition of this state of affairs, corresponding with each paroxysm of fever, in the ordinary cases, are in opposition to this statement.

Further, we cannot accept as a fact another consequence, derived from the following proposition of Golgi's, namely, that an examination of the circulating blood "may yield a diagnostic conception of the existence, but not of the degree of gravity of the malarial infection." This statement is not exact; pernicious fevers, in fact, in *the majority of cases*, present a characteristic parasitic condition of the blood, which permits of the diagnosis and prognosis of the gravity of the infection. In order to arrive at such a conclusion, however, it is necessary not only to estimate the result of one examination, but at times of several, in order not only to ascertain the number of the parasitic forms, but also of their state of development, and of other facts, to which we have already called attention in treating of the parasitic finds in severe fevers, and of the prognostic value of other signs. In the second Appendix we have spoken of, and dwelt upon, the considerations suggested by the exceptional cases of pernicious fever in which there are but few traces of parasites in the blood and in the internal organs. At this point we beg to state that, as in the cases to which we refer, not only the blood, but also the internal organs contain only small numbers of parasites; the fact in itself is no more opposed to our view than it can sustain Golgi's interpretation.

However, if the altered state of the circulating blood be accidental, what becomes of the small amœbæ that appear during every paroxysm of fever? In his earlier publication, already cited at the beginning of this chapter, Golgi states as a fact that the small amœbæ do not develop to maturity, but disappear, *probably in consequence of granular degeneration.* He does not exclude the possibility that in exceptional cases they may develop *into tertian and quartan forms* (!). In the publication at present in question we, however, find contradictory views. On page 32 we note the following :—"The small amœbæ in the circulation bear no relation to the pathogenesis of the febrile process; they are merely the first phases in the process of development." However, on page 34 he expresses a certain doubt in stating, "I do not wish to enter into the question whether a part of these young amœbæ, at a certain stage of their development, may not become arrested in the internal organs, and here continue their evolution up to complete maturity, or whether these circulating amœbæ are destined to perish." Again, on page 36 the author expresses a similar reserve.

Now we have always held that part of the circulating amœbæ are arrested in their process of development, and perish together with the red corpuscles which envelop them; we allude particularly to those found in the red blood-corpuscles having undergone so-called "brassy degeneration." But we have no reason to doubt that a great part of them do continue up to full development after becoming arrested in the internal organs. A conclusive confirmation of these facts has recently been obtained by Bignami and Bastianelli in a series of experiments with regard to inoculation. They have demonstrated that the inoculation of the blood of a subject suffering from malaria, even in the smallest quantity (*e. g.* two drops), into the circulation of a healthy individual will, after a varied period of incubation, produce fever; furthermore, that the blood of the individual inoculated, *from the very first attack of fever*, demonstrates the presence of new generations of young amœbæ.

The opinion, accordingly, that everything found in the circulating blood is accidental, is in part due to allowing a mistaken value of some exceptional factors, and in part to holding a preconceived idea. Taking for example that the temperature course in certain cases of typhoid fever is entirely irregular, would it be logical to affirm that in these cases the course of temperature is *accidental?* One can find numerous analogous examples in all infectious diseases.

In contradistinction to Golgi's view we affirm the following:—*That in summer-autumn fevers, whilst a great portion of the development of the parasites, especially segmentation, does take place in the internal organs, there occurs, in a determinate relation with the course of the paroxysm of fever, an invasion of young amœbæ into the circulating blood. The presence of forms of advanced development and in the state of segmentation in the blood is a certain indication of gravity.*

Now to Golgi's second proposition, "The entire process does not take place in the circulating blood, but in the internal organs." If Golgi were only to change the position of the word "entire" in this sentence, and thus were to say, "*the process does not take place entirely in the circulating blood, but in the internal organs,*" it would indicate exactly the position we have occupied in this and other publications in treating of this question.

To sustain his view, Golgi details the results of the expedient of puncturing the spleen in those affected with these fevers. He begins with the affirmation that the blood of the spleen invariably presents a positive condition or state as regards the parasites (l. c., p. 35). We were aware of this, and it is in perfect accordance with our observations and our views. If the young amœbæ are in the general circulation, it is quite natural to find them (and in great quantity) in the spleen. Further, if at a certain phase of their development they are arrested in the internal organs, and here complete their cycle of life, as we have always held that they do, as thus in the internal organs an accumulation of amœbæ at the stage of maturity and segmentation is found, it follows, as one can readily understand, that the examination of the blood of the spleen will always yield positive results.

In treating of the cycle of life of the parasites the author distinguishes three phases.

The first phase "is represented by young unpigmented amœbæ, or by those containing but few granules of pigment, such as are usually described and depicted as the amœbæ circulating in the blood." This phase corresponds to the first and second phases of our description of the summer tertian.

The second phase is "represented by the small amœbæ with a central accumulation of pigment, up to a more or less advanced invasion of the red blood-corpuscle, sometimes with complete destruction of the hæmoglobin, at others with a portion of it remaining" (l. c., p. 37). In treating of this form, Golgi insists upon the variation in size of the structures containing a pigmentary accumulation, which may be small, or instead may assume a *relatively very large size*, he regarding the larger forms as being derived from the smaller ones. We also have observed and depicted this variation in size. Further, we have also noticed most minute forms of sporulation originating from very small amœbæ with a central pigmentary accumulation (see the sporulation of the quotidian), and larger forms with many spores derived from larger parasites containing the central pigment. All the forms of segmentation, however, be they of larger or of smaller type, if recognisable with certainty as such, are developed within the confines of the red blood-corpuscles, the latter possibly presenting a profoundly altered aspect. It is only in consequence of a later change that they are liberated. Golgi does not fix the length of time necessary for the development of the second phase, but believes it must be a long one. He is led to this by the question of size they may arrive at. This reason is hardly a valid one. Do we not observe, perhaps, that the parasites of tertian in the space of two days attain a notably greater size than those of the quartan in three?

"The third phase is represented by parasites in advanced stages, endoglobular or free, *modified in various modes* by the *later development*, and above all by the processes of reproduction.

In the description following, one in vain seeks to find out which are the forms "*changed in various modes by the later development.*" On the contrary, much attention is devoted to the types of multiplication. Regarding these, Golgi makes the following distinctions:

(*a*) "A form of reproduction, which one may call, that by total segmentation, and which takes place with a regularity of phases and of forms, comparing with sufficient exactness with that which one observes in classical intermittent fevers." This type of fission corresponds with that observed and described by us. Golgi, however, adds that he has observed some segmenting forms belonging to this class of an exceptionally large size, containing as many as from forty to fifty spores. We have counted from twenty to thirty spores, or even a few more, in these forms of multiplication. We have never been able to meet with a much greater number, not even in stained preparations, in which it is impossible to mistake other forms for those of fission (as, for example, degenerative, disintegrating forms), and it is easier to count the individual spores. If new researches confirm this statement, it will be the sole new fact in Golgi's work.

(*b*) "A form of reproduction which points to *a process of endogenesis* through an internal differentiation of the protoplasm, and which takes place in such a manner that the periphery of the parasitic form is surrounded by a membrane-like stratum of its substance."

However, terming this form of segmentation "*endogenous*" would lead one to suppose that the other processes of fission were not so. Now all observers agree in affirming that segmentation of the parasite of malaria *always takes place by endogenesis*,—that is, by the formation of a varying number of most minute chromophil bodies, the latter gravitating toward the periphery of the body of the parasite, to become surrounded by a part of the protoplasm. Also, in this relation, the study of specimens stained with hæmatoxylin, demonstrating that there are no fundamental differences in the process by which segmentation of the parasites takes place, has resolved the argument in question. It does not appear that Golgi, in his researches, availed himself of those methods which alone permit of a careful study of the structure.

(*c*) As a third division, Golgi treats in a very doubtful manner of the segmentation of particular forms of greatly varying size, of which he admits "*the still distant possibility of establishing their biology.*" According to Golgi, "the contours of these bodies are irregular, often markedly tuberous or berry-shaped, and are capable of changing their forms. Apparently they reproduce in a different manner."

If we do not err, which is possible, considering the vague description, we incline to the belief that these forms correspond to those which we have alluded to in the text, and which we have looked upon as the bodies containing masses of pigment, and which, being free in the plasma, are in a state of degeneration. This metamorphosis may take place by a process of vacuolisation or of hyaline disintegration. As long as Golgi himself admits *that he is far from being able to establish their biology*, we do not push our view.

As seen by this summary but careful review, any newly ascertained facts which may prove of fundamental importance are entirely wanting in Golgi's memoir. In concluding his own observations he sustains the view *of the continuous development of the parasites in the internal organs*. Further, he inclines to the belief that the forms of segmentation which occasionally are found in the circulating blood have *casually* escaped from the viscera in a similar way to that indicated by the presence of young amœbæ in the circulation, which also must be looked upon as *accidental*. It is almost useless to repeat here that this conclusion is contradicted in the most absolute manner, by the fact *that a very large proportion of the circulating amœbæ is capable of mature development up to segmentation*. We have already shown that it is partly based on an erroneous estimate of exceptional facts, and partly on a preconceived idea.

In referring to this, Golgi, in order the better to elucidate his view, resorts to the arguments of analogy; he compares the condition of the circulating parasites in these fevers to that of the nucleated red blood-corpuscles found in the circulation in cases of pernicious anæmia, of severe common anæmia, and of leukæmia. While, in fact, the nucleated red blood-corpuscles are found in the greatest number in the bone marrow and in the spleen in these pathological conditions, *yet it is only on rare exceptions that these are observed in the circulating blood* (l. c., p. 33).

We do not know to what extent investigators engaged in hæmatology, who are specially interested in these questions, would agree in the estimation of this fact *as a rare exception*. If, for example, in pernicious anæmia the state of the nucleated red blood-corpuscles, specially certain types of them (megaloblasts), are looked upon as characteristic, and constant, and necessary for the clinical diagnosis of certain forms of progressive anæmia, and if the same applies to certain medullary cells in medullary leukæmia, on what authority may one speak of *accident?*

We have felt impelled to dwell so long upon this argument merely from our dread of the harm which may accrue to medical practice if Golgi's error, in deference to the authority of the observer, should be accepted. In fact, if there can be cases of pernicious infection with regular absence of circulating parasites, and if the condition observed in the blood be purely *accidental*, naturally the utility of a clinical examination of the blood will prove of much lessened value, and even with the microscope, certainty in arriving at a decision must be lacking. Under this state of affairs some physicians may abandon this valuable means of diagnosis, which in certain cases, in the absence of clinical criteria, is the only means which permits of the recognition and proper treatment of malarial diseases.

The acceptance of this preconceived view would thus manifestly be harmful in its effects, and we can never oppose it too warmly.

A few more remarks. In treating of the observations already quoted, regarding the forms of segmentation in this group of fevers, Golgi again gives us to understand that our knowledge of these segmentations is almost entirely based upon the results of autopsies in cases of pernicious fever. We have already demonstrated the inexactness of this assertion. Moreover, although Golgi on this point is not clear, he seems to express the view that the condition of the parasitic forms may vary according to the longer or shorter period ensuing before the autopsy is performed (l. c., p. 39). In alluding to this, our observations do not permit of the slightest doubt. We have examined the structure of the spleen immediately after death, and again after many hours and even days, it hardly need be added, as it is self-evident, in the same case, and never have we been able to detect any modification in the state of development of the parasite,—so much so that we are ready to affirm with certainty that *after the death of the patient the development of the parasite becomes arrested.* Moreover recent researches have demonstrated that after death the parasites, as best seen in preparations stained with hæmatoxylin, rapidly undergo structural alterations. The young amœbæ, studied in the blood during lifetime, on being stained appear as a more or less delicate ring, whilst those examined but a few hours after death take up the colouring matter in so diffuse and general a manner as to resemble in certain cases large micrococci. In all probability the parasites are profoundly affected and killed by those intimate changes in the blood and tissues following death. Bignami and Bastianelli will shortly treat of this subject at greater length in a forthcoming publication.

Another point meriting attention is the hypothesis, hazarded with reserve, of the development of the parasites of malaria within the leucocytes and tissue elements, and "of the exceptional protection which these hidden sites may afford them" (l. c., pp. 34 and following). The author also supposes that this hypothetical intercellular position may explain the intractability of many fevers to the action of quinine. Even accepting this hypothesis, it would always remain to be demonstrated that a parasite enclosed in a white blood-corpuscle or in a splenic cell offers a greater resistance to the action of drugs than one in a red blood-corpuscle. The unqualified acceptance of this primary possibility would, to say the least, be rather arbitrary. Besides, even according to Golgi, to attribute to phagocytosis the inclusion of parasites in the white corpuscles may be considered as a proper interpretation in *the majority of cases.* Accepting this, how is it possible to explain, by means of an exceptional fact, the greater resistance to drugs which, according to Golgi, is a most common occurrence?

The hypothesis of a possible development of the parasites within the white corpuscles, or the cells of the tissue of the spleen, is based upon the well-known fact that parasites, having all the appearances of forms capable of development, may be found within the white corpuscles, and upon another feature, also demonstrated by us, of necrotic degeneration of many white corpuscles containing many parasites. We have called attention to this latter fact, constructing upon it an hypothesis to explain the recurrences so common in these fevers. We have supposed that at least a part of these enclosed parasites escaping destruction, and continuing to exist in latent vitality after the necrosis of the white corpuscle, renew their course of development and give rise to new recurrences. If we have, above all, treated of included spores, it is not that we are influenced by the hypothesis that the spores of the parasites of malaria are analogous in their powers of resistance to external agents with those of bacteria, but by facts observed by us. We may mention that we are perfectly aware that the terms "spore" and sporulation, in speaking of malarial parasites, are made use of by Leuckart, Bütschli, and others in a special sense for other similar structures. In preparations stained with hæmatoxylin one may often succeed in observing spores perfectly preserved in structure embedded in the leucocytes, and these more often than other forms of development in the same state.

Regarding Golgi's hypothesis of a possible development of the malarial parasites of this group, not only in the red, but also in the white blood-corpuscles, we may state that this would be a contradiction of the general laws of endocellular parasites, which as a rule are parasites of fixed histological elements in determinate animal species, and not at the same time of other elements.

Another question of importance touched upon by Golgi, but which we can only now allude to, is that of the genesis of black pigment in enlargement of the spleen. However, in order not to dwell on it, we must refer the reader to a recent publication of Bignami's[1] on this subject, noting that in this as well as in other places the author shares our view.

But let us hasten to a conclusion. We have shown that the critical part of Golgi's essay can be easily refuted; and, moreover, that the part devoted to original research contains nothing new that has as yet been firmly established, but it contains merely a repetition of well-known facts, which the reader can find in our various publications. Golgi, in parts of his work, confirms the results of our observations: *e.g.* he admits that pernicious fevers are due to the parasites of this group; he shares our view that the semilunar variety does not form a species or group by themselves, as Grassi and Feletti claim for them, but belong to the same parasitic variety. He recognises the importance of the parasitic state in the internal organs, and confirms the fact that the forms of advanced development and in segmentation are almost exclusively found in the viscera. He agrees with us in the main regarding the known facts of the special morphology of this variety of parasite, and of the characteristic alterations which they produce in the red corpuscles. Furthermore, in treating of phagocytism, of the manner in which it takes place in these fevers—in brief, of facts—he simply confirms our views.

Regarding the "varying special localisation of malarial parasites in different viscera," we have described and commented upon not a few examples in our latest as well as in preceding publications. Alluding to the semilunar variety, and their derivation from the endoglobular amœbæ, Golgi states that "if this can only exceptionally be observed in the blood, it is easily demonstrable by verifying a succession of their phases in the bone marrow and in the spleen in cases of fatal pernicious fever." This is a complete confirmation of what had already been observed by Bignami and Bastianelli. Golgi, however, forgets that these latter had described this succession of phases principally in patients in whom puncture of the spleen had been resorted to. The divergences of opinion are mainly due to varied interpretations of facts. There are still

[1] "Studies on the Pathological Anatomy of Chronic Malarial Infections," 'Bullettino della R. Accad. Med. di Roma,' 1893.

many lacunæ in the biology of this variety of malarial parasite, and to these we have called attention in the course of our investigations. *None of these have been filled in by Golgi's researches.* He does not accept the cycle of parasitic life as we describe it, but he himself offers no alternative one. He says it is irregular, without determining the limits of irregularity. No one who has had any experience in the natural sciences will believe that there are not determinable limits, or that it is impossible to find in this class of facts a regular order. These limits of irregularity are fixed, according to our researches, by the cycles of development which take place in from twenty-four to forty-eight hours, and which correspond to the various types of fever.

In concluding this lengthy discussion, we simply insist upon the correctness of the results of this our last publication as well as of our previous researches.

The parasites of summer-autumn fevers are parasites exclusively involving the red corpuscles. In the red corpuscle they continue their process of development up to the period of segmentation. The young endoglobular amœbæ circulate in the blood. Those more developed and in the phase of segmentation become arrested; *they take up a position* in the vascular areas of the viscera (spleen, bone marrow, brain). Regarding the localisation of the parasite, there is probably a difference in what occurs in cases of median gravity and in more serious (pernicious) cases. There is reason to believe that "in the first cases the parasitic forms specially accumulate in those organs which serve ordinarily as places of deposit for the contaminating matter of the blood (the spleen), and in the second instances other organs may become involved, as the brain, &c."[1] The last will explain the various special localisations in pernicious fevers. The forms circulating in the blood are capable of complete development. Their presence in the circulation can be verified by the laws we have established, and is not at all *accidental.* Segmentation of this group of parasites takes place always by *endogenesis* in various ways, but by a process which is fundamentally the same in all cases.

[1] Bignami, 'Pathological Anatomy of Pernicious Fevers,' p. 34 of the reprint.

POSTSCRIPT.

Our views regarding the malignant tertian have been severely censured by authoritative critics. It has been said that we have created new clinical types solely on the basis of parasitological observations, and that we have done wrong in adopting the term "summer-autumn or malignant tertian," forcing the meaning of the word "tertian" to describe a febrile type altogether different from that to which custom has consecrated this name. We are unable to accept either the first or the second of these criticisms as just. The clinical differences between the two forms of tertian are as great and as manifest as the differences between the parasitical varieties that produce them: we repeat, so remarkable are they that some of the ancient authors had recognised these differences merely from clinical observation, and had made them the basis of a division of tertian fevers. We have already quoted the words of Sydenham; but the clearest and most exact description of the two clinical types of tertian fevers are to be found in the works of Celsus, who after having spoken of the quartan says, "Tertianarum vero duo genera sunt: alterum eodem modo quo quartana et incipiens et desinens; illo tantum interposito discrimine, quod unum diem præstat integrum, tertio redit: *alterum longe perniciosius quod tertio quidem die revertitur, ex octo autem et quadraginta horis fere sex et triginta per accessiones occupat, interdum etiam vel minus vel plus; neque ex toto in remissione desistit, sed tantum lævius est.*" &c.

All will find in these words the clearest allusion to that type of fever termed by us "summer-autumn tertian." That fever is described almost in the very words used by us, but unfortunately at the time of the publication of our work we did not know of this passage in Celsus, in which is clearly acknowledged both the tertian type and the gravity (*genus perniciosius*). With regard to the question of the name, we hope that those according to whose dictum we cannot adopt the name of tertian for this type of fever, because classical writers use the same word with a different meaning, will consider the classical authority of Aulus Cornelius Celsus as sufficient.

Of unknown and forgotten observations, as well as of those which more frequently recur in ancient writings, and which are so exact and keen as to rouse great wonder and satisfaction in those who are acquainted with the recent researches, there are found not a few round the history of malaria. Not only in the ancient, but also in recent authors we find opinions expressed which coincide as if by happy inspiration with the most recent discoveries. For instance, Rasori speaking of the intermittent fevers, during an interview with Agostino Bassi of Lodi, thus expresses himself:— "For many years I have held the opinion that the intermittent fevers are produced by parasites which renew the paroxysm by the act of their reproduction, which recurs more or less rapidly, according to the variety of the species."[1] It is interesting to note that the same idea of the probable relation of the febrile paroxysm to the multiplication of the parasites has also been expressed by Tommasi-Crudeli. He, indeed, thought that the febrile paroxysm might coincide with the multiplication of the bacilli, which he believed to be the cause of malaria; he held that the parasites had their seat in the spleen, and that in the act of the production of the young generation, which leaving the spleen enter the blood, the febrile attack might arise.

Rasori alluded also to the multiplicity of the species of the malarial parasite, supposing that the intermittence more or less depended upon the varying duration of the cycle of development.

[1] 'Discorsi sulla Natura e Cura della Pellagra, &c.,' Milano, tip. Chiusi, 1846. Citato da S. Calandruccio, 'Agostino Bassi di Lodi il fondatore della teoria parassitaria e delle cure parassiticide,' p. 70, Catania, 1892.

PLATE I.

Figs. 1—14. The amœba of the quartan fever. (Figs. 1—9. Progressive endoglobular development of the quartan amœba. Figs. 10, 11. Endoglobular forms of fission. Fig. 12. Free spores. Figs. 13, 14. Free pigmented forms in a degenerative condition.)

Figs. 15—33. The amœba of the tertian fever. (Figs. 15—24. Progressive endoglobular development of the tertian amœba. Figs. 25—27. Endoglobular forms of fission. Figs. 28—30. Free sporulating forms. Figs. 31—33. Free pigmented forms in a degenerative condition.)

Figs. 34—55. The amœba of the quotidian fever. (Figs. 34—50. Endoglobular development of the quotidian amœba. Figs. 42—48 and 49. Amœba in brass-coloured, shrivelled red blood-corpuscles. Figs. 51—55. Endoglobular forms of segmentation.)

N.B.—All the figures of this plate, as well as those of the following, are taken from fresh moist preparations. Only the Figs. 50 and 55 are drawn from a preparation of bone marrow in a case of malignant quotidian. The marrow was dried according to Ehrlich's method on a glass cover, and coloured with methylene blue.

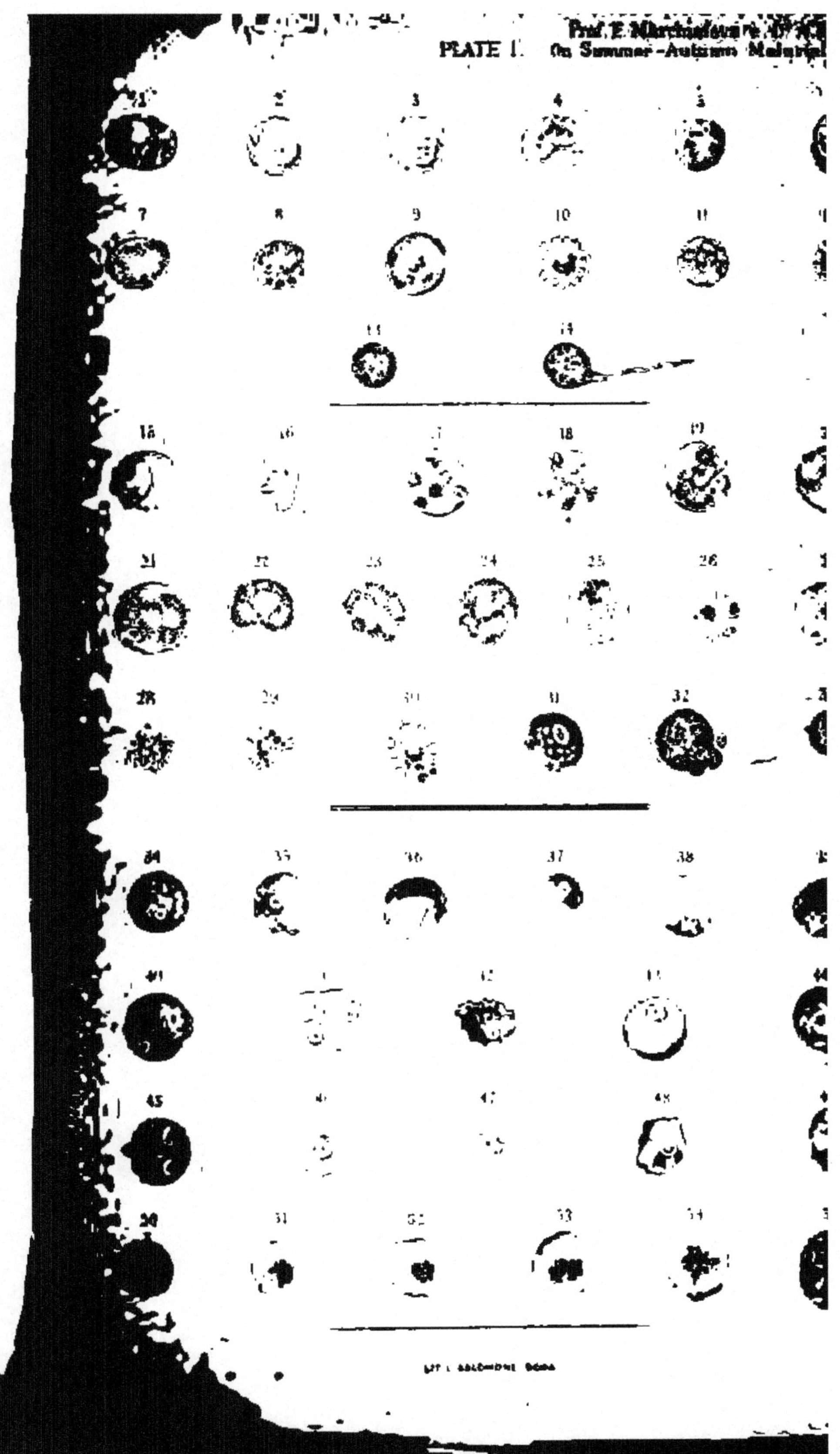
Prof. E. Marchiafava ...
PLATE I. On Summer-Autumn Malaria...

PLATE II.

Figs. 1—45. The amœba of the summer-autumn tertian fever. (Figs. 1—9. Young non-pigmented amœbæ. Figs. 10—32. Amœbæ in course of development with pigment at the circumference. Figs. 33—42. Amœbæ ripe for multiplication, with the pigment collected at the centre. Figs. 43—45. Forms of spore production. In Figs. 8, 9, and 30—42 are represented the various changes in colouring and form of the invaded red blood-corpuscle.)

Figs. 46—67. Various forms belonging to the group of crescent-shaped bodies. (Figs. 46—56. Endoglobular forms, spindle-shaped, ovoid, and round. Figs. 57—60. The same forms in a free state. Figs. 61, 62. Crescent-shaped bodies properly so called. Fig. 66. A free crescent-shaped form in process of forming vacuoles. Fig. 67. A form with flagella.)

Figs. 68, 69. Accumulations of free spores around masses of pigment in the cerebral capillaries in a case of comatose malignant infection.

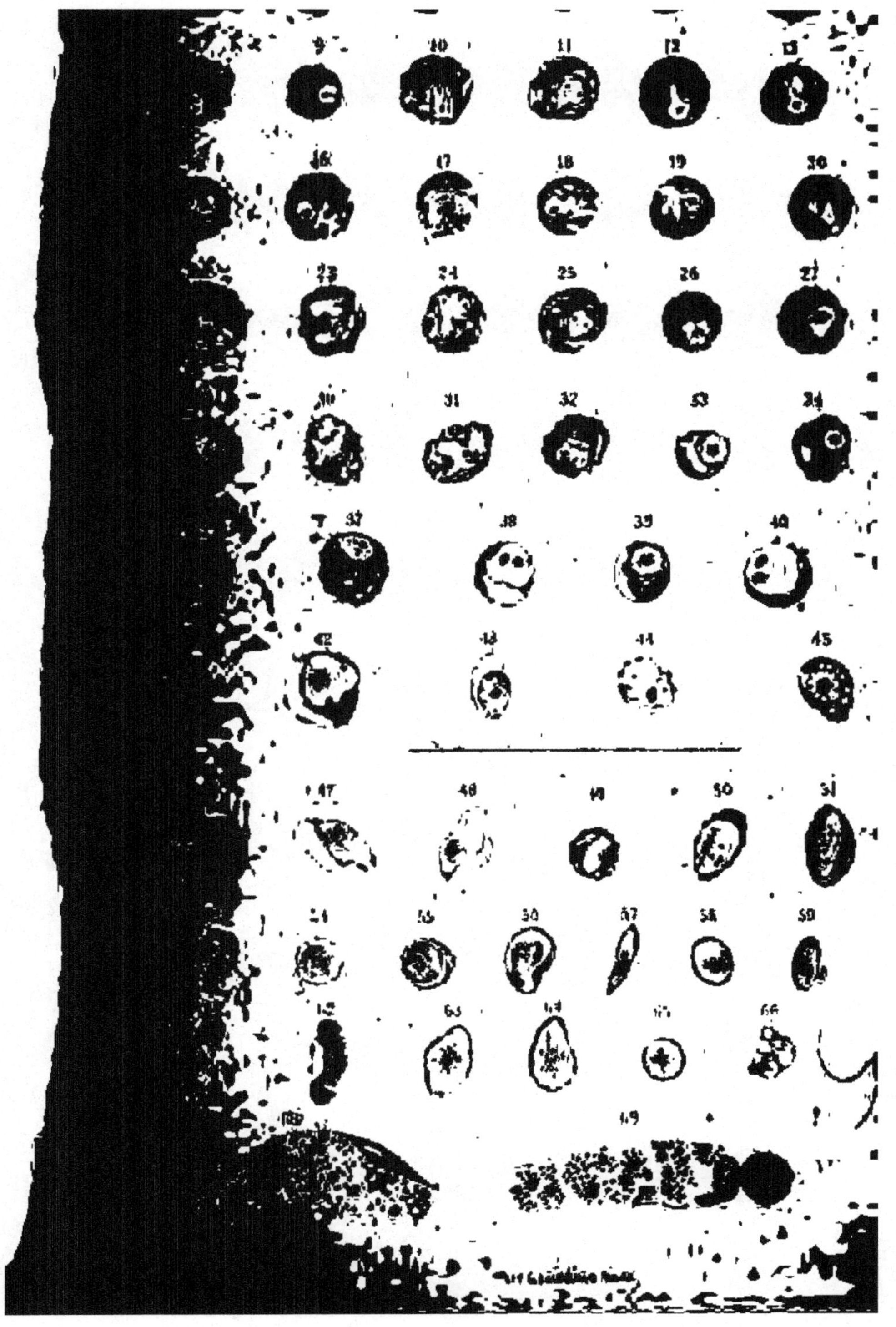

15

7th day. AUGUST 9th PERNICIOUS FEVER

E	M	E	M	E	M	E	M	E	M

41

40

39

38

37

36

A SEPTE

M	M	E

41

40

39

38

37

36

19

SEPTEMBER 18

MIXED MALARIAL INFECTION SUMMER A

M	E	M	E	M	E	M	E	M	E	M	E

41

0

39

38

37

36

E

41

40

39

38

37

36

EXPLANATION OF THE CHARTS.

CHART I.

1. Summer-autumn quotidian.
2. Irregular quotidian. (See Case 2 in the text.)
3. Irregular quotidian. (See Case 1.)
4. Irregular quotidian. (See Case 3.)
5. Summer-autumn tertian. (See Case 4.)
6. The same. (See Case 7.)
7. A tertian attack followed by another which is modified by the action of quinine. (See Case 6.)

CHART II.

8. Summer-autumn tertian with remarkable pre-critical elevation. (See Case 5.)
9. Summer-autumn tertian. (See Case 10.)
10. The same: a prolonged attack. (See Case 14.)
11. Summer-autumn tertian. (See Case 9.)
12. The same: a subcontinued fever changed to an intermittent after treatment with quinine. (See Case 26.)
13. The same: a subcontinued fever. (See Case 25.)
14. Summer-autumn tertian with relapse. (See Case 8.) In Chart I the phrase "quotidian or summer tertian" is sometimes adopted in place of "quotidian or summer-autumn tertian."

CHART III.

15. Comatose malignant fever. (See Case 27.)
16. The same. (See Case 22.)
17. The same: quotidian attacks. (See Case 23.)
18. The same: post-malarial fever. (See Case 28.)
19. A summer and quartan mixed infection. (See Case 11.)
20. A summer and spring tertian mixed infection. (See Case 12.)
21. A spring tertian.
22. A quotidian of quartan origin.

ABBREVIATIONS USED IN THE CHARTS.

Pl. w. p. Plasmodia without pigment (young forms).

Gr. pl. Plasmodia with granules of pigment at the circumference (forms in course of development).

Gr. pl. br. Plasmodia with granules of pigment in red blood-corpuscles which have become brassy.

Pl. m., or simply *m.* Plasmodia with a small mass of pigment at the centre (forms ripe for multiplication).

Spor. Forms of sporulation.

Pl. q. $\frac{1}{2}$, $\frac{2}{3}$. Quartan plasmodia, the $\frac{1}{2}$, $\frac{2}{3}$, &c., in size of the red blood-corpuscle.

Pl. q. spor. Quartan plasmodia in sporulation.

Pl. tert. Spring tertian plasmodia.

Semil. b. Semilunar bodies.

P. w. gl. Pigmented white blood-corpuscles.

N. p. f. No parasites found.

Qu. Quinine.

In., or simply *I.* Hypodermic injection.

P. o. Per os.

The amount of the parasites found is marked underneath, or denoted in different ways in accordance with the relative quantity of the forms. Thus a black line indicates a moderate number of parasites, an interrupted (dotted) line a rather scanty amount.

THE

MALARIAL PARASITES.

A DESCRIPTION BASED UPON OBSERVATIONS MADE BY THE AUTHOR AND BY OTHER OBSERVERS.

BY

JULIUS MANNABERG, M.D.VIENNA.

ILLUSTRATED BY FOUR LITHOGRAPHIC PLATES AND SIX CHARTS.

TRANSLATED FROM THE GERMAN

BY

R. W. FELKIN, M.D., F.R.S.E.,

LECTURER ON DISEASES OF THE TROPICS AND CLIMATOLOGY, EDINBURGH MEDICAL SCHOOL; SENIOR PHYSICIAN TO THE COWGATE DISPENSARY, EDINBURGH.

PREFACE.

In the following pages I have set forth the knowledge I have gained during a study of the malarial parasites extending over several years. The material upon which my investigations were based consisted to a certain extent of the sporadic cases of fever which I had the means of observing in the clinic of my much-respected chief, Herr Hofrath Nothnagel, but chiefly of severe forms of malaria which I had the opportunity of studying in the summer and autumn months of 1890, 1891, and 1892, in the fever districts of the Austro-Hungarian monarchy, Istria, Dalmatia, Croatia, and Slavonia.

I have to sincerely thank the College of Professors of the medical faculty in Vienna for stimulating me to undertake this study by awarding me a prize from the "Oppolzer-Stiftung," with the commission to take up the etiological study of malaria (which up till this time had been almost exclusively in the hands of French and Italian investigators) in the fever districts of our monarchy. It is to me a pleasing duty to express to the College of Professors my respectful thanks.

I also thank the Imperial and Royal Ministry for the Interior for their favorable support, they having instructed the respective officials in different places to aid my work.

Lastly, I recall with the warmest thanks the friendly help which has been shown me everywhere by numerous colleagues.

The discovery of the malarial parasite has revolutionised the whole of our conception of the malarial process in all directions and given rise to new ideas, so that I have felt it desirable to submit the etiology of malaria in monograph form. In doing this my idea was on the one hand to offer aid to the general practitioner by enabling him to make use of the results of the new discovery in the sphere of his work, and on the other hand, to submit to specialists those particular facts which have resulted from my investigations. I have endeavoured to set forth in a strictly objective manner the historical development of the subject.

I hope that my work may contribute in some measure to arouse, if possible, a still deeper interest in Laveran's important discovery.

In conclusion, I have to warmly thank my publisher for the highly satisfactory way in which he has produced my book.

THE AUTHOR.

VIENNA;
April, 1893.

TRANSLATOR'S PREFACE.

Few words are needed to introduce Dr. Julius Mannaberg's work. It has taken a high place upon the Continent, and it may with confidence be asserted that it adds considerably to our knowledge of the malarial parasites. The Author has not only given with great acumen the results obtained by other observers, but he has clearly defined those obtained by himself after much experience and painstaking observation.

The book forms an admirable supplement to Professor Laveran's 'Paludism,' a translation of which has been recently published by the New Sydenham Society.

I have endeavoured to reproduce accurately the Author's views, and have avoided as far as possible a slavishly literal translation.

R. W. F.

EDINBURGH;
March 15*th*, 1894.

CONTENTS.

CHAPTER I.

HISTORICAL INTRODUCTION.

The discovery of the malarial parasite was made on the 6th of November, 1880, by the French military surgeon A. Laveran, professor at the Val de Grâce Medical School. This investigator was at that time in active service at Constantine, a military station in Algiers, where malaria is exceedingly rife. Using the opportunity, he undertook the task of making a new revision of the pathological anatomy of malaria. He began this work by investigating, in the first place, the formation of pigment in the organism. A thought, as logical as it was happy, led him to observe the pigment in the blood obtained from patients, in order by this means to augment the results already obtained from post-mortem material. Although before him many other investigators had examined the blood of malarious patients microscopically, and had recognised certain pigmented bodies in it as being pigment-carrying leucocytes of the malarial blood, it was Laveran who first conjectured the parasitic nature of these bodies and who thoroughly convinced himself of the correctness of his conjecture by long-continued observations. This new conception of a well-known condition, which numerous observers since Heinrich Meckel had passed by without appreciating its importance, contributed so much the more to Laveran's fame because his discovery came at a time when the Klebs-Tommasi-Crudeli's *bacillus malariæ* appeared to have cleared up the etiology of malaria, and to have met with very general acceptance.

As I have often met with many misleading remarks in German, French, and Roman authors in this connection, I take the opportunity here of referring to previous statements made concerning the pigment in blood.

Heinrich Meckel [1], in 1847, was the first to find and to describe pigment in the blood and in the organs of the dead body of an insane patient. The results of the post-mortem (slate-coloured staining of the grey substance of the brain, very large spleen, enlarged liver, œdema) permitted no doubt that the patient had suffered from malaria, although in the history given, probably on account of faulty observation (for the insane patient had been for many years in an asylum) there is no reference to the subject. I do not think it superfluous to give a quotation from Meckel's original report, because it shows that this distinguished observer recognised clearly the difference between lymph cells and pigment cells. On page 205 [1][1] he says: "This blood (from the heart), as well as that obtained from all parts of the body, either lying in the capillaries or squeezed out of the vessels, contains black pigment. . . . *Invariably a more or less great number of black, irregular granules were united by a colourless substance to a globular, egg-shaped or fusiform body; the size of these bodies amounted to ·002 to ·007 of a line. In them no other structures could be made out but a transparent connective tissue with 1, 2, 4, and more pigment granules. Even in the larger bodies no particles except pigment granules could, as a rule, be seen. But in several bodies one noticed between the pigment granules a clear, roundish space left free, so that one was obliged to imagine that the nucleus lay there, although not clearly recognised. In rare cases single complete pigment cells could be seen in which there was a distinct nucleus. A distinct cell membrane was not distinguishable, and the granules never had molecular movement. The bodies were most numerous in the vessels of the grey matter of the brain.*"

Meckel reported quite independently during the subsequent progress of his work with regard to the behaviour of the lymph-cells, so that no doubt can be entertained that he differentiated clearly between the pigment cells, *the malarial parasites of to-day*, and the leucocytes. Almost simultaneously with Meckel, Dlauhy in Prague observed pigment in the organs of the body of a person who had died suddenly with "typhus-like symptoms." Virchow was present at the post-mortem examination of this body, and reported its results in a letter to Meckel. Virchow [2] had later in Berlin the opportunity of personally making a post-mortem on the body of a patient who had died from fever, and he confirmed the occurrence of pigment cells in the blood. Illustrations of these cells are to be found in the different editions of his *Cellular Pathology* [3].

At this time also attention was directed in Vienna to the pigment in the bodies of persons who had died from malaria. Heschl [4, 5], at Rokintansky's suggestion, made a series of observations in this connection. Lastly, Planer's [6] work must be mentioned

[1] The numbers in brackets refer to the bibliography at the end of the book.

here, in which also the hyaline, non-nucleated, pigmented bodies were distinguished from the lymph-cells, and for the first time the possibility was considered of *the pigment being formed, not, as Meckel and Virchow considered, in the spleen, but in the circulating blood.* Planer also appears to have been the first who began the practice of examining the blood of patients and saw the pigmented bodies in fresh blood. Later investigators have added nothing to our knowledge of the "pigment cells," so that we now return to Laveran, who has at one stroke placed in a new light the importance of these bodies.

Laveran found his opinion confirmed that these hyaline pigmented bodies in the blood of malarial patients were parasites when, on the 6th of November, 1888, as he was occupied in examining the blood from one such body several long flagella suddenly made their appearance, and thereupon commenced lively lashing movements in the blood. At first, on account of these flagella, he held these bodies to be forms belonging to the genus Oscillaria, and suggested, therefore, the name of *Oscillaria malariæ* for them. It soon, however, became evident that they must be placed in the species of the Protozoa, about which more details will be given later on. Laveran published his observations in a short note to the *Académie de Médecine* in Paris (at a meeting on the 23rd of November, 1880) [7]; soon after (at a meeting on the 28th of December) he published a second note [8] to the same Society giving the points in which the bodies found by him were differentiated from melaniferous leucocytes.

Just a year later (1881) he published a small monograph with illustrations [9], and at the same time reported to the *Académie des Sciences* in Paris on the most important points in his results. As we shall subsequently often have to refer to the contents of this, Laveran's first publication, I think it will be convenient to quote several sentences from it, and I give the text of his communication to the *Académie des Sciences* on the 24th of October, 1881 [10]. Laveran writes, "There exist in the blood of patients suffering from malaria certain parasitic elements which present themselves under the following aspects:

"1. *Cylindrical elements* fringed at their extremity, and almost always curved in the form of a crescent. The length of these bodies is ·008 mm. to ·009 mm.; their average breadth ·003 mm. Their margin is indicated by a very fine line. The body is transparent and colourless, save at its middle, where there is a darkish spot formed by pigment granules of a very dark red colour.

"One often observes on the concave side a very fine line, which seems to cause the ends of the crescent to stand out in relief. These elements do not appear to be capable of movement. They are occasionally oval in form, and when the oval is but slightly elongated, and the granules of pigment are arranged in a circle, the bodies closely resemble the following:

"2. *Transparent spherical elements* of the average diameter of a red blood-corpuscle, containing pigment granules, which in a state of rest are often arranged in a tolerably regular circle, while in motion these granules are briskly shaken and their arrangement thus becomes irregular. Further, one often observes at the margin of the transparent spheres very fine flagella which seem to be inserted in it, and which are animated by the most rapid movement in every direction. The length of these mobile flagella may be stated at three or four times the diameter of a red blood-corpuscle. I have often counted three or four around the same spherical body, to which they communicated an oscillatory motion, while at the same time they displaced the neighbouring red blood-corpuscles in every direction. The free extremity of the flagellum is slightly swollen. While at rest these flagella are invisible from their fineness and complete transparency. These mobile flagella finally detach themselves from the spherical pigmented bodies; after this separation they continue to move and pass freely among the red blood-corpuscles.

"3. *Elements of a spherical or irregular form*, transparent or finely granular, having a diameter of ·008 mm. to ·010 mm., containing rounded pigment granules of a fiery red colour, which are sometimes arranged fairly regularly at the periphery, at other times connected either at the centre or at some peripheral point. These bodies are motionless, as are also the pigment granules they contain.

"If one observe a transparent spherical body containing mobile pigment granules and furnished with moving flagella till the time that the movement ceases, one may see it take the appearance above described, whence one may conclude that these elements only represent, as it were, the cadaveric form of the preceding ones. These elements have no nucleus, and are with great difficulty stained with carmine, which seems to distinguish them from the melaniferous leucocytes, with which they have up to this time been confounded.

"4. *Spherical transparent elements* containing pigment granules, either moving or motionless, like those described above, but of a diameter much less than that of these bodies. The smallest of these elements are barely a sixth of the diameter of a red blood-corpuscle, and only contain one or two pigment granules, while the largest approach the diameter of a red corpuscle. These bodies, sometimes single, sometimes joined together to the number of four, at times free in the blood, at others attached to the red corpuscles or the leucocytes, only appear to represent a certain phase in the development of the parasitic elements above described.

"The living character of these spherical bodies containing pigment granules is indisputable. I suppose it is a question of an organism which exists in the state of agglomeration, of encystment, and which in its perfect state becomes free and in the form of moving flagella. Among the Protista there are numerous examples of these different states of the same organism.

"In addition to the elements described above there are often seen in the blood of patients suffering from malarial fever—(1) Red corpuscles which appear vacuolated at one or more points, and which contain pigment granules. (2) Melaniferous leucocytes. (3) Pigment granules of various sizes free in the blood; these pigment granules are probably derived from the destruction of the parasites; they are taken up by the leucocytes, as happens to all granular matter entering the blood.

"It is now a year since I discovered the parasitic elements above described in the blood of patients suffering from malarial fever. Since then I have collected observations of 192 patients suffering from different forms of malaria, intermittent or remittent fever, pernicious complications and malarial cachexia. I have ascertained the existence of the parasitic elements in 148 of these patients."

At the conclusion of this communication Laveran develops the idea that the parasites are killed by quinine, and that in this way the specific action of this drug is to be explained.

We shall subsequently see that, even in this early publication, Laveran refers to all the forms of the malarial parasite which had hitherto become known, except the completely unpigmented forms, which, however, he comes very near to, when he mentions the frequent occurrence of the very smallest bodies containing very little pigment (one granule). This accuracy of the observer is all the more remarkable because Laveran worked with a relatively small magnifying power (400 to 500 diameters). It must, however, be admitted that the importance of these results were later subject to various alterations through the work of Laveran himself, as well as of that of other investigators.

The missing, perfectly unpigmented, stages were almost imme-

"One often observes on the concave side a
seems to cause the ends of the crescent to
These elements do not appear to be capable
are occasionally oval in form, and when the
elongated, and the granules of pigment are
the bodies closely resemble the following:

"2. *Transparent spherical elements* of the
red blood-corpuscle, containing pigment gran
of rest are often arranged in a tolerably reg
motion these granules are briskly shaken an
thus becomes irregular. Further, one of
margin of the transparent spheres very fine
to be inserted in it, and which are anima
movement in every direction. The le
flagella may be stated at three or four ti
red blood-corpuscle. I have often count
the same spherical body, to which they
tory motion, while at the same time t
bouring red blood-corpuscles in eve
extremity of the flagellum is slightly
these flagella are invisible from the
transparency. These mobile flagella
from the spherical pigmented bodies
continue to move and pass freely am

"3. *Elements of a spherical or i*
finely granular, having a diameter
taining rounded pigment granules
sometimes arranged fairly regula
times connected either at the
point. These bodies are motio
granules they contain.

"If one observe a transparent
pigment granules and furnis
time that the movement ce
appearance above described, w
elements only represent, as
preceding ones. These elem
great difficulty stained with
them from the melaniferous
to this time been confounde

"4. *Spherical transparen*
either moving or motionles
diameter much less than

ri
m
or
rep
hold
coalescing
rightly apprec

the larger bodies; further, that the pigmented bodies in all probability indicate retrograde metamorphosis of the red blood-corpuscles, and that this peculiar *degeneration* is combined with the transformation of hæmoglobin into melanin. This opinion was still held by both authors in 1884 [17], in which year Laveran [18] thoroughly discussed the malarial parasites in his "*Traité des fièvres palustres*" and illustrated them with numerous figures, availing himself of the material obtained from the microscopical investigation of 432 cases. About this time Marchiafava and Celli published in the "*Archives Italiennes de Biologie*" a paper with the title "Les altérations des globules rouges dans l'infection par malaria et le genèse de la mélanémie," in which once more the pigmented and unpigmented minute body (Körperchen), stained by methylene blue, was described. On page 166 the authors write, "Maintenant, quelle est la nature de cette altération des globules rouges? Il est hors de doute que cette altération doit etre regardée comme de nature regressive, ou, plutôt, elle peut etre définie avec Tommasi-Crudeli *comme une nécrobiose du globule rouge, dans laquelle s'opère la transformation de l'hémoglobine en mélanine,*[1] et par laquelle il ne reste du globule qu'un cadâvre circulant." The authors do not specify the causes of this "*degeneration,*" but they appear to consider it due to the points which are held to be cocci. Laveran's "filaments mobiles" were considered by them as similar to Schultze's, which were the products of decomposition of the red blood-corpuscles due to the action of heat, the same artificial products which had three years earlier been held by Marchiafava and Cuboni to be bacilli.

This opinion of Marchiafava and Celli found strong support in Tommasi-Crudeli, who could not give up the idea of the "*bacillus malariæ,*" and it was he who, at the International Medical Congress at Copenhagen in 1884, both in his own name as also in that of both the Italian authors, gave expression to the term "degeneration-hypothesis."

In 1885, Marchiafava and Celli suddenly changed their opinion in regard to these matters, for in the communications which now appeared from both authors the bodies which only a short time ago they had considered to be degeneration products of the red blood-corpuscles were now suddenly called parasites. The reason for this change of front was due to observations made upon fresh blood in which the small unpigmented bodies were seen to possess lively amœboid movements. As is clearly expressed in Laveran's former publications, he had from the first recognised and described

[1] The italics are not in the original.—AUTHOR.

this movement, at least in the pigmented forms. and Celli arrived at the true appreciation of the m by this roundabout route because they at first stained preparations of blood, which they also desc which it was perfectly impossible for them to see t which they held for degeneration products were organisms. It was first in 1885, after they had of the mobile and heterogenous appearances of fresh blood, that they came upon the fact of the tru malarial parasite, long previously discovered by from this time the investigations of both author knowledge of this organism.

It was henceforward to the credit of both obs assumed the method of reproduction of the mala in the segmental bodies, and thus the developme the first time sketched. It was they, too, who valuable information concerning the diagnosti importance of the unpigmented varieties. Als *modium malariæ*"—which, if not very hap one at present most usually employed for —must be ascribed to Marchiafava and C suggested it originally for the unpigmented of which they still ascribed to themselves, claims which Laveran has made to its pri

From 1885, more and more numerous discovery, which had been at first so d from the most various malarial districts greater part of these reports brought served to confirm the facts already disc were valuable, however, in that they malarial parasite, and increased the i diagnostic purposes. The most note Sternberg [21], Councilman [22], [25], Sacharoff [26], Paltauf [27] Jaksch [30], and Chenzinsky [31] who proved the general and exc hæmatozoon in malaria, numero themselves with the elucidation the question of malaria had assu covery. It was E. Metschnikoff

[1] I avoid entering into details on dispute, and refer the reader who graphy.

who first sought to classify the blood parasite. He classed it with the Coccidia near to the *Klossia soror*, and suggested for it the name of *Hæmatophyllum malariæ*. This has, however, up to the present, not obtained general usage. Metschnikoff also discussed the relation of the "Hæmatophyllum" to the Phagocytes, but this is referred to in Chapter IX.

From the clinical point of view, we have to thank C. Golgi [33—37] for very valuable observations to which we shall subsequently pay special attention. It was Golgi who endeavoured to establish the relation between the symptoms of fever and the various stages of development of the hæmatozoon, on the one hand, and between the types of fever and the form of the parasite on the other. He has ingeniously brought into clear and natural relation the confusing number of varieties which other observers, without respect to biological and clinical value, had brought to light. Following his track, especially in the methods adopted with reference to the quartan and tertian fevers, Marchiafava and Celli [38], P. Canalis [39], and others sought to bring Golgi's rules also to bear upon the pernicious summer and autumn fevers.

Golgi's investigations further brought up the question as to the unity or multiplicity of the malarial virus; whereas the majority of the Italian observers took the view that different types of fever required different hæmatozoa, Laveran took the side of the unitarians, who believe that the many forms at present known are varieties of a very polymorphous but single organism. Notwithstanding the numerous weighty confirmations of the parasitic nature of malaria and of the pathogenic importance of "Laveran's bodies" (in the widest sense), there were still to be found some observers who tried to uphold the idea that these bodies were degeneration products and who supported this idea by fresh proofs. Among the representatives of the degeneration-hypothesis, we mention Tommasi-Crudeli [40], with whom are associated Maragliano [41] and Mosso [42—44]; in Germany also several opposing voices were heard. The objections raised by these observers were, on the one hand, disproved by experiment, as by Golgi [36] and his pupils Cattaneo and Monti [45]; on the other hand, by the accurate study of the structure of the hæmatozoon, they were disposed of once for all. The first thorough investigations into the nature of the structure of the hæmatozoon were made by Celli and Guarnieri [46], and were followed soon after by Grassi and Feletti [47], who studied the quartan parasite and published the first accurate histological investigation of the relation of the nuclear chromatin, the formation of spores, &c. In like manner the tertian parasite was next studied by Romanowsky [48] and myself [49].

Up to the present very little knowledge has been obtained from the pathological and anatomical point of view, but A. Bignami's [50] work deserves notice, for he has published valuable information respecting the distribution of the parasites throughout the general vascular system and concerning phagocytism, &c.

Although in the present study the intention is followed of discussing only the malarial parasite in man, still certain observations from the pathology of the animal world, which to some extent run parallel, cannot altogether be ignored, the less so because the extended development of our knowledge of the blood parasites in man requires a comparative, and possibly also an experimental, basis in the like blood parasitical conditions of animals. Hæmatozoa have formerly been often described in animals, especially in cold-blooded animals, by Gruby [51], E. Ray Lankester [52], Osler [53], Lewis [54], &c., but we are interested chiefly in Gaule's [55—57] examination of the "little worm" in frog's blood, a discovery which was made a short time after Laveran's, and which was immediately followed by Danielewsky's [74—77] numerous new discoveries in the blood of lizards, tortoises, and various birds; it is especially the hæmatozoa of birds from swampy districts which very closely resemble the malarial parasites, and give promise of being of much value in the elucidation of the same. It is, therefore, comprehensible that investigators of malaria, as Celli and San Felice [78], have devoted themselves to the study of this blood parasite in birds, and, on the other hand, that zoologists also pay attention to the malarial parasites in man.

The advantages to the therapeutics of malaria which have accrued from Laveran's discovery are also not to be despised, firstly, on account of the fact that the action of quinine can be defined with more precision than it has yet been possible to do with almost any other remedy or in any other internal disease; secondly, because it has now become possible to control exactly the result of our therapeutic measures, by examining the blood at short intervals during the administration of quinine, and by deducing therefrom the most favorable conditions for their success, as has recently been done by Golgi. The investigations which refer to the first point were already made by Laveran on the living subject, whereas later, by myself, and further by Romanowsky, by means of more accurate histological methods, the destruction of the parasites by the administration of quinine has been proved.

The questions, therefore, which C. Binz [79], by a sort of presentiment, asked himself in 1867, at the time of his investigations concerning the action of quinine upon Infusoria, have at last been answered, namely, *as to the nature of malaria, and as to the cause of the specific action of quinine.*

CHAPTER II.

METHODS OF INVESTIGATION.

For the investigation of the unstained malarial parasites, the general rules for the microscopic examination of blood are followed. The preparation of stained specimens, on the other hand, is carried out by a method specially suited to the hæmatozoon.

In order to examine fresh blood for malarial parasites, slides and cover-glasses are carefully cleaned with water and alcohol, and then perfectly dried. The blood is obtained from the tip of the finger or from the edge of the lobe of the ear (which has been previously cleansed with soap and brush), by pricking it with a needle, or, better still, with a small lancet. If the drop of blood so obtained is too large, it is gently mopped up with a linen pledget, and then the part is carefully, but as rapidly as possible, pressed, so that a very small drop of blood exudes. This is immediately caught upon the cover-slip, which is held by a pair of forceps, and placed upon the top of the drop of blood; after being thus charged, the cover-slip is placed upon the slide, and the drop of blood rapidly spreads itself out between the two glasses. I do not think it is advisable to aid its spread by either pressure or any other method, because I have often found that the blood-corpuscles undergo a change of form if any such mechanical interference is made. It hardly need be said that it is advisable on each occasion to make several specimens, so that if one is unsuccessful, others will be ready, but before a second or third is prepared one must not neglect to wash away the remainder of the blood from the finger, and to press out a fresh little drop for the next preparation. The necessary size of the drop is soon learnt by experience; beginners usually take too large a drop. It is especially necessary for the investigation of malarial parasites to have the least possible quantity of blood under the microscope, because in larger quantities the formation of rouleaux interferes with, or even renders impossible, the investigation.

Apart from the ordinary microscope slides, I have often used the one recommended by Hayem [80], which has in the centre a circular disc surrounded by a hollowed groove; the level of the disc is *not* sunk. This arrangement serves the purpose of preventing rapid evaporation of the blood, so that a longer observation is rendered possible. Although these slides are very advisable, they are not absolutely necessary. For the microscopical examination a good immersion lens is of great use and really indispensable when it is necessary to distinctly appreciate the structure of the hæmatozoon, although it is possible to see the various forms with a good dry lens (magnifying to 400—500 diameters), that is to say, if one has already some experience and knowledge of the subject. As is known, Laveran made his discoveries without a very high power, and even noticed the smallest parasitic forms.

The careful survey of the specimen under the microscope requires at times great patience; in severe cases of malaria it not infrequently happens that a whole number of parasites is seen in each microscopic field, so that the investigation is immediately successful, but in mild cases, especially the sporadic, as for instance those which occur in Vienna, it is often necessary to search through the whole of the specimens before a single parasite is found. Besides this, the stage of the fever in which the investigation is made has considerable influence, and for this reason it is customary to attempt to prove the presence of the parasites in the peripheral blood when they are most numerous, namely, from a few hours before the commencement of the attack until it has reached its height.

We now turn to the preparation of dried specimens; these serve for the preservation of the malarial parasites and for the more accurate study of their structure, but they can also, under certain circumstances, render considerable diagnostic aid.

The dry cover-slip specimens are obtained either by placing a cover-glass, upon which a drop of blood has been received, upon another, and then rapidly drawing the cover-slips apart, or by drawing the edge of a cover-slip transversely over the drop of blood upon the tip of the finger, whereby the edge receives a small rim of blood, and then drawing this cover-slip, held at an angle, over a second and third cover-slip. In both these ways—practice and rapidity taken for granted—equally good specimens are obtained. Here, again, it is necessary to manipulate with small drops of blood, because the film of blood should be so thin that the several blood-corpuscles should lie side by side of each other, so that each individual one presents its surface to the observer. It is very advisable during the preparation of the dry specimens to take hold of the cover-slips with proper forceps, such as those first employed by Ehrlich for this purpose; these forceps, after sufficient practice, prove of advantage in many ways; nevertheless, serviceable specimens may be prepared without them. The cover-slips, protected from the dust, are dried in the air, and their further treatment depends upon the object in view.

The malarial parasites can be fixed and stained in various ways.

Laveran mixed upon the slide a drop of blood with a drop of a solution of osmic acid 1 in 300, applied the cover-slip, and then permitted glycerine, in which picro-carmine was dissolved, to flow through. By this method the parasitic elements were stained a pale rose colour, whereas the nucleus of the leucocytes took on a thorough red colour. In certain bodies, of which we shall speak later, a double contour further appeared.

Marchiafava and Celli stained the products of degeneration, which they at first held to be parasites, with methylene blue and other aniline colours, but did not obtain any satisfactory results, on which account Celli and Guarnieri (loc. cit.) attempted to stain the living parasites by taking a drop of acetic fluid in which methylene blue was dissolved, placing it upon the finger-tip, and making the prick through the stain, by which method the unaltered blood came immediately in contact with the stain. This mixture was then placed between the microscope slide and the cover-slip, and the process of staining of the hæmatozoon was examined microscopically, either at once or after the preparation had been laid for a few hours in a moist chamber, and the staining completed.

The results of this method, as will be explained later on, are rather faulty; also the method of staining is inconvenient and produces no permanent preparations.

In order to obtain the latter, various modifications of Ehrlich's method of staining blood are appropriate, as specified by Sacharoff, Chenzinsky, Plehn, Romanowsky, and others, and also staining with hæmatoxylin, after fixing with picric acid, which I first brought into use for bringing out the fine details of structure.

For the common staining of dry preparations methylene blue and eosin are most useful. The cover-slip, with the dried film, is placed in a mixture of equal parts of absolute alcohol and ether for half an hour. It is then, after drying between blotting-paper, floated upon a half-saturated watery solution of methylene blue for half an hour, then washed with water, dried upon blotting-paper once more, and then stained with a 2 per cent. solution of eosin in 60 per cent. of alcohol for another half hour, washed in water, well dried, and then mounted in xylo-Canada-balsam. With this method the leucocytes and the hæmatozoa are stained blue, whereas the red blood-corpuscles and the eosinphile granules take on a red colour. It is possible to use both these stains at one time if the two solutions are mixed in equal parts. The formula for such a mixture would be—

Saturated watery solution of methylene blue .	. 40
2 per cent. solution of eosin in 60 per cent. alcohol	. 80
Water	. 40

Plehn recommends the following solution:

Saturated watery solution of methylene blue .	. 60
½ per cent. solution of eosin in 75 per cent. of alcohol .	20
Distilled water	. 40

Add twelve drops of a 20 per cent. liquor potassæ.

These mixtures should produce well-stained preparations in from five to six minutes.

The above-mentioned stains work rapidly and are useful for the general demonstration of the hæmatozoa. If, however, an intense stain is needed, or if one wishes to clear up the details of structure, more complicated or at least longer lasting methods of staining must be employed.

Malachowski [58] recommends Sahli's solution of borax methylene blue, which is prepared in the following manner:

Saturated watery solution of methylene blue .	. 24
5 per cent. solution of borax . .	. 16
Water	. 40

To be filtered after standing for twenty-six hours.

Preparations, after having been fixed in absolute alcohol for several minutes, are placed for twenty-four hours in Sahli's solution and then washed in water.

Malachowski also recommends the addition of a few grains of eosin to the solution of methylene blue, in order in this way to obtain a double stain.

According to my own experience, I can strongly recommend Malachowski's method of staining. It gives relatively quick images in which the nucleoli are generally well stained.

Romanowsky (loc. cit.) heats the dried preparation for thirty minutes at 105° to 110° C., and then lets them float for two or three hours in a stain consisting of—

Saturated watery solution of methylene blue	. 1
1 per cent. watery solution of eosin . .	. 2

then washes in water, or, if over stained, first in alcohol. The mixture is always made just before use. The two solutions used for this purpose can be kept for a long time, and indeed the solution of methylene blue stains best when the formation of mould is noticed upon its surface. The solution is filtered before use. When the two stains are mixed a heavy precipitate occurs; the solution, however, must *not* be filtered, but used together with the precipitate.

Romanowsky assumes that in his mixture a third neutral colour develops, to which the nuclear network of the hæmatozoon shows the greatest affinity. With this method the protoplasm of the malarial parasite is stained blue (Prussian blue), the nuclear cromatin (nucleolus) carmine violet; the results are often very beautiful; still thick precipitates often occur, and the formation of the neutral violet is not infrequently missing, in which case the nuclear chromatin is also stained blue like the protoplasm.

I have [49] suggested staining the parasites with hæmatoxylin after fixing them with picric acid. This method I employ at the present time with slight modifications in the following way:

The dry preparation is first floated for about five minutes upon distilled water, then dried between blotting paper, and then drawn several times through a very weak solution of acetic acid (one drop of acetic acid to 20 cm. distilled water) until it has completely given up its hæmoglobin. Thereafter the preparation, which is now almost completely colourless, is placed for two hours upon the following fixing solution:

Saturated watery solution of picric acid . .	30
Distilled water	30
Glacial acetic acid	1

from which it is transferred to absolute alcohol for another two hours.

Thereafter follows the staining during twelve to twenty-four hours in alum hæmatoxylin.[1] Lastly, differentiate (clear up) by means of acid alcohol (75 per cent. alcohol with 0·25 per cent. of hydrochloric acid added) and ammonia alcohol (three drops of ammonia to 10 c.c. alcohol, 75 per cent.), then wash in 80 per cent. alcohol and mount in xylo-Canada balsam. The washing of the preparation with water and acetic acid removes the albumen, which is apt to give rise to troublesome precipitates in the following

[1] I used a fairly old solution of 10 grammes of crystallised hæmatoxylin in 100 grammes of absolute alcohol. Just before use one part of this solution is mixed with two parts of a half per cent. solution of ammonia alum.

treatment by picric acid. Specimens prepared in the method which has been described show the parasites, as also the leucocytes, coloured blue; the red blood-corpuscles remain perfectly colourless. In successful preparations the details of the structure of the parasites are very clearly shown (see Plate III).

For staining blood parasites in tissues, Bignami Amico [50] gives the following directions:

Fix the finely cut sections of tissue in a 1 per cent. watery solution of corrosive sublimate with 0·75 per cent. NaCl and 0·5 to 1 per cent. acetic acid.

The sections remain in this solution from half an hour to several hours; they are then hardened, first in iodised alcohol, lastly in absolute alcohol.

Staining follows in saturated watery or alcoholic solutions of safranin, methylene blue, vesuvin, or magenta-red for five minutes, subsequently washing in alcohol.

Apart from the staining methods, there are further various attempts suggested with the object of retaining the hæmatozoa alive as long as possible, in order to observe any possible developmental appearances or modes of reproduction.

To attain this object it is necessary to prevent the coagulation of the blood, to avoid evaporation, and to keep the specimen at a constant temperature. To prevent coagulation, Plehn [28] recommends the adoption of Freund's [59] method. The tip of the finger, from which the blood is to be taken, is well smeared with vaseline, and then an ordinary microscope slide must be used, which by means of a flat ring of a spirit varnish has been converted into a hollow slide; a drop of fluid paraffin should also be placed upon the cover-slip, so that the blood is prevented from touching any substance which would favour coagulation. Plehn states that with such precautions the blood-corpuscles retain for two or three days their normal shape and their elasticity. To prevent evaporation, Hayem's slides (cellule à rigole), already mentioned, are used, or the edge of the cover-slip is ringed with paraffin; the hollow microscope slide, into which a small drop of water has been placed, is also useful for this purpose.

I often use with considerable success a hollow microscope slide which is at one and the same time a moist and oxygen chamber. It consists of a rather thick glass, having in the middle a deep depression, as is the case in the ordinary hollow slides. Into this depression two grooves are ground, into each of which a thin ebonite tube is cemented, projecting about 3 or 4 cm. beyond the end of the slide. The cementing must be very accurate, [illegible] at the point of juncture with the depression, and must [illegible] above the level of the slide. The apparatus is used [illegible] after smearing the edge of the depression with thick [illegible] a drop of sterilised water is placed in it, then the [illegible] upon which a drop of blood has been spread out as [illegible] by a swinging motion given to it, is accurately [illegible]. Then one tube is either connected with an [illegible] or the oxygen is led to it direct from the retort [illegible] in my journeys, use manganese with peroxide of [illegible]. The passage of the oxygen through the chamber [illegible] by holding a glowing match to the mouth of the [illegible]. In this manner, in addition to using a warm [illegible] been able to keep the hæmatozoa alive longer than [illegible] manner.

[illegible] an even regulated temperature one uses either the [illegible] (works with Reichert's table) or a hot chamber [illegible] constructed for the microscope. Investigations in [illegible] and in the moist chamber have no value for the [illegible], and even for the special investigator they [illegible] present of little real value.

[illegible] made with the warm stage, apart from the [illegible] are retained a little longer alive, and that [illegible] appear more lively, have rendered no note-[illegible] ordinary diagnostic purposes, and may, there-[illegible] dispensed with.

[illegible] which have been made to cultivate the [illegible] of the human body have been of little [illegible] attempts have been undertaken by most of [illegible] malaria under all the various methods [illegible] with often very fantastic modifications; [illegible] materials specially adapted to the [illegible] the hæmatozoa, but all have up till now been [illegible]. The questions, therefore, whether the [illegible] under any circumstances be cultivated, [illegible] external to the body, as saprophytic or as [illegible] are up to the present unanswered. The [illegible] investigators concerning these matters will [illegible] the course of the following chapter. After [illegible] think it unnecessary to give details concern-[illegible] cultivation attempts; whoever intends to [illegible] must invent new methods to reach the goal, [illegible] reached.

[illegible] general methods of investigation, a few

remarks may follow on others which are difficult to carry out and therefore seldom practised. To these belong transmission of the parasites to healthy human beings and animals, and lastly the extraction of blood from the spleen.

Since 1884, when Gerhardt [60] proved the possibility of inoculating healthy individuals with malaria by the subcutaneous injection of malarial blood, such experiments have not infrequently been repeated, especially by Italians. The object of such procedure is to ascertain whether the inoculated individuals suffer from the same type of fever from which the patient suffered from whom the blood was taken, or whether such is not the case. The experiments have further the object of answering the question as to the *unity* or *plurality* of the malarial virus. Up to the present time these experiments have led to no completely identical results, from which it is apparent that the different experimenters defend from different standpoints this question of unity or plurality. The reasons for this diversity in the results obtained from investigations of the blood will be discussed further on, and an attempt will be made to show that the differences of opinion are reconcilable.

The inoculations are always made with fresh blood, because the hæmatozoa are so exceedingly sensitive and any addition to the blood would be injurious to or even fatal to their vitality. Inoculations may be either subcutaneous or intra-venous, the latter plan being preferred by Italian investigators. Accidents have not yet been reported.

Marchiafava and Celli felt compelled to employ intravenous injections owing to the frequent non-success of the subcutaneons method. They operate as follows : ½ to 1 cubic cm. of blood is aspirated by means of a sterilised Pravaz syringe from a vein in the arm of the patient, and with the same syringe it is immediately injected into the vein of the subject inoculated. The veins are not exposed, the whole operation taking place through the skin. It is obvious that the strictest antiseptic precautions are employed during the operation.

Inoculations upon animals have been as numerous as have been the cultivation experiments, and like them with *negative results*, although animals of every species, both cold-blooded and warm-blooded, have been employed, so that at the present time it can be stated with the greatest probability *that the hæmatozoa of man cannot be transferred to animals*. The same thing happens with regard to the blood parasites of animals; they cannot be transferred from one species to another ; even the few records of transference between animals of the same kind and species are open to doubt.

Lastly, with reference to *drawing blood from the spleen*. It is obtained by means of a sterilised Pravaz syringe, with the object of obtaining some information as to the distribution of the hæmatozoa in the living organism. As a matter of fact, certain forms which are scantily found in the blood of the periphery are found in greater number in the blood taken direct from the spleen. Also several developmental forms (the spore-formation of the small unpigmented parasites) which are never or very rarely seen in blood obtained from the finger, may be demonstrated in splenic blood.

In my opinion, the abstraction of blood from the spleen is unnecessary, as well for diagnostic as for experimental purposes, whilst for the first purpose the examination of blood from the finger is completely sufficient, and for the second, splenic blood gives very meagre results as compared with those obtained post mortem. The operation is only indicated under exceptional circumstances.

CHAPTER III.

GENERAL AND SPECIAL MORPHOLOGY OF THE MALARIAL PARASITE.

The malarial parasites are unicellular living organisms which in their early forms show a more or less lively *amœboid motion*, whereas during their stages of development they lose it entirely and only show slight changes in form, probably caused by the contraction of certain strata of the body.

Whereas then we see in the developed parasite definite simple forms recurring, to which a relatively small scope is allowed, we find the young forms possessing the most various outward appearances. *As a rule, the immature parasites have a flattened disc-like form* which, according to whether it is at rest or in movement, may have a circular, oval, smooth, edged, or completely irregular shape. The mature parasites are globular or sometimes also flattened.

The predominance of the flattened forms is probably due to the site occupied by the malarial parasite, the red blood-corpuscle, which possesses a flattened form; the perfectly globular form is first assumed by the parasite when it has escaped out of the red blood-corpuscle.

The size of the parasite varies according to its age; its diameter measures $1\,\mu$—$10\,\mu$. *The parasites are mostly isolated*, but not infrequently several may be found side by side, and, as I shall later on explain, there are amongst the malarial parasites certain kinds which must take on the *sexual form* (copulationsformen); these consist of two single parasites, sometimes of four. The sexual forms possess in the developed stage a double-contoured membrane, which is absolutely wanting in the isolated parasite; they are therefore to be described as *cystic bodies*.

The *reproduction* of the malarial parasites takes place through a simple segmentation (spore-formation) in the developed condition, probably also by the formation of spores after previous conjugation and encystment.

MORE DETAILED DESCRIPTION OF THE SEVERAL ELEMENTS OF THE ORGANISM.

(*a*) *The external cell membrane* (Cuticula).—Hitherto it has not been possible to make out or to demonstrate, either in the natural condition or prepared by any method, a double-contoured membrane in an isolated hæmatozoon. This refers just as much to the developed bodies nearing spore-formation or to those in the act of spore-formation as to the immature forms. On a spore-forming body a single fine boundary line may be rarely seen, a double contour never.

Laveran's crescents alone show a cuticle as a perfectly recognisable double-contoured membrane, and those oval or round bodies which by means of change of form are able to proceed from them. This double contour was noticed by Laveran from the first, and he says that in those preparations which are treated by osmic acid (1 in 300) and stained with picro-carmine in glycerine it can be preserved. Later observers have not paid much attention to the presence of this membrane; even in 1887 Marchiafava and Celli [61] neglected the existence of a double contour, whereas two years later we see in the report which then appeared of the work of Celli and Guarnieri [46] that the crescents were mostly formed with double contours.

The importance of the double contour as a proof of the presence of a membrane is doubted by Antolisei and Angelini [62], these authors giving expression to the opinion that this double contour is caused by a layer of hæmoglobin being attached to the crescent.

This opinion was likewise adopted by Marchiafava and Celli, who since then always speak of a "hæmoglobin membrane" (hæmoglobin cuticula).

I also can confirm the fact that this membrane is often, though by no means always, of the colour of hæmoglobin, but it does not follow from this that it is nothing more than the substance of a blood-corpuscle, for it is clear that the crescent, as all other forms of the parasite, is nourished by endosmosis and that it must obtain the hæmoglobin necessary to its growth through the membrane; that the latter also may appear to be coloured by it is only natural. I have not infrequently seen fragments of undigested hæmoglobin even in the crescents themselves (see Plate IV, fig. 47). Further, the membrane is, as already mentioned, very far from being always coloured, indeed, it is very often completely transparent and colourless (Plate IV, figs. 63, 64; Plate I, figs. 57—66).

Further proofs for the existence of a true investing membrane round these bodies will be given subsequently. Even under high powers no proof of structure in the membrane is obtainable.

Lastly, it must be mentioned that Antolisei sometimes observed a double contour in the spores of the quartan parasites, and that the same author is of opinion that the spores in general have an investing membrane.

(*b*) *Plasmic bodies and their contents.*—Each hæmatozoon possesses a plasmic body which occupies a different amount of space in relation to the whole parasite; relatively it is least in the quite immature forms, because in them the size of the nucleus much predominates, whereas in the fully-developed parasite the relative size of the two is generally reversed. The bulk of the cytoplasm is excentrically situated with reference to the nucleus, as is seen in the illustration (see Plate III).

In the *living* parasites, especially in all immature forms, it is generally impossible to differentiate the plasma from the nucleus. Both constituents apparently form a homogeneous mass, and this explains why it was so long before the difference was made out.

In *stained preparations* the more or less markedly stained plasmic body projects itself quite clearly from the unstained vesicle which forms the nucleus (see Plate III).

As the amœboid processes of the immature forms proceed from the plasma, it is natural that in the stained preparation all possible forms are presented.

In the Protozoa, to which, indeed, the malarial parasite belongs, two layers of the plasmic body are in general distinguished, the inner and the outer layers of protoplasm (*Entocyte* and *Sarcocyte*). These layers are found clearly separated from one another in many developed Protista; the granules of the Entocyte especially present a marked difference in comparison with the hyaline construction of the Sarcocyte. In the malarial parasites it is not always possible to accomplish such a division of the protoplasm into two accurately differentiated layers, just as little as it can be done in a large number of the Rhizopoda, in the small single Gregarinida and the Coccidia. Celli and Guarnieri [46] were the first to use for the malarial parasites the expressions *Ecto-* and *Endo-plasm*, but they caused some confusion because they designated Endoplasm the unstained part of the hæmatozoa,—that part which represents the nucleus and which has, therefore, nothing to do with the protoplasm.

I observed, as did Grassi and Feletti, that in immature parasites the melanin granules are chiefly found in the *external* part of the protoplasm, whereas the inner, the part next the nucleus, contains little or no pigment. I have therefore suggested that the distinction of the two layers should be based upon this fact. In many of the illustrations in the plates the reader will notice the conditions mentioned well marked. As, however, especially in the larger forms, the opposite condition is also to be observed, or certainly no considerable difference in the distribution of the pigment is appreciable, I think that we shall do best in the meantime to consider the protoplasm of the malarial parasites as a body without any distinct differentiation. I must distinctly deny Romanowsky's [48] opinion that in healthy parasites, which have not been influenced by quinine, the marginal layer is always left free from pigment. A glance at the illustrations shows that just the opposite is the case; in young lively amœboid bodies, and, therefore, certainly in perfectly vigorous bodies, I have very often observed that the very few pigment granules which are present are found at the extreme periphery of the parasite (Plate II, figs. 12—14). Danielewsky finds that also in the blood parasites of birds pigment forms in the outer layer.

It is interesting to notice that this behaviour presents a contrast to the known fact that in the other Protozoa it is the inner protoplasmic layer (Entoplasma) which contains the granules, products of digestion, &c., while the outer layer (Ektoplasma) is free from them.

The protoplasmic substance appears to be chiefly homogeneous and hyaline, but in fully developed parasites it not infrequently shows a thick granulated appearance, which is made up of slight refractile granules. These granules also take part in the peculiar motion in which the pigment granules are found.

The most important protoplasmic contents are formed of melanin granules, the malarial pigment. It has already been mentioned in the introductory chapter that Heinrich Meckel was the first to see this pigment in the blood, and that Virchow first recognised the importance of the fact in regard to malaria. Virchow, as well as Meckel, then assumed that the pigment originates in the spleen and from there makes its way into the circulation of the blood, while Planer first thought of the possibility of the origination of pigment in the blood itself. Later observers divided themselves chiefly into two groups, one of which represented the view started by Virchow, for instance Frerichs [63], who, placing the principal source of pigment in the spleen, regarded the liver as a secondary source, and Mosler [64], &c., while the others pleaded for the formation of pigment in the blood itself; among the latter, Arnstein [65] must be specially mentioned, as he distinctly described the melanæmia as the first factor of which the melanosis is the result.

Arnstein and Kelsch [66] almost simultaneously took the side of the origin of the pigment in the circulating blood, bringing forward as the chief argument that sometimes, even in intense melanæmia, no trace of pigment is found in the spleen, and therefore that that organ cannot be considered the source of the new product.

C. Schwalbe [67] put forward a remarkable idea, namely, that, by the injection of carbon bisulphide and oxysulphide of carbon (also by inhalation of the latter) into animals, melanæmia could be produced, and therefore it followed that malaria was a poisoning with these substances and that they were present in the malarial atmosphere as gas.

B. Afanassiew [68] also had an idea which differed from the others in that he held the pigment granules, on account of their equal-sized grains, to be chromogen micrococci.

Marchiafava [69], on the other hand, as early as 1879 considered that the melanin was formed *within the red blood-corpuscles*, basing this opinion upon microscopical appearances in the marrow of bones and splenic pulp in malarial subjects (p. m.). In these he frequently saw altered red blood-corpuscles enclosed in the large leucocytes. To-day we know that these are blood-corpuscles infested by phagocytes.

Marchiafava and Celli [17] were of the same opinion whenthey wrote in 1884 that they believed the bodies stained by methylene blue (now recognised to be the malarial parasites) to be a necrosis of the red blood-corpuscles, "dans laquelle s'opère la transformation de l'hémoglobine en mélanine." With this expression both these authors indicated the place where the melanæmia originates from the hæmoglobin, only they could not then state the originating cause of this so remarkable a transformation. This last point is first clearly dealt with by Laveran [18], who likewise in 1884 writes as follows: "Il paraît très vraisemblable, en effet, que les grains pigmentés ne sont que des produits de destruction des hématies, des résidus de leur digestion par les microbes du paludisme, si j'ose ainsi dire, résidus qui s'accumulent dans l'interieur des corps cystiques" (l. c., p. 205).[1]

[1] It appears very probable that in reality the pigmented granules are only the products of the destruction of the hæmatin, the residue of its digestion

These words, indeed, indicate the standpoint we now take up concerning the formation of the malarial parasite and which we are not likely to have cause to relinquish.

The pigment therefore represents a product of digestion of the hæmoglobin. It is produced by the metabolism in the hæmatozoa, which are obliged to (*angewiesen*) obtain their nourishment from the substance of the red blood-corpuscle; it accumulates in the interior of the parasite as it grows in size.

The malarial parasite produces the pigment in the form of exceedingly fine dust-like particles, as coarse granules, and as distinct rods or spicules. The longest spicule measures about 1 μ. The agglutination (*zusammenbacken*) of numerous pigment fragments results in the coarser conglomerate forms of granular masses. *The colour of the pigment* is black in the masses just mentioned; in the fine spicules and granules it may have a shade of reddish brown. Laveran [9, p. 36] describes the colour as dark fire red ("rouge feu très foncé") and says that he has also sometimes seen light blue pigment which is said to come from the black pigment. Rosenbach [70] saw in one case granules which were less black than colourless or greenish and reddish.

Concentrated hydrochloric acid and sulphuric acid do not alter the pigment; on the contrary, it is markedly cleared up by alkalies and it appears soon after their action reddish brown, even yellowish.[1] It is dissolved by ammonium sulphide (Kiener). The chemical composition of the pigment is unknown.

All malarial parasites do not contain pigment. Firstly, all immature forms are free from it: there is, however, also a definite species of parasite which up till spore-formation has either no pigment or only shows slight traces of it. This important fact was noted by Marchiafava and Celli, but it must be qualified by the statement that the species of parasite referred to, if only it is allowed a few days' time, forms regular bodies which are always deeply pigmented (crescentic bodies), so that an attack of malaria can only exceptionally run its course without forming pigment, namely in those cases in which an especially severe infection with unpigmented parasites causes death within one or two days.

As well as these completely unpigmented forms, there are such as contain only few and most minute pigment granules. They

by the malarial parasites, if I may so say, residue which accumulates in the interior of the cystic bodies.

[1] For this reason in some of the drawings the parasites are shown less black in colour than is the case in vivo. The preparations in question have been passed through ammonia.

are so small as to be only just appreciable with the best objectives. The protoplasm looks as if "finely dusted." In other forms the pigment occurs in coarse particles, which are so numerous that when the parasite is nearly fully developed it seems to be perfectly crowded with pigment granules.

Golgi found that the quartan parasites have coarser pigment granules than the tertian parasites. As the finely or non-pigmented forms just described belong to the quotidian type, it may be said in general terms *that the size of the pigment granules increases throughout the evolution of the parasite.*

The movements and definite grouping of the pigment will be discussed under the heading of "Phenomena of motion."

The protoplasm also contains vacuoles; as Celli and Guarnieri have pointed out, these are to be seen as small, roundish or even oblong, clear interruptions in the protoplasm; *they are not contractile.* Usually small vacuoles and few in number (one or two) are seen in a parasite, but it happens sometimes that the whole of the protoplasm is riddled with them and looks like a sponge (see Plate III, fig. 32). Whether a parasite so affected can live long it is difficult to say.[1] I have often observed in certain specimens a remarkable number of such vacuolated parasites; in others very few or none were found.

It would appear that several authors have mistaken this vacuolation for spore-formation. I would here call their attention to the structure of the spores as seen by the light of improved staining methods. Vacuoles have no structure; they are fissures in the protoplasm which are filled by fluid, and therefore spore-formation and vacuoles have nothing in common.

The nucleus of some forms, again, is often erroneously taken to be a vacuole; so Marchiafava and Celli mistook the large central nucleus of the small form of parasite, which they later, as I think wrongly, considered to be a biconcave variety.

(*c*) *Nucleus and nucleolus.*—The nucleus of the malarial parasite has only recently been recognised as such. Laveran from the very first insisted that the hæmatozoa were differentiated from the leucocytes by the absence of a nucleus, and this statement seems to have placed the search for the nucleus for a long time in the background. Laveran was so far correct, for the malarial parasite does not possess a nucleus which can be stained like the nucleus of the leucocyte; with a simple carmine stain, which is quite sufficient for staining the nuclei of the white blood-corpuscles,

[1] It may be noted in passing that certain Gregarinida, for example *Conorhynchus echiuri*, are always quite vacuolar.

Th
conce
are

Th
ha mo
whic
the
inte

Th
ceed
tinct
1 μ.
fragm
masse
ment
shade
as dark
someti
the bla
which w

Conc
the pigm
lies and
yellowish
The chem

All
immature
species
pigment
was noted
the stater
allowed a
deeply pi
can only
namely
unpigm

As
as

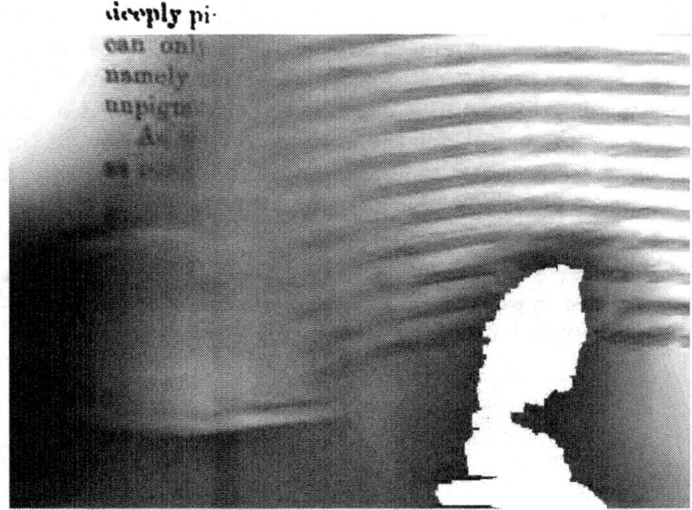

situated. This little body contains the largest mass of the nuclear chromatin—it is the nucleolus.[1]

Two nucleoli may also be present (see Plate IV, figs. 15 and 17). Sometimes several dark points are seen in the nucleolus, as is clearly shown in Plate III, figs. 8, 15, 16. They are, as a rule, very regularly placed little bodies; their *rôle* is unknown to me.

In my opinion, there is a stage in which the nucleolus disappears; it probably breaks up in the protoplasmic body (see Plate III, figs. 8 to 18), then only empty nuclei remain, as shown in Plate III, figs. 19 to 21; further, there is a second stage in which the nucleus contains chromatin, as in Plate III, fig. 21, and then the nucleus finally ceases to be recognised as such, as in Plate III, fig. 22, and Plate IV, figs. 5 to 10.

When dealing with spore-formation, details will be given concerning these matters. I only note here that Romanowsky, as also Grassi and Feletti, make no mention of the disappearance of the nucleolus and the nucleus, but that these authors assume the continuance of these cell contents till spore-formation, which, according to Romanowsky, takes place by karyokinesis.

I need hardly further insist on the importance which must be placed upon an accurate knowledge of the structure of the parasite. Through this alone all objections to the living and independent nature of hæmatozoa are once and for ever set aside; since the first contributions concerning these details have appeared no further doubts have been raised by the holders of the "degeneration hypothesis."

(*d*) *Phenomena of motion.*—It was this appearance which first gave Laveran proof that the pigment-bearing bodies were living organisms.

In fact, the movements of the malarial parasite, both the external (amœboid, lashing) and the internal movements (protoplasmic waves) present under the microscope as fascinating a picture as one could well wish to see. Laveran from the first differentiated three kinds of movement in the hæmatozoa.

1. *The amœboid movement.*
2. *The movement of the flagella.*
3. *The movement of the pigment.*

[1] Romanowsky does not speak of a nucleolus, but of the chromatin network of the nucleus, and speaks of the "clear areola" as the nuclear humour. I think that this contradicts the usual opinion. The Protista have, as far indeed as is known, large vesicular nuclei with one or more nucleoli; as we find the same conditions existing in the malarial parasite, we should do better to make use of the usual nomenclature.

he was unable to bring out anything that looked like a nucleus in the parasites.

Marchiafava and Celli, amongst their numerous drawings of the small unpigmented forms, have here and there perfectly distinct representations of structure, but they have given no special attention to the structural relations.

Celli and Guarnieri [46], first employed the methods of staining above referred to, but without much success, for they permitted themselves to be misled, and to take the nucleus to be a part of the protoplasm (their endoplasm). They were not fortunate enough even to get the nuclear chromatin sufficiently stained in the unpigmented bodies; at any rate there is nothing of the kind to be seen in the plates attached to their publications.

Grassi and Feletti [47] first gave accurate information concerning the nucleus and nucleolus of the quartan parasite. Soon after, I [49] and Romanowski [48] published similar information concerning the tertian forms. Since then I have become convinced of this, that the details of structure of the small pigmented and of the unpigmented forms are analogous to those of the large forms.

In fresh (living) preparations one can occasionally see at certain stages something of the structure of the parasite. These stages are the spore-forming stage of the quartan parasite and the fully-developed, large, so-called free forms. In the spores the nucleus appears as a bright, strongly refractile body, which forms the chief constituent of the spore, and on which a still smaller and more brilliant body (nucleolus) is to be distinguished (see Plate II, figs. 6 to 8). The nucleus is more rarely to be seen in the fresh spores of the tertian parasite [illegible] Plate II, figs. 22, 23). The nucleus of the large forms has [illegible] often seen and described by former observers; it forms [illegible] interior of the parasite a relatively large vesicle which [illegible] times waved hither and thither by the movement of the [illegible] plasmic waves. It is also noticeable that the pigment [illegible] stored up in it, but rebounds from its border as it were [illegible] II, fig. 24). In these nuclei of the large living forms [illegible] boundary contour is seen, so that a nuclear membr[illegible] spoken of. I have never been able to distinguish this [illegible] preparations, for in them the nucleus appears as a relati[illegible] more or less rounded *kind of vesicular structure* whi[illegible] usually *eccentrically* placed. The nucleus is not at [illegible] slightly stained, but at the periphery it possesses a [illegible] coloured body, around which a slightly tinged zone is [illegible]

Marchiafava and Celli added to these the presence of *an undulating rim.*

The amœboid movement of the malarial parasite consists in a more or less lively alteration in form, which is brought about by the projection and retraction of delicate or well-marked *Pseudopodia.*

Laveran observed this kind of movement both in the large and medium-sized bodies as well as in the smallest sparely pigmented minute ones; Marchiafava and Celli noticed that the unpigmented forms also showed amœboid movements of the most lively description.

The amœboid movement is most marked in the immature forms and gradually diminishes with the development of the parasite. According to Golgi, it is from the very commencement least in the quartan parasites, but, as Marchiafava and Celli have shown, it is very well marked in the unpigmented forms of pernicious fever. The activity displayed by the immature forms of the tertian type occupies a middle position.

Upon the warm plate the amœboid movement increases, though it is noticeable without this aid, but it must be mentioned that all the forms are not in movement at the same time, most being seen in a quiescent condition. As in the other forms of movement of the parasite, the amœboid movement shows certain moods, being sometimes active, sometimes sluggish, sometimes stopping completely, apparently without any reason.

There does not appear to be any special local change of position with the amœboid movement; it is chiefly to be recognised as a general alteration in shape; naturally in the close quarters of the red blood-corpuscle there is not much room for change of place.

Flagella.—The flagella are developed out of the large mature varieties. I find in the literature of the subject only a single note by Marchiafava and Celli [71, page 159], in regard to the observation of a flagellum in an immature endocorpuscular parasite. The development of the flagella out of the large spherical bodies can be very often seen under the microscope. In the spherical bodies of the crescent series it takes place as follows: the round body which has been quite quiescent, is suddenly seized with a very intensive jerking movement. This throws it backwards and forwards, and is accompanied by the production and withdrawal of the periphery. Soon after, from different points at the edge, finger-like projections are shot forth with great energy; *the projections are formed of the membrane of the body, which stands the pressure of the flagella for a time (sometimes continuously).* But lastly, the membrane ruptures, whereupon the projections sink back, and from them long thin threads shoot out, which lash so actively that their contours can only now and then be partially caught sight of. The violent way in which the flagella lash the red blood-corpuscles in their neighbourhood has often been described; they even cause marked depressions upon their surface, which, however, immediately disappear (see Plate II, figs. 62, 66).

Knot-like swellings are often noticed on the flagella; apparently they change their situation; their extremity is usually knobbed and a fine pigment granule may be seen here and there lying in their substance. The number and position of the flagella varies. One to five are noticed from one body, but owing to their exceedingly rapid movement they are difficult to count. They may project from one side or both sides of the spherical body, symmetrically or unsymmetrically. The movement of the flagella lasts from fifteen to thirty minutes; it becomes gradually weaker, intermits, and then comes to an end. Sometimes quiescent flagella can be seen attached to the bodies; sometimes, however, they become detached, and then swim about in the protoplasm like eels; *these freed flagella are the only form of the malarial parasite which possesses the power of changing its locality.*

The picture which these flagella present is a very startling one, especially to pathologists who are not used to like appearances, and it is therefore not surprising that Laveran gave the greatest attention to the flagellated bodies, and attributed to them an especially important place in the biology of the malarial parasite.

Laveran *had from the first the impression that the flagella represented the highest developmental stage of the parasite.* They appeared to be developed in the cystic bodies, and to escape from them when mature. If so, this would also explain the method of reproduction of the parasite.

A second condition might have influenced Laveran considerably in forming this opinion, namely that the flagella are usually to be found in the blood at the time of, or shortly before, an attack, whereas they are rarely seen in the intervals of apyrexia.

Laveran's statement with reference to the flagella was soon confirmed by Richard. The Italian investigators at first did not mention them, and later considered that they but rarely occurred. In Marchiafava and Celli's first communication nothing is mentioned of these bodies, for this reason—these observers at that time only worked with stained specimens, in which the flagella are seldom seen. In 1886 they [61] saw flagella four times in forty-two severe cases of malaria, in 1887 not once in 120 cases; it is, therefore, comprehensible that they saw in them the rarely attained final stages of development [19].

Apart from French observers, Councilman [22] was the first to call attention to the frequency of these bodies.

Since the method of the reproduction of the parasite has been found to occur in a different way, one is on the whole inclined to depreciate the importance which Laveran attributed to the flagellum, and at the present time its importance is, as I believe, very under-estimated. Grassi and Feletti [72] saw only the "appearance of agony" in them, and Marchiafava and Celli are now of the same opinion, as appears from their last joint report [73]. Grassi and Feletti base their opinion on the fact that the flagella are first developed in the specimens some time after the blood is taken, that they are not present in the circulating blood, and that they vary in number and in arrangement.

Danielewsky [75] alone at present agrees with Laveran in the opinion that the flagella are to be regarded as organs of the parasite. He calls attention to their constant presence in the *Polymitus avium*.

During the course of my investigations I have given the flagella special attention, and have arrived at the following conclusion. *The flagella appear in all the species of the malarial parasite.* They are most frequently observed in the spherical bodies of the crescent series, almost as often in the tertian parasites, less frequently in the quartan parasites. The frequency of their presence, which, however, is only to be proved by a repeated and accurate observation of the blood, convinces me that *the flagella are to be considered a necessary attribute in a distinct stage of the development of the parasite.* As already mentioned, it is the large developed spherical bodies which send out the flagella. It is also clear that the flagella are more frequently to be found during the paroxysms of fever in which the large forms are most numerous than during the period of apyrexia.

In many species of parasites, as in the tertian parasite (Golgi), the flagella may be regularly demonstrated, and often in great number, a few seconds after blood has been drawn. A longer time (about ten to thirty minutes) passes before the spherical bodies of the crescent series appear. *In nearly all cases of malaria* in which there has been to any extent an abundance of parasites found, and whose persistence has permitted several observations, *I have found flagellated bodies.*

In my opinion these appearances are, as already mentioned, certainly not to be considered as "agony products." For why should they only be exhibited in a relatively small number of parasites, when certainly all of the bodies in the preparation die within a short time? There must also be here and there flagella to be seen in the circulating blood, in which, as I shall later on prove, an enormous number of parasites perish at the time of the paroxysm, and therefore great numbers of forms "in agony" are present. One ought to expect the same thing to occur after the administration of quinine. But none of these expectations are confirmed. Lastly, the extraordinary activity in the movements tells convincingly against the supposition of an "agony-phenomenon."

My idea is that we have to regard the flagella as organs which *enable the parasite to adapt itself to a saprophytic condition.* I imagine that the flagella shrink in at the first commencement of life outside of the human body, and that the death of the young saprophytes takes place in consequence of the unsuitable soil. This explanation makes it comprehensible why flagella are only formed by developed organisms. It is only the strong, well-nourished, large bodies which are in a condition to bring them forth; they alone are called upon to change into the saprophytic condition in suitable soil.

A proof of the correctness or otherwise of this supposition is only to be obtained by successful cultivation experiments; still I believe that at the present time there are more facts in favour of it than for Grassi and Feletti's idea.

The flagellum can only be stained if a cover-glass film is immediately placed in a moist chamber for about a quarter of an hour, that is to say, the flagella must be permitted an opportunity to form. As soon as they are present they can be stained, as is the protoplasm.

The third kind of movement is that which takes place within the parasite, and which finds expression in the more or less active intermolecular movement of the pigment. When the movement is slower the pigment granules lazily but hardly recognisably alter their position, but when greater they are whirled about like a swarm of midges. Laveran has compared the latter condition very happily to the disturbance of boiling water. His opinion is that the movement is caused by the flagella enclosed in the interior of the parasite, and that the pigment granules are thereby set in motion. *Other authors* see in this pigment movement a Brownian phenomenon. One is obliged to contradict this latter view when one sees in what tortuous ways the pigment granules whir about amongst one another. It is no vibrating motion, but a continuous, if frequently repeated, change of position. Against Laveran's proposition it has been rightly objected that the movement of the pigment is noticed in the immature forms which send off no flagella.

I think that it has to do with a wave-like motion of the protoplasm, which drives the pigment granules with slower or more rapid pace through each other, according as surrounding conditions favour or retard it.

This movement is best seen in the mature pigmented forms of the tertian parasite, and in the spherical bodies of the crescent series. The quartan forms have usually quiescent pigment, whereas it is nearly always found in movement in the tertian parasites. The crescents often show, so long as the pigment lies scattered in them (*i. e.* in the immature crescents) a slight movement of pigment; if the pigment is a concentrated heap in their centre, it remains still. In the spherical bodies which arise from the crescent the pigment remains quiet for a time, then, under the microscope, it is often seen to be moving, and gradually attains the most violent motion. At this time the flagella usually break forth, whereupon the pigment may come to a standstill, but not invariably.

The movement of the pigment is also to be seen in some of those forms which I shall afterwards describe as "*quinine forms.*"

The duration of this movement varies; in all cases it continues the longest of the three movements which have been mentioned. I have been able to observe it for from twenty-four to forty-eight hours in my moist oxygen chambers.

It is not yet certainly decided whether the movement continues or not in the parasite cadavres; the answer to this question depends upon the definition of what a cadavre is. One very often sees, for instance, how from a large spherical body single small balls containing pigment, which we believe to be perfectly unable to reproduce owing to their non-nuclear character, free themselves, and in them the pigment continues active movements. The "quinine-forms" are at any rate very reduced in their vitality and yet they show pigment motion. On the other hand, the fact must be recognised that the cadavres of all parasites contain quiescent pigment. After all, one will not be much in error if one takes for granted that parasites in which the vitality is deeply injured (unhealthy parasites) can still contain pigment motion, whereas dead ones do not possess it. By saying this,

However, it does not imply, as will be seen from what has just been said, that all forms with quiescent pigment must be dead.

Marchiafava and Celli [19] have described the occurrence of an *undulating edge* in various spherical bodies (as appears from their description of those of the crescent series); Councilman once saw a crescent with a wave-like movement of its edge.

I have several times observed the undulating movement of the edge of the spherical bodies of the crescent series, but I got the impression that this phenomenon was caused by the flagella which had not been able to break through the relatively strong membrane of the spherical bodies. If the eruption of the flagella is often observed, it is not infrequently noticed that in the preparation for this process the "undulating edge" is noticed for several seconds. A similar, if not exactly the same, opinion appears to be held on this subject by Danielewsky [75]. He writes: "It appears to me that this undulating form can produce itself from the one described above by the gradual drawing in of the flagella." After this I do not think it justifiable to consider "the undulating edge" as a movement in a special category, but I perceive in it only a modification of the flagella movement, which is produced by the resistance of the membrane; *it is a flagella movement within the membrane.*

(*e*) *Concerning the relation of the parasite to the red blood-corpuscles.*—From the time of his discovery onwards, Laveran was of the opinion that the parasites existed, partly free in the liquor sanguinis, partly adherent to the red blood-corpuscles or pressed into ("accolé") their upper surface, and he holds to this opinion to the present day. Richard [11], on the other hand, was of the opinion at the commencement of his investigations that the parasite was developed within the red blood-corpuscles, and that after becoming large in them they left them by rupture of the membrane. Later [81] he gave up this idea and returned to Laveran's opinion of the extra-corpuscular existence of the parasite.

Among the Italians it was Marchiafava and Celli who most strenuously defended Richard's first view that the parasites existed within the red blood-corpuscles and that they are therefore endo-corpuscular parasites. As chief argument they brought forward the fact that the amœboid parasites never overlap the border of blood-corpuscles, which must sometimes occur if they lie upon them and are not held fast to their substance. ...ier, they noticed in this connection the consideration that ...veran's view were correct a parasite must occasionally come the object. This method of illumination renders excellent service when one wishes to see the bodies in plastic relief. In this way shadows are produced, which is not the case when the specimens are illuminated directly from below. By this oblique illumination with an open Abbé, the umbilication, for instance, of the red blood-corpuscles appears remarkably plastic. If the infested blood-corpuscles are now found, it is seen that in the places where the parasites were observed, distinct impressions in the substance of the blood-corpuscles are noticed, and that the margin of this so-formed depression is perfectly sharp. I have made this observation innumerable times, and I found it confirmed in all the small varieties (also in the immature varieties of the quartan and tertian parasites), so that I do not scruple to consider it to be the rule. In face of the fact just mentioned, we must doubt to some extent the assurance given by Marchiafava and Celli that the amœboid forms are endoglobular. If these bodies were within the substance of the blood-corpuscles, one cannot understand how the observed depression in the upper surface of the blood-corpuscle takes place. One would, on the contrary, expect it to be evenly expanded. It seems to me, also, that in regard to these forms Laveran's opinion is correct, whereas the endoglobular situation of the large pigmented bodies is to be held as proved.

I should not have dwelt so long on these histological details if the Italian authors had not gone too far in claiming to be the discoverers of the parasite by their discovery of the endoglobular growth (which, indeed, as has been mentioned, has already been discovered by Richard). For the biology of the parasite and for its pathological importance it is just the same whether surrounded on all sides (endoglobular) or only on one side (extra-globular) with the nourishing substance of the blood-corpuscle.

Against Marchiafava and Celli's opinion given above that all the free bodies are degeneration forms, it is further to be noticed that the spores which have become free, and are swiming in the protoplasm, are often to be demonstrated in enormous numbers. The way in which their structure takes on stain is so striking, that one is prevented from suspecting them to be "degeneration forms," as also from mistaking them for other elements of the blood (see Plate III, figs. 27 to 30). The amœboid bodies, too, which are developed further than their spore-forming stage, are not infrequently to be found free in the liquor sanguinis fully retaining their structure. With reference to the other free varieties, especially the large pigmented bodies, I refer to the special description of the quartan and tertian parasites (see Chapter VI).

Under the influence of the parasite the red blood-corpuscle undergoes various changes; under the influence of the pigment-producing parasites they lose more or less rapidly their colour, so that the blood-corpuscle débris which is present is often hardly distinguishable. Again, alterations in the size and shape of the red blood-corpuscles are frequently seen. In tertian ague the infested blood-corpuscles are often very hypertrophied, sometimes growing to three or four times their normal size (see Plate II, figs. 15 to 20). Probably this hypertrophy is analogous to other cellular hypertrophies which have been observed in infested Gregarinida, for instance in the *Klossia soror*, which feeds upon the renal epithelium of the snail and often causes an enormous increase in the size of its cells. On the other hand, a decrease in size and also a shrinking of the infested red blood-corpuscle has been observed, for instance in the very interesting "*Globuli rossi ottonati*" first described by Marchiafava and Celli. They are shrivelled blood-corpuscles, having a copper colour (see Plate II, fig. 49). They are infested with the small unpigmented or slightly pigmented parasites (quotidian or malignant tertian parasites).[1]

In the more deeply pigmented small species of parasites, small ones are sometimes seen lying, as it were, in a folded veil, which is formed of shrivelled and completely decolorised blood-corpuscles. These appearances are extremely delicate, and are to be counted amongst the most beautiful microscopical objects.

After some experience the shrivelled blood-corpuscles cannot be mistaken for the ordinary "morning star form."

Of the diminution in red blood-corpuscles in consequence of the malarial infection, as also of phagocytosis, mention will be [illegible] subsequently (see Chapter IX).

(*f*) *Mode of reproduction.*—The reproduction of the [illegible] parasite occurs by spores which are formed in the [illegible] bodies. Celli and Guarnieri endeavoured to add to this [illegible] reproduction that of proliferation of the spherical [illegible] crescent series. It appears, however, that these [illegible] this idea, and rightly so, for those "buds" possess [illegible] and cannot therefore be spores.

From Laveran's first publication it appears that [illegible] at that time seen and described the spore-forming [illegible] failed to recognise their importance, holding them [illegible]

[1] I designate these shrivelled and darkly coloured blood-[illegible] "Messing-Körperchen" (translated, copper-coloured bo[illegible] by the author to have the colour of old brass).

...ad, broken-down bodies. As has been already mentioned, ...averan then recognised in the formation of the flagella the ...ethod of reproduction of the parasites.

It is to Marchiafava and Celli's credit [20] to have first ...ought of the importance of the spore-forming bodies, but they ...re first definitely recognised, fully appreciated, and described ... Golgi [34].

Golgi first made clear the process of development of the ...uartan ague parasite, then that of the tertian. A year later Marchiafava and Celli [61] were also able to demonstrate the formation of spores in the parasites of the summer and autumn fevers to which the pernicious fever belonged.

The spore-formation consists in the appearance, in what had been up to this time a single organism, of a larger or smaller number of little bodies, each of which, on account of its complete cell-structure, possesses the power of individual life, growth, &c. These little bodies are the spores, and they represent the first immature stage of the parasite.

The spore-formation takes place as a rule in mature organisms, that is to say in fully-grown large specimens, but here and there one does come across some which generate spores without yet having reached medium size.

Spore-formation closes the existence of the spore-forming bodies; there remains lying side by side of the newly-formed young bodies a smaller or larger number of *dead residue*, the *débris* of the original mother parasites. These quiescent bodies consist chiefly of pigment, which is taken up by leucocytes and is deposited in the spleen, the liver, or in the marrow of bones.

The process of spore-formation differs in the various kinds of parasites, as also to a certain extent in one and the same species.

The spore-formation proceeds with least variation in the parasites of the quartan fever. Golgi, whom we have to thank for the most accurate information respecting the formation of spores, shows that the parasite, fully filling the blood-corpuscle and ripe for division, gradually produces delicate radiating streaks, and that the pigment, hitherto distributed throughout the protoplasm, concentrates itself in the middle of the body in globular form. The stripes become well marked, and suddenly the body of the parasite is divided by them into from six to twelve oblong divisions grouped round the central pigment mass. This stage Golgi compares to a "*daisy*," and, as a matter of fact, in the quartan fevers spore-forming bodies are often seen which do permit this comparison (see Plate II, figs. 6 to 8).

The several divisions then begin to round themselves and suddenly break apart as rounded bodies, leaving the dead residue behind. *Each of these bodies, having now become independent, is a spore.*

The starting apart of the spores can be observed under the microscope. It occurs probably through the gradual increase of the germs, which at length causes the rupture of the delicate residue of the blood-corpuscle.

In the spores of the quartan fever a brilliant body representing the nucleus may be already often seen in the unstained condition.

In like manner the spore-formation in the parasites of the *Febris tertiana* takes place, although, as Golgi has proved, it is modified in a characteristic manner. The pigment here also becomes concentrated, as a rule, in the middle of the parasite preparing to spore; still the concentration may just as well take place at the edge, or it can be omitted altogether, in which case the pigment forms an even network in the meshes of which the spores are formed. According to Golgi, the residue of these parasites retains more protoplasm than those of the quartan forms; also sometimes it may be enclosed in a membrane. According to the same observer, the division into spores occurs in two or three circular rows around the residue, and there are produced, not six to twelve, as in the quartan variety, but fifteen to twenty spores, which are smaller and unpigmented, and in most of them no nucleolus can be recognised. The grouping of the tertian spore-forming bodies is compared by Golgi with a "*sunflower*" (see Plate III, C and D).

According to my experience, as indeed is mentioned by most observers up to the present, considerable differences occur in the shape of the spore-formation of the *Febris tertiana*. It forms only seldom and exceptionally a typical sunflower shape. Usually the spores are irregularly arranged; their number is greater than in the quartan parasite, but occasionally spore-forming bodies are seen with less numerous spores (see Plate II, figs. 22, 23). I have not yet been able to convince myself that I have found the larger sized residue with its membranous envelope.

It is of practical importance to know that to differentiate the [illegible] types of spore-formation by Golgi's signs, and therefore to [illegible]le to diagnose the character of the fever, is not difficult.

[illegible] spore-formation of the *small parasites* of the pernicious [illegible] occurs, as Marchiafava and Celli have proved, chiefly in [illegible]ernal *organs*, and indeed in the capillaries of the brain and spleen; these spore-forming bodies are only exceptionally to be seen in blood obtained from the finger.

These small parasites invariably form spores at a time when they only occupy a fractional part of the red blood-corpuscle.

The pigmented small forms concentrate the pigment before spore-formation into a relatively large mass (see Plate II, fig. 35), and then fall into six to eight or more spores which are exceedingly small. The unpigmented smaller forms separate in like manner into a smaller number of the smallest spores (see Plate IV, fig. 66).

The finest histological details of the formation of spores have not yet been described with complete agreement; the minuteness of the objects and the difficulty of staining them are probably to blame for the diverging views.

Grassi and Feletti [47], who have studied the details of the structure of the quartan parasites, state that the nucleolus of the parasite enlarges itself, often takes on a rod-like form and thereafter falls into numerous pieces, each of which is said to form a nuclear membrane and nuclear humour; *it comes to be, indeed, an endogenous reproduction by direct nuclear division.*

I [49] found in the tertian parasites that the nucleolus in certain stages dissolves into the protoplasm of the parasite, and that soon after the non-chromatic nucleus contains chromatin, whereupon a stage follows in which the parasite contains neither nucleus nor nucleolus. Thereafter dark points appear in the protoplasm, which gradually increase in distinctness and represent the position of the nucleoli of the spores (see Plate III, figs. 23 to 25; these are drawings of specimens from which I have taken this description).

Romanowsky [48], lastly, finds that the formation of spores occurs by means of karyokinesis. He admits himself, however, that he has "not been able to follow all the phases of the typical figures of karyokinesis."

With regard to Romanowsky's view, I must assert that in very successful preparations, stained by any method whatever, numerous mature parasites are found possessing neither nucleus nor nucleolus and which cannot be considered offhand as cadavres, especially if the preparations are not from the blood of patients who have been treated with quinine. These non-nuclear varieties (they are invariably large, fully-developed specimens) Romanowsky ignores (as do also Grassi and Feletti), I think unjustifiably. I would call special attention to the drawings (see Plate III, figs. 8 to 18) in which the transformation of the nucleolus into the protoplasm is visible, and which confirm me in the supposition that the spore-formation is commenced with the destruction of the nucleolus and the nucleus.[1]

According to my descriptions, the nucleolus is the first part of the spore which is formed; this receives a protoplasmic mantle, often even before the vestige of a nucleus is to be seen (see Plate III, figs. 1 and 25); it is only rather later that the formation of the nucleus itself occurs (see Plate III, figs. 2, 24).

A spore is, therefore, only then to be recognised as such when a nucleolus with a protoplasmic envelope, eventually also with a nucleus, is present. Products of segmentation which do *not* possess this structure, are therefore *not spores but residual bodies;* they are often to be observed under various conditions (in fever, owing to quinine, spontaneous cure) and, in consequence of non-attention to the details of structure, they have often been erroneously taken to be spores (as by Celli, Guarnieri and Plehn).

In fresh specimens of blood the spores can only be recognised with certainty if they lie together in heaps, whereas single spores floating in protoplasm are only possible to diagnose by means of the requisite staining.

(*g*) *The process of development of the parasite in general.*—In the previous sections so many stages of the parasite have already had attention that it is now easy to forge them into a continuous chain. This construction of the process of development of the parasite is chiefly Golgi's work, even though it must be admitted that before him Marchiafava and Celli, as well as Laveran and Richard, gave isolated hints of the same.

Golgi arrived at his results by repeated observations of the blood at relatively short intervals of two or three hours, and by comparing the single results with one another, whereby he was able accurately to follow the progressive alterations of the parasite.

The developmental cycle of the parasites of the quartan and tertian fevers, as clearly shown by Golgi, is shortly as follows: "The small escaped, invariably unpigmented spores, float for a time free in the liquor sanguinis and grow in it, if only slightly, as I think may be assumed. Hereupon they attach themselves, possibly in consequence of their adhesive nature, to a red blood-corpuscle, and so gain the soil for their further development. Here the

[1] Romanowsky's drawing must, further, certainly not be taken as representing karyokinesis, for two or more nucleoli are not at all rare in the malarial parasites, nor indeed in similar organisms, unless this appearance proves the presence of karyokinesis.

spore become a small parasite, without any real morphological change being demonstrable during this change except the growth. The immature parasite possesses, as already explained, more or less amœboid movement, and makes use of this within its limits, these being the red blood-corpuscle occupied by it. With the growth, the products of digestion—the melanin produced out of the hæmoglobin—commence to collect in the external layer of the protoplasmic body. Lastly, the parasite arrives at the height of its individual life; in the quartan species it fills the whole of the red blood-corpuscle, which has remained unaltered, (in the tertian variety it remains rather less than the size of the blood-corpuscle in consequence of its hypertrophy), and then follow the phenomena of spore formation which were described in the previous section. We have, therefore, again arrived at the point of commencement of development.

The parasites of pernicious fever carry out the same process, with a new element added, namely, the bodies of the crescent series, to which we must give special attention.

(h) *Laveran's crescents, and the fusiform and spherical bodies belonging to them (spherical bodies of the crescent series).*

Laveran's crescentic bodies, and the spherical and fusiform bodies respectively which proceed out of them, have formed since their discovery the object of much investigation. Their perplexing behaviour in various directions, and their morphological divergences from the other varieties of the malarial parasites already described, aroused the interest of investigators.

However easily the material is obtained, and however easy of solution the questions raised as to the origin and importance of these bodies may *a priori* appear, the widely divergent opinions of observers prove that we have here to deal with a body which is most difficult to comprehend, whose peculiarities have not yet become clear to us in all respects, but which pressingly require further study.

Before turning to the examination of the importance and origin of the crescentic body, we will take a view of its general morphology.

The typical crescent-shaped body possesses the form which is expressed in the name given by Laveran ("corps en croissant"). It is slightly built, very delicate looking, rather strongly refractile, and sometimes rather glittering. Its length is some 8—10 μ and its breadth in the middle amounts to 2—3 μ. Within this body pigment is *always found*, even if in varying quantity; sometimes only a few pigment granules are seen in it (see

Plate IV, figs. 40, 41), but oftener large masses of pigment. The pigment is either scattered throughout the whole of the body or limited to one part of the same, usually the middle, more or less thickly grouped. I have found that this grouping often takes the form of the figure of 8 (see Plate IV, figs. 35, 36, 46—48), and that its final concentration into two masses or into two rows may take place. To this I shall return later.

The concentrated pigment is invariably quiescent, whereas the scattered pigment granules often show a slight vibratory movement, added to which there may be a slight changing of place.

I look upon the crescents with scattered pigment as immature forms, and upon those with concentrated pigment as the mature developed forms. This opinion is chiefly based upon the ground of analogy with the appearances which we have learnt to associate with other forms of parasites, and it therefore does not require any further description. The crescentic-shaped bodies do not possess amœboid movement, but possibly they have the power of slowly altering their shape. Laveran has already observed how under the microscope a spindle-shaped, an oval, or, lastly, a completely round body may gradually be formed from some crescents (see Plate II, figs. 57—61). This alteration in form takes place in an almost unrecognisable manner, and requires for its demonstration an observation extending often over several hours. It appears, indeed, that only definite crescents possess this power (it is probably a certain step in development), for specimens can be seen that have been kept in the moist chamber for days, in which most of the crescents have not changed their form.

In perfectly fresh preparations very few fusiform or oval bodies are seen; therefore, as a rule, very few such bodies are seen in the dry preparations which show best the condition of fresh blood. In consequence of this I incline to the idea that the alteration in form of the crescent is almost if not entirely coupled with its removal from the human body, and that the change never, or only rarely, occurs within the blood-vessels.

Just as the crescents may be drawn out into a fusiform or cigar shape in order afterwards to form oval or spherical bodies by gradual distension of their diameter, so also one not infrequently finds Laveran's bodies,[1] whose limbs (Schenkel) form a smaller angle, considerably modifying the appearance of the crescent (see Plate IV, fig. 51).

[1] Under the expression "Laveran's bodies" is understood at present the crescents in general.

The change of the crescent into the spherical body is followed by further remarkable changes. The pigment, hitherto lying quiescent, which for the most part forms a fairly regular circle within the body, begins gradually to carry out the well-known tremulous and "swarming" movement which has previously been discussed. After a time the pigment circle is dissolved, and the now scattered pigment granules actively tumble about throughout the whole body. Soon after the projection of the flagella occurs, as has been previously described in detail. Before calling attention to certain details of this process we must first clearly show the relation between Laveran's crescents and the red blood-corpuscles.

Laveran himself held the crescents to be floating free in the protoplasm, and reported in his first communication that they only here and there leaned upon the red blood-corpuscles, from which they could easily be again detached. It must, however, be remarked that Laveran mentioned in his first communication a *fine line* which connected in a bow the limbs of the crescent, and which, after further observation, proves to be nothing else than the *contour of the blood-corpuscle* in which the parasite has developed itself. The recognition of this endocorpuscular development of the crescent is to be credited to Marchiafava and Celli [20]. The drawings (see Plate IV, figs. 34—50) show that the crescents are either completely enclosed by the blood-corpuscle, or that they at least lie for the most part in it; a fine, sometimes smooth, sometimes markedly crenated line is seen upon them, which represents the contour of the blood-corpuscle, and which can hardly be missed *in vivo*.[1]

I have already given expression to the opinion that the crescents and the spherical bodies of this series respectively possess a true membrane, in proof of which I have referred to the appearances of the flagella at the moment of formation. I have still to add here that the membrane is not always coloured, but is often completely colourless. That Antolisei and Angelini [82] have confused blood-corpuscle *débris* and membrane is illustrated by the contradiction which exists in their declaration that the "hæmoglobin-coloured cuticula" cannot be stained. It is known to every one who has been occupied with staining blood that particles of red blood-corpuscles containing hæmoglobin, however little, can always be well stained with eosin. Also

[1] In some of the drawings nothing is to be seen of either the blood-corpuscles or the bow-line; this is because the treatment of the preparations with acetic-picric acid renders the red blood-corpuscles almost invisible.

the presence of a crenated inner line on the cuticula, which Antolisei and Angelini mention, and of which, unfortunately, without drawings no one can form a conception, has never been seen by me, and this makes me imagine that there exists a confusion between two things, *i. e.* membrane and blood-corpuscle residue.

The membrane is not to be seen in all, but only in a relatively small number of specimens. Together with it there may be a broad blood-corpuscle residue which is sharply defined from it (see Plate II, figs. 57—65, and Plate IV, figs. 63, 64). It remains also during the transformation of the crescent form into the spherical body, and gives to these bodies a peculiarity which differentiates them from the large spherical bodies of the previously described forms (tertian and quartan parasites.)

It has been already mentioned that these spherical bodies can very often be observed on their escape out of the red blood-corpuscles. The disappearance of the membrane can also be connected with this occurrence, which probably takes place through rupture, or, indeed, the two processes may be separated from one another in point of time, and it is then seen how the torn membrane shrinks together into either a loop or a ring, whilst the remainder of the blood-corpuscle is left immediately after by the spherical body. Even when these spherical bodies do not any longer possess a double contour, that is when the membrane has ruptured, they are not always very sharply defined, so that it is easily possible to mistake them for other spherical bodies. This mistake, however, can be guarded against, especially if the formation of flagella has occurred, by noting the little balls and ringlets which are often found at the periphery of the spherical bodies of the crescent series, and which, as we have seen, proceed partly from the residue of the blood-corpuscles, partly from the membrane which is rolled together, or also from a bit of protoplasm which has become separated. These little balls, which are found on the edge of the spherical bodies of the crescent series, were first described by Celli and Guarnieri (see Plate II, fig. 66), and said to be a budding—an idea which, as we have seen, was not accurate, and which has already been given up by the authors themselves. Lastly, these bodies very often send out flagella, thereby arriving at their last change. The procedures just described do not always occur with the same regularity; many deviations in the order and in the method of escape from the capsule, &c., are observed, which present in part inexplicable appearances; for instance, I have often observed that the quiescent perfectly colourless residue of the blood-corpuscles is suddenly distended and coloured by hæmoglobin, as if a stream of fluid from the parasite is driven into the empty sac of the blood-corpuscle. The margin of the blood-corpuscle is folded, and then soon becomes tensely distended until it quite unexpectedly disappears, and nothing remains of the form but a few hardly appreciable light yellowish droplets (see Plate II, figs. 62—65). I will not describe the numerous modifications under which I have observed the escape of the spherical bodies; they are details which up to the present are not explicable, and of which it is questionable whether they are to be considered as vital to the biology of the parasite. In any case, however, it is interesting to follow these changes under the microscope. It is difficult to fix them by means of drawings, for the alterations take place quite suddenly and with great rapidity.

Apart from the metamorphosis of the crescent-shaped bodies into oval, spherical, and flagellated bodies, the *segmentation* of the crescents must be mentioned. *This occurs transversely,* and usually through the middle of the body (see Plate IV, fig. 52). Grassi and Feletti [83] first mentioned this occurrence. I shall return presently to its probable significance, and the detailed structure of the crescents will also be dealt with subsequently.

In fresh preparations appearances are sometimes seen in the crescents which must be considered to be processes of degeneration. They consist of the appearance of clear circles and spots, which alter their shape under the observer's eye; they are often erroneously considered to be spores (see Plate IV, figs. 55, 56).

Now that we have discussed the general morphology of the crescents, we will endeavour to answer the questions how the crescents arise, what they indicate, and what becomes of them.

In order to comprehend these matters it is absolutely necessary to know the views of different investigators. We shall therefore go through them shortly in due order.

Laveran, the discoverer of the malarial parasite, who gave in his very first publication an extremely good description of the crescent, did not express an opinion concerning their biological position, just as he chiefly elucidated the other varieties more from the morphological side. It must, however, be remembered that Laveran [18], in his book published in 1884, spoke of the crescents as "corps kystiques No. 1, ou en croissant," and at another place in the same publication (page 109) inferred that they belonged to the protozoa because the malarial parasites occurred in free and in *encysted* conditions. We can therefore summarise Laveran's view of the crescents thus—that he held them for cysts in which eventually the flagella were formed (which Laveran considered from the first to be the highest phase of development of the parasite).[1]

Councilman [22] took up another view of the crescents, chiefly on account of their marked *resistance to quinine*. He imagined that they were *spores*. This view was held for a long time without any objection being raised, and gained strength because of its being known that in the coccidia there are germs which resemble the crescents in form (the so-called "sickle-shaped germs").

In the meantime Marchifava and Celli advanced the idea that this form of the parasite also, just as all the others, arises in the red blood-corpuscles, and, indeed, out of small amœboid parasites. These authors once observed under the microscope how a small parasite, lying at the margin, developed into a crescent-shaped body, by which process the blood-corpuscle gradually lost its colour.[2]

So far as I know, no other investigator has been fortunate enough to observe this occurrence under the microscope; general confirmation, however, was given to the discovery of the endo-corpuscular origin of the crescents, through which the importance of the line spanning over the concavity of the crescent described by Laveran was cleared up as being the decolorised red blood-corpuscle.

Councilman's view was attacked by Antolisei [82], who found in the pigmented contents of the crescent a definite proof against the view that these bodies are spores. He considered, quite in opposition to Councilman, that the crescents were mature forms, whose fate it is to perish. Bignami and Bastianelli [85], building further upon this idea, expressed the opinion that the crescents are sterile deviation products of the amœboid parasites, which perish without spores, and to which therefore no pathological importance can be attributed. It appears that Marchiafava and Celli [73] have adopted this view.

A view which contradicted the opinions hitherto put forward is expressed by Canalis [39], for this author, who allows that the crescent proceeds out of the amœboid form, appears to have asserted that the spherical bodies of the crescent series produce spores. A drawing of one of these spore-forming figures can be seen in his work. However, no other observer has seen this mode

[1] Also see Laveran [84], p. 284. He there writes, "Les corps en croissant ne sont vraisemblablement que des formes enkystées."

[2] Quoted from Celli and Guarnieri [46].

of spore formation, though so much effort has been expended in the search for it. My own efforts also in this direction have been in vain.

There was much opposition to this view, especially since Marchiafava and Celli have given their view, explaining the spore formation of Canalis to be degenerative segmentation.

While the authors so far mentioned are agreed on the single point that the crescents originate from the small amœboid parasites, which on their part may fall directly into spores (they are described under their special heading as pigmented and unpigmented quotidian parasites, and as malignant tertian parasites), Grassi and Feletti [86] consider that this is not the case, but that the crescents originate from the amœboid parasites *which are not capable of direct spore formation, but can only form crescentic bodies.* They are, indeed, not to be distinguished morphologically from the amœboid bodies above mentioned, though they are to be regarded, together with the crescent series, as a distinct genus. Grassi and Feletti distinguished this genus by the name *Laverania,* and the species of it appearing in man specially as *Laverania malariæ.*[1]

I now turn to my own investigations. This short sketch shows sufficiently that the views concerning the origin, importance, and fate of the crescentic bodies are diametrically opposed to those of Laveran, and that further information concerning them is needed.

From Laveran, Marchiafava, and Celli it is already known that several of the small amœboid unpigmented or slightly pigmented parasites are frequently found in a blood-corpuscle. Two or three of these parasites are very often seen lying in one blood-corpuscle, sometimes even five or six of them (see Plate IV, figs. 24, 26). They may occupy the blood-corpuscle either separated from one another, which is by far the most usual condition, or, as I have observed, two, or more rarely three, of the parasites may lie closely adhering to one another (see Plate IV, figs. 27—32). In fresh blood these conglomerate parasites, consisting of two to four specimens, cannot be recognised as such, for in these preparations one takes them to be large but single parasites, and it is only in properly stained preparations that the structural relations and the conditions of the bodies are cleared up. For in them we recognise clearly two nuclei, two nucleoli, and the protoplasmic bodies lying close

[1] The following pages, as far as Chapter IV, are taken from a lecture which I [87] gave at the *XI Congress für innere Medicin* in Leipzig in 1892.

together. And it is probable that on this account this frequently occurring conglomerate form, has up to the present not been mentioned by any investigator. These *paired parasites* occupy usually the edge, less frequently the centre of the blood-corpuscle. They consist sometimes of large, sometimes of quite immature forms, and sometimes one also sees unequal-sized forms adhering to one another. In some pairs the protoplasmic membranes are clearly to be seen lying close to one another; at other times they are hazy or hardly to be recognised, so that in the latter case one gets the impression that through coalescence the two parasites have produced a new form, which in its structure betrays its origin.

The question now arises, what are these paired parasites to be considered? Are we to regard it as accidental that the hæmatozoa form pairs in this way, or have we to seek a biological fact in this formation?

If we glance at those classes of the animal kingdom into which different investigators seek to place the malarial parasite and such like blood-parasites of certain animals, especially if we look at the sarcodina, sporozoa, and flagellata, we find the *process of conjugation* very frequent, two or more units lying close together, and either completely or partially coalescing. Thereby the original structure of the single body is more or less lost, the nuclei especially, as a rule, entirely disappearing. Sooner or later a membrane forms itself around the fused bodies, by which they are encapsuled or encysted. The further changes which these conjugation products (called by zoologists syzygies) undergo is usually the formation of spores, so that it appears to be justifiable to look upon the syzygies as a species of sexual mingling of the protozoa. The further fate of the syzygies has in many cases remained unexplained up to the present, and it is for further investigation to ascertain whether the conjugation is always followed by reproduction or not.

Returning now to the paired amœboid malarial parasites, the analogy of the zoological facts just mentioned must lead us to the opinion that we have possibly here to do with a process of conjugation, or with the formation of syzygies. A glance at two partially developed forms thus conjugating brings us still nearer to a resemblance to the crescents, especially when the pair, as is generally the case, is situated at the margin of the blood-corpuscle: the outer contour of both parasites frequently coalesces without interruption, and falls together with the edge of the blood-corpuscle; the innercontour is often of a concave shape. To this may be added that the length of the conjugating bodies often completely coincides with that of a crescent, and then, further, the fact that the chief mass of the protoplasm is to be found at both poles, whereby the well-known polar staining of the crescent would be explained; in a word, if *only a few pigment granules were present the conjugation form might be an immature crescent.*[1]

Notwithstanding this similarity, one could hardly maintain that the crescentic bodies were syzygies of the amœboid varieties if other forcible grounds for this view did not endorse it. But the following points I consider conclusive:—1. *The membranous formation of the crescent.* 2. *The structural details of the crescent.* 3. *The formation and distribution of the pigment in it.* 4. *Segmentation.*

1. With reference to the membrane of the crescent, and to the spherical body belonging to it, I have already in another place sought to bring forward the proof that such is present; it has also already been pointed out that this is the only variety of the malarial parasite which possesses a membrane, and I believe that this fact alone points to the biological difference of this body from all other varieties. Now we have seen above that the formation of syzygies is also invariably followed by encystation.

2. The structure of the crescent does not vary much from the structure of the amœboid varieties out of which it springs; and, on the other hand, crescents are often found which by their structure clearly point to their origin out of two component parts.

Celli and Guarnieri have pointed out that the crescents only stain slightly and diffusely, and that only at the poles; further, that here and there one or two granules near the middle of the body take on a darker stain. In regard to this, my investigations show as follows: the immature crescents—that is to say, those in which the pigment in the finest granules is distributed along the whole of the body—take on an even pale stain in the interior; whereas the poles and also the peripheral zone are stained somewhat more darkly. In *mature parasites*, known as such because the pigment is concentrated into one or two masses, either in the middle of the crescent or chiefly at a pole, *we see with hardly any exception the bipartite character again indicated*, because, apart from the stained poles and edge, there is now also a transverse portion over which the pigment lies, which is stained deeply, and which divides the crescent into two symmetrical parts. To this may be added that the interior of both limbs remains almost colourless, and

[1] In Plate IV, fig. 32, is a drawing of a syzygy in which there are already several pigment granules; the resemblance to a crescent is here very great.

that underneath the pigment in the transverse bridge two darkly stained points appear. These points are not often seen in ordinary preparations because they are usually hidden underneath the pigment, but if this is dissolved by placing the preparation for several hours in a weak solution of ammonia, it can then be demonstrated in numerous mature specimens, which in consequence of this treatment are more slightly stained (see Plate IV, figs. 33 and 34). Such a mature crescent, freed from pigment, looks remarkably like the conjugation form with which we started; the small difference between the two appearances consists in the fact that in the crescent the protoplasmic mass, especially at the boundary of the two units (transverse bridge), has become thicker, and that the nucleoli have lost both in size and chromatic properties.

3. *Concerning the origin and arrangement of pigment in the crescentic bodies*, I am of the opinion that by the conjunction of the two conjugating parasites a really heightened vitality is developed in them, which manifests itself in the rapid formation of pigment, and the corresponding decolorisation of the blood-corpuscles. Whereas the amœboid forms are faintly, if at all, pigmented, more or less pigment is always found in the crescents; it appears in single scattered grains and rods, just as in the forms of the tertian and quartan fever types. In the fresh condition these scattered pigment granules are seen to make a slight tremulous motion within the crescent; they often also slowly change their position in consequence of protoplasmic waves, and form thereby ever-changing groups. In the concentrated pigment, however, movement is never seen. The pigment becomes concentrated in the mature crescents, corresponding to the conditions seen in the forms of the regular type; this takes place, indeed, in a way which once more proves the bipartite nature of the crescent. The granules withdraw from both limbs towards the middle in such a way *that at a certain point of time they form a figure of* 8. If the concentration proceeds further two little heaps are formed correspondingly in both limbs, which very often remain lying separated from one another, or may be at length compressed into a single heap.

The figure of 8 arrangement of the pigment is such an exceedingly prevalent one that it cannot be doubted that in each limb of the crescent the grouping is caused by separate waves, *so that this circumstance again indicates the bipartite nature of the crescent.*

In regard to those crescents in which the concentration of the pigment is not in the middle of the body, but is situated nearer to one or other pole (see Plate IV, figs. 42 and 50), it may be taken for granted that this arrangement proceeds from the conjugation (as described above) of two units unequal in size.

4. I have often been able to observe *the transverse segmentation of the crescent*, which has also received attention from Grassi and Feletti. The segmentation is especially frequent through the middle of the body, as if produced by constriction, so that before complete separation the two parts of this body hang together like a pair of sausages; to each part some of the pigment remains attached.

These segmented bodies possess dark-coloured granulated contents. It is in the highest degree probable that the segmentation and the dark-coloured granules, which are often present in great number, have some connection with reproduction, but up to the present time this has not been proved.

I only draw one conclusion from the segmentation of the bodies, —that *through it the bipartite character of the crescent is again proved.*

From all this we see that the process of the crescent-shaped bodies from two or four conjugated amœboid parasites receives substantial support in the morphological as well as in the biological behaviour of the different phases of development; and I believe, on the ground of the facts brought forward, that the crescents may be described as syzygies of the malarial parasites.

With this conception much with regard to the mysterious behaviour of these bodies becomes clearer than before.

The size and form of the crescent as opposed to that of the amœboid varieties are by this means at once rendered clear, the somewhat later entrance into the blood becomes comprehensible, as also the long and apparently unchanged continuance after the attacks, the resistance to quinine, and, lastly, the fact of the inner structure being so totally different from all other forms of parasites.

The fact that the crescent throughout its entire existence retains the bipartite character leads to the assumption that there must be a so-called "pseudo-conjugation" when no thorough coalescence of the conjugating bodies takes place, but only a limited interchange. Further investigation remains to be carried out in order to learn the details of this process, namely, the fate of the segmented bodies.

Clinical experience also agrees much better with the supposition just brought forward than with all other views on the nature of the crescent hitherto held.

We know that patients who have these bodies in their blood appear to be free from malaria during long intervals (although they are always anæmic), but that they from time to time, at periods of from two to three weeks, have fresh attacks (relapses).

This fact, which has been corroborated in many cases, does not agree with the opinion of Bignami and Bastianelli that the crescents are "degeneration forms," and therefore these authors are compelled to accept the idea that from the directly formed spores (first cycle of *Canalis*) of the amœboid varieties a number *remain latent* in the marrow, and after two or three weeks *awake to new life*, having been in the meantime absorbed by macrophagi and liberated again. This hypothesis appears very improbable.

The resistance of the crescent to quinine is also very unfavorable to the degeneration hypothesis; and so is, lastly, the circumstance that crescents are so seldom to be found in phagocytes, whose function it is to clear away all dead residue from the circulation as quickly as possible.

Professor Metschnikoff, to whom I had the honour of demonstrating some of my preparations at the *Congress für innere Medicin* at Leipzig, was kind enough to call my attention to the fact that one need not consider the paired amœboid little bodies as necessarily the conjugation between two single units, but that one must also consider the possibility of the division into two halves of a larger parasite. In consequence of this suggestion I gave, during this last summer, very careful attention to fresh preparations, especially to the double invasion of the blood-corpuscles, viewing them for long periods in order to see whether one could not observe the process of coalescence of two parasites. My efforts were successful, for I was able to see repeatedly how two parasites coalesced and formed a larger body. In Plate II, figs. 53—55, such a process is depicted.

After this there can be no further doubt that the amœboid parasites coalescing with each other can form larger bodies; that these latter become the crescents also seems to me, after the foregoing arguments, as in the highest degree probable.

CHAPTER IV.

CONCERNING THE UNITY OR PLURALITY OF THE PARASITE.

Species of Parasites and Fever Types.

THE questions around which the chief interest of the investigators of malaria has been concentrated during the past few years, and which still divide them into two groups, are that of the *unity and plurality* of the malarial virus—that is to say, the malarial parasites,—and that of *the relation of the form of the parasite to the type of the fever.*

The one party, headed by Laveran, defend the view that the malarial parasite is an individual species whose various shapes are brought about by polymorphism, and that the different types of fever are not caused by different species of parasites, but by a changing individual condition of the organism attacked, the cause of which is not yet known. Laveran [88] writes in his monograph, in 1891, regarding this (page 130), "Le parasite est unique, mais son évolution est variable." He supports his view by the microscopical results obtained from numerous cases of malaria in which there did not appear to be any parallel between the type of fever and the form of the parasite.

The other party, which may be called the Italian party, believe in the presence of several genera or species and varieties of parasites, and hold fast the opinion that each type of fever (with certain limits to be mentioned presently) corresponds to a definite species. In details the individual investigators of the Italian school differ, and that considerably.

Golgi, to whom the great credit belongs of having brought order out of the chaos of the forms described by earlier observers, and who confronted the clinical symptoms of disease with the cycle of development of the parasite, considers that a definite type of fever is invariably based upon a definite variety of the parasite. He seems, however, on the other hand, to allow the possibility that one variety may transform itself into another, thereby recalling Laveran's theory of polymorphism. Marchiafava and Celli, as well as their pupils, cannot give up the belief in a single polymorphic organism, and they support this view chiefly by the difference in the forms of the parasites according to climate, to season, and to the occurrence of a change of type.

Grassi and Feletti take up a decidedly radical view, dividing the malarial parasites of man into two genera—*Hæmamœba* and *Laverania*—and into five species (allowing, however, the occurrence of variations); but they energetically deny the possibility that a definite species can be transformed into another, either through climatic or telluric conditions, or by any kind of individual predisposition of the patient attacked.

If we would judge of the correctness of these various points of view, we must examine the proofs given by the representatives of the diverging views for the facts and reasons they bring forward.

The comprehension of these somewhat complicated *pros* and *cons.* will be substantially facilitated if we first of all learn which groups they are which are regarded by the one set of investigators as independent species, and by the others as the polymorphism of one species.

Golgi, as already mentioned, was the one who, out of the confusing multitude of bodies described by Laveran, Richard, Marchiafava, and Celli, which appeared to have hardly any relation to each other, distinguished three groups which evidently differ from each other, and which appear to produce three different types of fever. Together with this division into three "varieties," and their relation to the type of fever, Golgi also first gave a picture of the development of two varieties with most minute accuracy, and so by means of this explanation of two questions an important simplification of the case was obtained.

Golgi [34 and 89] first studied a large number of quartan fevers, and found that in all cases the same form of parasite always recurred, that its process of development proceeded regularly, and that the febrile paroxysm each time corresponded to the production of a new generation of parasites (segmentation or sporulation). Soon after, Golgi [90] became convinced from three cases of tertian fever that the parasites there present, and identical with each other, were nevertheless considerably different from the parasites which he had previously studied in the quartan fevers. He later on, after repeated confirmatory observations [37], gave an accurate description of these differences, and also described the whole cycle of the development of the tertian parasite. Together with these two groups, Golgi described [91] another group, *the parasites of the irregular fever, or the fever with long intervals*, which is represented by Laveran's crescentic bodies.

Golgi, therefore, differentiates the varieties of parasites of the quartan, tertian, and irregular (or long intervalled) types of fever. A general review of the characteristics of this group has already been given in previous sections; it will be dealt with in detail below. It must be further mentioned that Golgi refers the quotidian fever to the presence of either two generations of the tertian or three generations of the quartan type of parasites, which in their development are twenty-four hours distant from each other; and that he further faces the possibility that, through the infection of blood with several generations of the one or the other variety, or of both varieties at the same time, divided from each other by not twenty-four hours, but by longer or shorter intervals, an irregular fever can take place, the ætiology of which must not be confounded with the irregular fevers of the third variety.

Marchiafava and Celli [71] confirmed Golgi's statements, in so far as they refer to the tertian and quartan parasite, in all details, but they later [38] gave as the *special parasite* of the irregular fever the *small amœboid forms* from which the crescents are produced, which they have studied for long and have repeatedly described. The *irregular fever* can be either of a continued or subcontinued type; *it may also occur in the form of a true quotidian.* As Golgi described the cycle of development of the parasite of the tertian and quartan fevers, so in like manner Marchiafava and Celli have now described that of the small parasite of the pernicious fever called by them the summer or autumnal Roman fever. Very soon after this Canalis [39] followed with a like description of the same variety of parasite, but with more attention to the crescentic bodies.

In his later publication Golgi [91] confirms the small amœboid parasites of the pernicious fever, and allows that they can also produce a quotidian fever, although much less frequently than the tertian and quartan parasites.

Marchiafava and Celli [92] in various places clearly enunciate their view that the various forms belong to a polymorphic parasite. Amongst others they quote Celli [93], who gave his experience in this connection at the Tenth International Medical Congress in Berlin, that "according to our present knowledge it may still be assumed that the single, clinical, and epidemiological depiction of malaria is based upon a uniform individual parasite."

E. Antolisei [82] first strongly supported the view, upon the basis of inoculation experiments, that from a definite form of parasites only the same kind invariably proceeds; and soon after this opinion was taken up by Grassi and Feletti, since which time it has been energetically defended.

As mentioned already, Grassi and Feletti differentiate *two genera*, namely, *the genus Hæmamœba* and *the genus Laverania*. To the first genus they reckon four species—*H. malariæ* (quartan fever), *H. vivax* (tertian), *H. præcox* (small amœboid pigmented forms of pernicious fever; by the name "pernicious fever" the summer and autumnal fevers produced by the parasites which form crescents will be indicated in the sequel), *H. immaculata* (small amœboid unpigmented forms of the pernicious fever); to the genus *Laverania* the species *Laverania malariæ* (crescentic bodies). As is seen, Grassi and Feletti not only divide the known varieties of parasites into eight species, but they separate also the small amœboid and spore-forming bodies which are met with in the pernicious fevers from the crescents. This will be referred to later on in detail.

If we inquire for the reason of these various opinions about an apparently simple matter, we must consider in the first place that the different authorities have had different material to investigate, and that their conclusions do not result from a perfectly homogeneous base. Whereas Laveran in Constantine had at his disposal severe tropical fevers, of which he says in his book [88, p. 127] that it was very difficult to separate the regular and irregular fevers from one another, and that nearly every malarial attack commenced as a continued fever, Golgi had in Pavia almost exclusively only slight forms of typical tertian and quartan fevers before him, and for a long time he found no opportunity of confirming the results obtained from pernicious fever, because the material at his disposal only provided him with such cases very occasionally. The Roman authors have material which may be characterised as being between that available at Constantine and that at Pavia, so that they have opportunity to observe both typical and excedingly irregular and pernicious fever types.

The results of this variation in the material investigated are clearly shown by the reports which Laveran and Golgi give of their cases; while Laveran found in the blood of Algerian patients every possible form of parasite all together, in a complete mêlée, Golgi had the good fortune to obtain regular and typical results from his regular and typical fever material, so that we can understand how it was that he and not Laveran was destined to recognise the grouping of the parasitic forms, and to determine their relation to the type of fever.

I find that I am in a better position than my colleagues to estimate the differences between Laveran and Golgi, because, on the one hand, I had opportunity in Vienna of observing exclusively the mildest regular forms of fever, and those not few in number; and on the other hand, through repeated and long residence in malarial districts, I was able to study a very large number of the severe forms of fever. For instance, I have never seen a crescentic body in a single case occurring in Vienna, whereas I have found them daily in numbers in the malarial districts. When one reads the observations made by colleagues in the German Empire (as far as they refer to malaria contracted locally), one fails to find in them any mention of the crescents or of the small amœboid bodies. By this one fact—the absolute non-appearance of the crescents and of the small amœboid bodies in mild intermittent cases—an important division is indicated between the parasites of a regular mild intermittent ague and those of the pernicious fevers, whether of medium or of great severity or irregular, and this division can hardly be bridged over with the polymorphism of an individual species. But I will not anticipate, but will endeavour to give the remaining reasons for the diverging views.

Let us now ask the question—in what way can the definite character of certain parasitic forms, that is their character as a true species, be proved? Our answer must be,—by a pure cultivation of each individual form with numerous inoculations, in order to fix definitely their morphological behaviour under different external conditions of life; in fact, by the method which, in bacteriology, clears up such questions with certainty, and from which we might also expect a definite solution in this case.

But, unfortunately, the numerous efforts at cultivation which have been made with the malarial parasite have so far remained unsuccessful, and therefore proof has been robbed of her sharpest weapon and referred to surrogates, the use of which leaves much to be desired. The next best method to the saprophytic pure culture is cultivation in the human organism, that is the inoculation of patients from patients (the inoculation of malarial blood from men into animals has also been unsuccessful); and we will now consider the inoculation experiments which have been undertaken chiefly by Italians, and which are of importance in elucidating the point at issue.

The table on page 300 shows the results of nineteen inoculation experiments made by different investigators; the forms of parasites, as well as the types of fever from which the patient suffered from whom the blood was taken, also the duration of incubation

TABLE I.—*Experimental Inoculations with Malaria.*

No.	Experimenter.	Form of parasite and type of fever of the source.	Period of incubation.	Form of parasite in the inoculated patient.	Type of fever in the inoculated patient.
1	Gualdi and Antolisei [107]	Quartan	10 days	Small unpigmented amœboid, later also crescentic bodies	Relapsing, irregular, sometimes subcontinuous, sometimes quotidian fever.
2	Do.	Do.	12 "	Unpigmented amœboid bodies, very slightly pigmented	Slight irregular fever.
3	Do.	Do.	15 "	?	Quartan fever.
4	Do.	Do.	12 "	Same form as at source . .	Do.
5	Antolisei and Angelini [108]	Tertian (anticipating)	11 "	Do. . .	Anticipating tertian, then quotidian.
6	Do.	Do., do. (same case as No. 5)	11 "	Do. . .	At first irregular, then tertian.
7	Gualdi and Antolisei [109]	Crescentic bodies (apyrexia)	13 "	Small amœboid bodies, 8 days later crescents	Irregular fever for 10 days, then 8 days' apyrexia and relapse.
8	Di Mattei [95]	Crescentic bodies	?	Crescentic bodies . . .	Irregular.
9	Do.	Quartan	?	Same form as at source . .	Quartan.
10	Calandruccio [96]	Do.	?	Do. . .	Do.
11	Do.	Crescentic bodies	?	Crescentic bodies . . .	Irregular.
12	Bein [101]	Tertian	12 days	Same form as at source . .	Quotidian.
13	Do.	Do. (fever type, quotidian)	12 "	Do. . .	Do.
14	Do.	Do., do.	9 "	Do. . .	Tertian
15	Do.	Do., do. (same case as No. 14)	9 "	Do. . .	First tertian, then 6 days' apyrexia, later relapse of quotidian fever.
16	Baccelli [124]	Quartan	11 "	Do. . .	Quartan.
17	Do.	Tertian	6 "	Do. . .	Tertian.
18	Gerhardt [60]	Quotidian (parasite unknown)	7 "	. . . .	First irregular, then quotidian.
19	Do.	Do., do.	12 "	. . . .	Quotidian.

and the resulting forms of parasites and types of fever produced in the inoculated patients, are clearly shown.

We will first consider the parasitic forms which were found in the blood of the inoculated individuals, together with the forms found in the patients from whom the blood was taken (and injected either hypodermically or into a vein).

In seven experiments with quartan fever and the corresponding parasites (after Golgi), there were found in four cases in the blood of the inoculated patients, solely identical forms, but in two cases, instead of these, there were found small unpigmented amœboid bodies (in one case with crescents, in the other with a few pigmented bodies). In the seventh case (No. 3 in the table) the microscopical investigation of the blood was not made. In seven inoculations of tertian parasites, the same forms were exclusively demonstrated in each of the seven inoculated patients; the same results occurred in three experiments made with crescentic bodies, in which were found, in the blood of the inoculated individuals, crescents with their immature forms, the small amœboid bodies. To sum up, *in the sixteen accurately performed experiments, there was in fourteen a complete resemblance between the forms of parasite in the source of the blood and those found in the inoculated individuals; only in two cases were forms present which were not present in the source.*

If one takes these results as they stand as a basis for further considerations, the result would be that the transformation of one form of parasite into the other (especially the quartan parasite into the small amœboid bodies)—indeed, the polymorphic nature of the parasites—is proved. These experiments were, in fact, used by Laveran to lend an apparently irrefutable support to his view. With a closer knowledge of the circumstances, however, they lose much of their weight. Gualdi and Antolisei [94], in their later publication, say with regard to one of their cases of experimental quartan fever (Case 4 in the table) that the patients whose blood was used by them for three experiments (Cases 1 to 3 in the table) were not suffering for the first time from malarial fever, but that they had already suffered from very various types of fever. They had therefore taken the material for inoculation from a source which, according to our clinical as well as our parasitological experience, could not in any way be considered as a pure source. It has, indeed, been known for a long time that persons who have once acquired a severe form of malaria may, even after a long period and under the most favorable climatic conditions, be attacked again. These relapses in localities free from malaria are to be explained only by the persistence of parasites possessing certain powers of resistance (probably the crescentic bodies) within certain tissues. It was very likely that those patients used by Gualdi and Antolisei as the source of their material, and who had continued to remain in a fever district, still retained in their blood a few crescentic bodies from their former infections. This fact became apparent at the inoculation, when these bodies came into a favorable soil in the healthy inoculated individuals.

That these few crescents which are supposed to have been present might have been overlooked by Gualdi and Antolisei is a view which does not reflect upon their conscientiousness, for I and many other investigators of malaria have only been able, after repeated examination of long series of preparations, to find isolated crescents in cachectic patients who have long recovered from fever.

Further, it appears that Gualdi and Antolisei, in ignorance of the critical nature of the experiment, did not subject the patients from whom they took the blood for a sufficiently long time to that very strict microscopical control which, as we now know, is in such cases absolutely necessary; at any rate, nothing appears in their report on this point.

There still remains one more circumstance to discuss, which increases our doubts as to the correctness of the views brought forward, namely, the very remarkable fact that the few crescents (or small amœboid bodies) supposed to be present should be able so entirely to suppress the numerous quartan varieties, whose presence is well proved.

Anyone practically experienced in bacteriology will not find this objection very convincing. It frequently occurs that in inoculations of what are supposed to be pure cultivations, results are obtained which deviate considerably from what was expected. A very few germs of an impure species may choke the numerous examples of another species which are present. How this occurs must be ascertained in each individual case, but such an occurrence would lead no one to think in the very least of polymorphism. Again, we can point to another very remarkable fact which has been stated by Di Mattei [95]. He injected a man who had suffered for months from a quartan fever, and whose blood, as proved by repeated daily observations, contained only quartan parasites, with the blood of a patient who had been infected for two months solely by crescentic bodies and their immature forms; *the result was that the quartan forms disappeared completely from the blood of the inoculated man, and in their place the crescents and the corresponding fever appeared.* Di Mattei attempted in two other cases the reverse experiment. He injected into a patient with crescents in his blood, quartan parasites, and in this case again the new arrivals supplanted the parasites which were formerly present. These are facts which give rise to various suggestions, and which stimulate to fresh experiments. I have referred to them here, only to show that we are perfectly justified in doubting the weight of evidence provided by the first two experiments of Gualdi and Antolisei, and that we cannot in the meantime accept the conclusions which Laveran has drawn from them. To prove the polymorphism of an organism, we must go as critically to work as was once done in the experiments with reference to spontaneous generation. The source of the inoculation material must be absolutely pure; before the inoculation is undertaken the blood of the patient who is to form the source must be examined with the greatest care daily for weeks; the same must be done with the blood of the patient to be experimented upon, and finally every suspicion of infection through the atmosphere must be avoided; experiments which are undertaken in a place which is free from fever, as were those of Bein's, are doubtless the most valuable.

We conclude from all the experiments mentioned here that they offer a highly unfavorable support to the idea of polymorphism; but, on the other hand, they do prove it to be very probable that the individual forms of parasites present true species which do not undergo a transformation into other forms.

I do not need to remark that a perfectly certain decision of this question can only be based upon numerous experiments, and those experiments must be undertaken under the strict conditions mentioned above.

Apart from these inoculations, which are almost as valuable as experiments by pure cultivation, there are *clinical and epidemiological facts* which indirectly, and with considerably less certainty, provide us with data on which to decide the question concerning the polymorphic or multiple nature of the virus.

Clinical observation can aid us in this question, for it is possible to examine for long periods the blood of a patient who is not subjected to a fresh infection, in order to ascertain if the form of the parasites in the blood changes, or if they belong constantly to the same cycle of development. It is clear that only such patients can be chosen for this investigation who are suffering for the first time from malaria, and in whose blood from the first only the one kind—be it the quartan parasite or the crescent—is demonstrated. These observations of blood throughout weeks

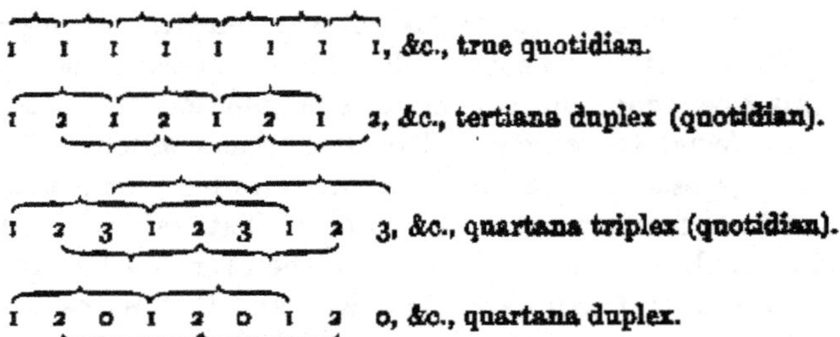

This differentiation of the quotidian fevers was made when the single attacks were of varying intensity, the attacks belonging together (in the series above, the attacks 1, 2, 3), being equally severe, or when the attacks occurred at different times of day, (for instance, the attack 1 before noon, the attack 2 after noon). Concerning the theories which have been built up to explain the typical attacks often occurring with the punctuality of a well-regulated clock, we will not enlarge here. They were not satisfactory at the time of their origin, and since the discovery of the malarial parasite they have hardly been discussed at all. They are now only of historical interest.

Golgi explains the origin of a type in this way—that the tertian parasite completes its cycle of development in twice twenty-four hours, the quartan parasite completes its cycle in three times twenty-four hours, and that the paroxysm of fever itself coincides with the breaking down of the parasite into spores, which, according to the variety of parasite, occurs either every forty-eight or every seventy-two hours.

If two generations of the tertian parasite are in the blood, or three generations of the quartan parasite, which in their development are always separated from one another by twenty-four hours, then a regular quotidian ague occurs; if the generations, however, are present either at irregular intervals or in greater number, then the fever will be as irregular in type as are these conditions. As already mentioned, it has been found by Marchiafava and Celli that there is a true quotidian fever, that is to say a fever resulting from parasites which complete their cycle of development in twenty-four hours, sometimes still faster; now several generations of these parasites can also be present in the blood simultaneously, and cause in that case respectively, either a remittent, continued, or irregular fever. Lastly, Marchiafava and Bignami [99, 100] have reported quite recently that there is a still further species of parasite which produces a true tertian fever, and that it is differentiated from the ordinary tertian

(Golgi), and can take on a pernicious character. The parasites of this malignant summer tertian fever differentiate themselves from those of the mild tertian, amongst other things, in that they form crescents, as do the quotidian parasites.

In the following table the assertions brought forward by the Italian investigators are clearly shown.

But before we commence to examine how far Golgi's statements are confirmed or disputed, we must mention a fact which it is necessary to know, especially in connection with the cases of mixed infections; this is that certain forms of parasites, even in considerable numbers, may be present in the blood without necessarily, at any rate for a short time, producing fever. These forms are the crescentic bodies. As long as only crescents are in the blood the fever is usually completely absent. Indeed, I have even met with cases in which, as well as the crescents, there have been quite a number of small amœboid bodies (immature forms of the crescent) without the patient experiencing the slightest fever. I mention this fact here because it does away with quite a number of objections which Laveran has held against Golgi's views. Whereas the Italian investigators have, almost without exception, confirmed the discovery concerning the relation between the forms of parasite and the types of fever, Laveran maintains a decided opposition. He brings forward a large number of results as the reason for his opinion, which we have now to some extent to elucidate.

TABLE II.—*Variety of Parasite and Type of Fever.*

Type of fever.	Can be ascertained by the species of parasite found in the blood.
Quartan	Only and alone by one generation of the quartan parasite (Golgi).
Tertian	1. By one generation of the tertian parasite (Golgi). Light form of tertian fever. 2. By one generation of the malignant tertian parasite (Marchiafava and Bignami).
Quotidian	1. By one generation of quotidian parasites (Marchiafava and Celli). 2. By two generations of tertian parasites (with a 24-hour interval). 3. By three generations of quartan parasites (with a 24-hour interval).

TABLE II (*continued*).

Type of fever.	Can be ascertained by the species of parasite found in the blood.
Continuous fever	1. By several generations of quotidian parasites. 2. By several numerous generations of quartan and tertian parasites (very rarely from malignant tertian parasites).
Irregular fever	1. By several generations of quotidian parasites. 2. By several generations of quartan and tertian parasites, which do not stand in a 24-hour interval to one another. 3. By the presence of several species (for example, tertian parasites and quotidian parasites of one or more generations); also by *mixed infections*.

We turn in the first place to the quartan fever, which, as is seen in the table, can, according to Golgi, be produced solely from the quartan parasite. In connection with this, there obtains amongst all the Italian investigators a clear decided opinion. I myself have little experience with the quartan fever, because it belongs to the rarities in the fever districts which I have visited, whilst the tertian and malignant fevers are very numerous; the few cases in which I have found quartan parasites were cases of mixed infection with irregular types of fever or multiple infection with quartan parasites, so that I am not able to give from personal experience a definite opinion on the point under consideration. On the other hand, detailed histories of patients of Golgi's are to hand which show the mechanism of the quartan fever to be the simplest and most punctual of all types of fever.

Laveran quotes in his book [88, p. 140] five cases of quartan fever. In three of them he found spherical bodies (in two also segmentation bodies), in the fourth spherical bodies, crescents and flagella, in the fifth crescents only. Unfortunately Laveran gives no detailed description of the characters of the "spherical bodies," and this is a great omission, for spherical bodies occur in all species of parasites, and it requires a detailed description of their appearance (movement, arrangement of the pigment, double contour) in order to form an opinion as to which species they belong. In the first three cases this omission is of less importance, for in them only spherical bodies were present and they may well be considered as belonging to the quartan parasite; the fourth case (crescents and spherical bodies) is only, according to the history, a case of quartan fever [loc. cit., p. 254]; Laveran himself had only observed a single attack. I therefore hold this case as inconclusive. In the fifth case (crescentic bodies) an attack was observed on the 19th of November in the afternoon, when the temperature reached in the evening 38·8° C. (101·8° F.). A second attack occurred on November 22nd in the morning (with the same temperature). It must be agreed with me that this case also cannot be recognised as a typical quartan fever, especially when we hear that the patient in question had suffered five weeks previously from a *Continua typhosa*; it is far more probable that it was an irregular relapse, as often happens in pernicious fevers and which in this case for once took on a type resembling quartan fever. With such hazy cases Golgi's reports, which are based upon classical typical cases observed for days and weeks, in no case are depreciated.

Turning now to the discussion of the tertian fever, as the table shows, it is, according to Golgi, produced solely by tertian parasites; Marchiafava and Bignami recently report that still a second species exists with crescents which can likewise cause a tertian fever with pernicious symptoms. I have myself described, out of thirty cases of simple tertian fever, twenty-three in which I saw Golgi's tertian parasites and seven in which I found small pigmented amœboid crescent-forming parasites, which Marchiafava and Bignami describe as the cause of the malignant tertian fever.

Marchiafava and Bignami's pernicious tertian parasite has not yet been confirmed by other authors, and for this reason we shall here turn our attention solely to Golgi's mild tertian parasite.

In Italy Golgi's views regarding this form have received complete confirmation. In Laveran's work, on the other hand, we find only a series of cases with differing results noted. In thirteen tertian fevers Laveran found in six cases spherical bodies with flagella and no crescents (probably Golgi's tertian parasite), in three cases crescents with spherical bodies, and in two crescents only. I pass over the first six cases, as they do not contradict Golgi's views. The five cases with crescents and "spherical bodies" are difficult to judge of, because we are again left in doubt as to what kind of spherical bodies were present. The report of the cases shows us, however, that here again the diagnosis does not rest upon his own observation but is obtained from the history of the case, a proceeding which is perfectly unreliable, because the patients themselves cannot judge whether they have fever or not. I have very frequently seen malarial patients who expressed themselves as perfectly well with a very high temperature, even indeed denying that they were feverish.

In reference to the two cases in which Laveran only saw crescentic bodies, the same remark applies. In the one (Case 28) there was a single attack (without the temperature being given); in the other (Case 30), as long as the crescents were present no single attack had been observed.[1]

After all this, we must admit that Golgi's views regarding the tertian fevers have not been depreciated.

In quotidian fevers the correspondence between the species of parasite and the type of fever is more difficult to demonstrate, because, as the table shows, this fever may originate in three different ways; in this case one must not only have the species of parasite in view, but it is also necessary to ascertain how many generations of the parasite present each time are circulating in the blood. The presence of several generations is recognised by the fact that the individual parasites do not keep equal pace in their development, but that, for instance, whilst part of them are already occupied in spore-formation, or are near to it, another portion is only filling up a third part of the red blood-corpuscles; when this occurs in relation to the tertian parasite, as it does in fact in Plate I, fig. *b*, then we have to do with two generations of this parasite circulating in the blood, namely, with a form of quotidian fever—the double tertian.

In a great number of double tertians I have been able to confirm the condition which Golgi has described; the slight apparent variations which occurred here will be discussed later.

The irregular fevers, still less than the quotidian, give a suitable material for the solution of the question engaging our attention, for these fevers can originate in very many ways (see the table); *they have just as little as the quotidian fever a specific character, and can only then be measured in their importance when an accurate microscopical investigation of the blood has been made. We have seen, so far, that the quartan fever is always produced by one and the same species of parasite, that the tertian fever, in the majority of cases, is called forth by Golgi's tertian parasite, but that still a second species may cause it.*

The consideration of the results of inoculation of blood of fever patients into healthy persons, as shown in Table I, is just as important as is the direct correspondence of the form of parasite and type of fever. Omitting the first two cases because, as has been explained, they are not reliable, we find in the remaining seventeen cases the following results:—From five cases of quartan

[1] It is, indeed, not impossible that both these cases, as also the other five cases, might have been caused by malignant tertian parasites.

fever, all five inoculated individuals suffered from quartan fever; from four tertian sources, twice tertian, once quotidian, and once mixed (tertian and quotidian alternating) resulted; from five quotidian cases, three times quotidian, once tertian, and once a mixed type (quotidian and tertian) occurred; and from three cases with crescentic bodies, irregular types resulted three times.

It is clear from these results that the quartan and irregular types have always given the expected results; varying results have been obtained by inoculations from quotidian and tertian fevers. These variations we shall at once recognise as *only apparent* when we see that the three quotidian cases from which Bein [101] inoculated had tertian parasites, that they were therefore really double tertians, the most frequently occurring combination; in the one inoculation (No. 13) the inoculated individual received into his blood two generations, and there consequently followed the quotidian type; in the second case (No. 14), in consequence of the inoculation one generation was evidently destroyed, and therefore only a tertian fever was produced. The third case with a mixed type (first tertian, then quotidian), is to be explained by the fact that the one generation was becoming enervated. In like manner the results from the two cases of tertian fever (Nos. 5 and 12) are to be understood.

If Bein, by his experiments, intended to upset Golgi's laws, he has therefore completely failed, and has indeed only confirmed them by further proofs. Only if he from a pure quartan could have produced a pure tertian, or *vice versâ*, would the result have been fatal to Golgi's theory.[1] Bein's error is all the more strange because Golgi has repeatedly and precisely published his views on the subject of the relation of the quotidian to the tertian as well as to the quartan. Bein would certainly not have fallen into this error if he had accurately investigated the number of the generations in the blood of the patients. In this respect the history of his patients is unfortunately without any information.

From the results and experiments here discussed, we may draw the conclusion that between the types of fever and the species of parasites an indisputable relation exists; it is especially striking that the quartan fever is always caused by the quartan parasite, the tertian fever most frequently by Golgi's tertian parasite.

The quotidian and the regular fevers, as well as certain details concerning their relative bearings, will be considered at length subsequently.

[1] Such a result from an inoculation has, up to the present, not been forthcoming.

CHAPTER V.

POSITION OF THE MALARIAL PARASITE IN THE ZOOLOGICAL SYSTEM.

NOMENCLATURE.

No unanimous opinion has yet been formulated as to the position of the malarial parasite in the zoological system; not, indeed, because the decision of this question has been in the hands of medical investigators who were not specially qualified to deal with the question, for zoologists of prominence, such as Metschnikoff, Danilewsky, and Grassi have worked with the parasite, but because the malarial parasites, and with them the hæmo-parasites, which have been discovered during the last few years in cold-blooded animals and birds, possess peculiarities which, although nearly related to already known and classified species, are, notwithstanding, differentiated from them in such a characteristic manner that it would be straining a point if they were put into the class of any of these different species. The first who gave an opinion as to the position of the malarial parasite was Metschnikoff [32], who placed it among the *Sporozoa*, in the genus *Coccidium*, in close relationship with *Klossia soror*, a *Coccidium* inhabiting the epithelial cells of the snail's kidney. He proposed for it the name of *Hæmatophyllum malariæ*. Laveran agreed with Metschnikoff, and in his last publication fully upheld his views. In the meantime an opposition arose to this idea in Italy, for Antolisei [82] denied that the parasite belonged to the *Sporozoa*, and classed it with the *Gymnomyxa* (*Proteomyxa*, Ray Lankester). At the same time, Grassi and Feletti [47] expressed the idea that the parasite was an *Amœba* belonging to the Rhizopods.

Danilewsky found in the blood of birds endocorpuscular parasites which are in some respects like the malarial parasites of man. He did not give a definite opinion as to their systematic place, but thought that they were best classed with the *Sporozoa*, and proposed to form for them a new group—*Hæmosporidia*.

Kruse believes that the malarial parasites belong rather to the genus *Gregarina* than to the *Coccidium*.

Among the difficulties which were created by the characteristic peculiarities differentiating the malarial parasite from every other known species, the circumstance that the second half of the life of this organism, namely that which it passes external to the human or animal body, is completely unknown, is of great weight, and it will hardly be possible to obtain all the requisite information for the purposes of classification before this is ascertained.

At this place, therefore, I shall avoid dealing with the general question of the classification of the malarial parasite, and shall limit myself to considering the most important points of view which are at the present held by different investigators.

Let us ask first what grounds there are for placing the malarial parasite and the similar parasites in the blood of birds and amphibians, as do Grassi and Feletti, among the *Sarcodina*, and more particularly among the *Rhizopoda*, sub-class *Amœbæa ?* First, their amœboid movement; second, their reproduction by the formation of naked spores which as such, without undergoing alteration in contents or form, represent the immature stage of the mother organism, and commence a new cycle of development.

The *amœboid movement* characterises, however, only some varieties of the parasites and only at a certain stage; as has already been pointed out at the proper place, a well-marked movement is only shown in the immature forms of the tertian and quotidian parasites, whereas in the quartan parasite it is only seen when upon the warm stage; in the parasites of birds only a slight movement is to be demonstrated, and this is often completely absent.

It is even of greater importance to note that the crescentic bodies in man show no movement whatever; they can only alter their form in a limited manner by straightening or bending themselves or by appearing as fusiform or spherical bodies; these alterations occur exceedingly slowly, without ever showing amœboid movement (projection of pseudopodia). Those parasites of the amphibians and birds which, at any rate in their external form, resemble the crescentic bodies of man, and which therefore have been compared to them, possess, if any movement at all, a worm-like one, known well in the *Gregarinæ*, and not observed in the *Rhizopoda*.

We see already, therefore, that the reason for classifying the blood-parasites with the *Amœbæa* falls to the ground. Also the supposition that reproduction by formation of naked spores takes place in the malarial parasites is open to several objections. So far no one has observed that a freed spore, either of the tertian or quartan parasite, has become amœboid; I have kept mature spore-forming bodies, in which the spores had already separated from one another under favorable conditions (warm stage, oxygen and moist chambers) for forty-eight hours and longer under the microscope, and I have never succeeded in noticing a movement in the spores. The possibility may still be admitted that the spores, before they form young amœboid parasites, pass through an intermediate stage. As above mentioned, Celli and Guarnieri (later also Plehn) believed they saw spores in the protoplasm which swarmed by means of the flagella; these forms recall the swarming spores of *Protomyxa,* which Haeckel has observed, or the zoospores of the *Myxomycetes,* but no nucleus has been stained in them, wherefore I rather look upon them as products of degeneration of the large varieties. It must be further called to mind that Antolisei has observed in the spores of the quartan parasites a double contour, that is a thicker membrane, which renders the naked character of this spore less probable.

This, as we have seen, rather meagre argument for the parasites of the blood-corpuscles belonging to the amœbæa, has other facts to contend with which still more militate against its probability. The weightiest of these facts is that the malarial parasite is necessarily a cell-parasite, whereas none of the amœbæa are known to be such, although one frequently finds such amœbæa as free living parasites, for instance in the intestinal canal of warm- and cold-blooded animals.[1]

This circumstance forms a fundamental difference between the parasites of the blood-corpuscles and the amœbæa, and this could only be overcome when in all other aspects a perfect agreement from a morphological point of view was arrived at, which is by no means proved. We have already stated why we cannot consider the flagella of the malarial parasite as non-characteristic "agony products," as do Celli, Grassi, and Feletti. The flagella also do not accord with the appearance of the amœbæa, which do not possess them, at any rate in the form in which they are present in the hæmoparasites.

When we weigh the facts brought forward in favour of and against the amœboid nature of the blood-corpuscle parasites, we find that the balance is rather in support of the latter,—that is

[1] I only once came across such an observation noted. It is taken from von Waldenburg (103), who once saw an amœbæa within an epithelial cell in the intestinal canal of a rabbit.

to say, against Grassi and Felletti's opinion, and that, at any rate, it remains doubtful whether the bodies in question are to be reckoned amongst the *Sarcodina.*

The majority of authors are inclined to consider the blood-corpuscle parasites as *Sporozoa,* indeed *Coccidia,* and we will now try to ascertain how far this opinion is justifiable.

The attribute of intra-cellular life is very widespread in the *Gregarinæ* and *Coccidia,* and hence these forms agree very closely with the hæmoparasite in this important biological character. The movements shown by the malarial parasite, even to the flagella, agree with those of the *Gregarinæ,* which in their immature condition may also be amœboid, whereas the developed forms are either immobile or only possess the power of alteration of shape (which may be accompanied by the power of progression).

There are, however, differences which must not be overlooked in morphological characters and in the method of reproduction. With regard to the first, the *Sporozoa* are distinguished by a more or less developed cuticle. In the malarial parasites we can only demonstrate this distinctly in the crescentic bodies and in the spherical bodies which are produced by them; mention must also be made of Antolisei's observation regarding the double contoured spores. We must, however, state generally that in the immature, and for the most part also in the developed, forms of the malarial parasite no vestige of a cuticle can be made out even with the highest powers. Only in specimens ready for sporing, as well as in those already mentioned, have I often seen a fine contour line, which, however, was always *single,* and therefore indicated an exceedingly thin cell membrane.

The reproduction of the *Gregarinæ,* and especially of the *Coccidia,* occurs after they have become encysted by the formation of more or less hard-shelled spores (so-called pseudonavicellæ or psorosperms), which in smaller or greater numbers are formed in the interior of the cysts. In the spores one or more sickle-shaped embryos develop, which, after creeping out, represent immature units, or the contents of the spore roll themselves together into an amœboid-like moving embryo.

When we examine the method of reproduction of the malarial parasite, we miss much of this typical spore-formation of the *Sporozoa.* To what extent an encystment is to be observed in the malarial parasite has just been indicated; excepting the crescents and their spherical bodies, one can hardly speak of cysts. So far as is already known, the formation of spores takes place *directly* without any previous formation of corticate psorosperms or pseudonavicellæ. Although there are not wanting statements concerning the direct spore-formation of non-encysted *Sporozoa*, as by Claparède, Lieberkühn, and Gabriel [105], these are not yet considered proved.[1]

The want of sickle-shaped embryos (that the crescents, notwithstanding their sickle-shaped form, have nothing to do with this has already been explained) can form no absolute objection to the malarial parasite having the nature of a *Gregarina*, i.e. *Coccidium*, because in numerous species of this class the sickle-shaped bodies are also wanting.

Further, I believe that we are not justified in asserting definitely that the malarial spores do not form sickles; for we do not yet know the method by which these spores become new immature units, and it is just possible that they pass through a sickle stage. In this place also must be mentioned Bein's [101] observation of an extra-corpuscular, worm-like crawling form in the blood of malarial patients, for it may be that these are wandering germs. The report, however, requires confirmation, and above all the structure of the wandering form must be elucidated.

We do not know what bearing the flagella of the malarial parasites has upon this relationship with the *Sporozoa*, because such organs have not been observed in that class.

Without wishing to solve the question of the systematic position of the malarial parasite, we must, after the previous statements, allow that many very important points of resemblance exist to favour the belief that the blood-corpuscle parasites are the *Sporozoa*, especially the *Coccidia*; but that, on the other hand, there are facts, although as would appear of a less weighty nature, which oppose this classification.

We will now shortly notice two of the sub-classes of the *Sporozoa*, namely the *Myxosporidia* and the *Sarcosporidia*, in regard to their points of resemblance and differences when compared with the hæmoparasites.

The *Myxosporidia* or the so-called fish-psorosperms are found in nearly all the organs of fish (fresh-water and marine) infested by them, especially in the skin and the head, in the bladder, gall-

[1] Just recently R. Pfeiffer [104] has found in the *Coccidium oviforme* a method of reproduction which he terms endogenous spore-formation, and which consists in the young parasite, either within or without the epithelial cell, falling direct into a great number of sickle-shaped embryos, without being previously encysted; the embryos are arranged like the segments of an orange. If this fact finds confirmation, teaching concerning the *Sporozoa*, especially *Coccidium*, will be thoroughly modified, and the placing of the malarial parasite into this class favoured.

bladder, in the kidney and spleen, &c. They form cysts or naked protoplasmic masses in which Bütschli [106] first demonstrated a great number of very small cell nuclei. This peculiarity appears to be characteristic of the *Myxosporidia*. According to Bütschli their reproduction takes place by the endogenous formation of clear protoplasmic bodies (*sporoblasts*) in which sickle-shaped spores are developed. The *Myxosporidia* appear not to be cell parasites, but only to attach themselves externally to the cells, thus differing from the blood parasites; their mode of reproduction occurs in a similar way to that of the *Coccidia*. *The numerous nuclei which the* Myxosporidia *contain form an essential difference from the blood-parasites, for the malarial parasites have a single nucleus.*

Those bodies with many nuclei are also termed by zoologists plasmodia, but this was a misnomer which has led to errors and to the confusion of heterogeneous ideas, so that Marchiafava and Celli have taken this name for the amœboid immature forms of the malarial parasite; this unsuitably chosen description is at present so widely used, that its elimination and replacement by a more scientific appellation is hardly now to be expected.

The *Sarcosporidia* (Miescher's or Rainey's "tubes") are fairly widely distributed parasites which are found in the primitive bundles of various striped muscles. They are specially found in the diaphragm, abdominal muscles, psoas, muscles of the eye, œsophagus and cardiac muscles of numerous animals, such as the pig, cow, sheep, goat, and deer. They are tubes which are surrounded by a membrane, and contain a large number of germs; the formation of these germs occurs continuously, and even begins in the youngest tubes. *From this description it will be seen that there is no great resemblance between the* Sarcosporidia *and the malarial parasites;* the chief resemblance consists in the fact that both are cell parasites. Active movement has not been proved with certainty in the *Sarcosporidic* germs.

We must also refer to the parasitic tubes of Crustaceans, the *Amœbidium parasiticum*, Cienkowsky. They are ectoparasites which are found attached to small fresh-water Crustaceans, insect larvæ, &c.; they have usually an elongated shape, and they also form tubes which possess a thin membrane; a number of germs is seen in their interior. Their reproduction takes place either by the formation of fusiform bodies which subsequently divide into several amœboid bodies or become *in toto* amœboid, or *by the direct division of the contents of the tube into a large number of amœboid bodies*, the so-called *zoospores*. These then form cysts which are surrounded by a very delicate membrane and then divide into fusiform bodies, or they pass for a time into a quiescent stage in which they are surrounded by a thicker envelope; later the contents of this form also divide into immature organisms. These *amœbidia* deserve our attention, because *they divide directly into zoospores* and because they have a double cycle of development—a procedure which also occurs in the malignant tertian parasites.

On the contrary the *Amœbidia* are not cell parasites, but they only attach themselves to the bodies which they infest; they are thus ectoparasites.

If we finally shortly review the characteristics of the different classes and sub-classes, we must come to the conclusion that the malarial parasites resemble all more or less, but that they are not to be identified with any of them without straining. The greatest resemblance we find nevertheless between them and the Coccidia, *both in a morphological and especially in a biological relation, for both are necessarily cell parasites.*

It will be for specialists to fix the systematic place of the hæmoparasites when they have given still further careful study to the subject and, where possible, to their condition as external parasites, or to the second half of their parasitic life, for it is possible that these parasites have considerable importance, and that they generally have not a saprophytic existence. According to present knowledge, however, it may be with some certainty supposed that for these hæmoparasites, which daily become more important in number and character, a sub-class of their own will have to be formed called *Hæmosporidia*,[1] which will be most suitably placed in the class *Sporozoaida* near to the sub-classes *Gregarinida*, *Coccidia*, *Myxosporidia*, and *Sarcosporidia*.

We have before repeatedly called attention to the parasites in the blood-corpuscles of animals; they present such special resemblance to the malarial parasites of man that several of them have been identified with these, as, for instance, the *Polymitus avium* by Danilewsky. If this identification has not been accepted by other authors, all are at any rate at one as to the near relationship between the animal and human parasites; recently zoologists and several pathologists have occupied themselves in investigating the hæmoparasites of animals with the hope that these researches would be of service in the study of human pathology.

[1] This name was first proposed by Danilewsky on account of the analogy with the terms *Myxosporidia* and *Sarcosporidia*.

Although this hope has not yet been fulfilled, because the attempts at transfer from animal to animal have been in nearly all cases unsuccessful, and also because the conditions of development of various forms, notwithstanding the ease in procuring the material, do not appear to be perfectly cleared up, nevertheless the direction followed promises to be fruitful in the future; and we must also not neglect to give our attention to the blood-parasites of animals, but only so far as it lends itself to the purposes of this book. To give a thorough explanation of all the discovered facts and the ideas coupled with them I do not think to be at the present time opportune, because the work done at present is only fragmentary, and because no agreement has been come to even in apparently primary questions, so that if I referred to all the individual opinions it would tend rather to confuse than to aid my readers in the study of malaria.

The first *Cystozoa* were discovered in 1874 in the blood of the rat by Osler [53]; a like result was subsequently attained by Lewis [54]. General interest, however, was first taken in these bodies when Gaule [55—57] found his "little blood-worms" in the blood-corpuscles of frogs, and soon after also in the blood-corpuscles of tritons and tortoises. These "little blood-worms," which Gaule did not consider to be independent organisms, and to which he, as the "most active elements of the cell," gave the name of *Cystozoa*, were later and more thoroughly studied by Ray Lankester, and named by him *Drepanidium ranarum*. They are elongated, worm-like bodies, rather pointed at the ends, lying within the red blood-corpuscles, sometimes in pairs, wandering out from them under certain circumstances, and then actively bustling about in the protoplasm. Danilewsky [74—77] succeeded in finding similar bodies in the blood of *Lacerta viridis*, *Lacerta agilis*, and in the *Emys lutaria*. He found also in the red marrow of the thigh of the Emys the reproductive bodies of the *Drepanidium*; they consist of endocorpuscular cysts in which the protoplasm divides into a large number of small sickle-shaped bodies; these are said to represent the immature forms of the *Drepanidium*. On the ground of this result Danilewsky speaks of the infection of the animals as of a psorosperming of the red blood-corpuscles.

Soon after, Danilewsky [77] discovered endocorpuscular parasites in the blood of birds, and their extraordinary resemblance to the malarial parasites described by Laveran led him to compare the two, and to identify them in certain respects with one another.

Danilewsky, like Laveran, was not able at first to form a

consecutive biological chain of the various phases of development of the different parasites which he so often met with at the same time in the blood, and in consequence he divided his discoveries in a way which took no account of the association of the forms in one cycle of development, and referred only to the passing external form of the body. I would not refer to the nomenclature, already for the most part abandoned by Danilewsky,[1] were it not that in the discussion in which we are at present engaged concerning the parasites of animals it will frequently recur.

This division is as follows:

1. *Pseudovermiculi sanguinis* (*Hæmatozoa sporozoica*).—Under this description Danilewsky understands worm-like bodies in the blood which are either completely formed or which grow out of the spherical bodies; the former possess a nucleus, are mostly thicker at one end than at the other, and show a similar movement to the *Drepanidium ranarum*, which, indeed, they very much resemble. Danilewsky found them in the blood of the small woodpecker and the owl. In these birds a second form, the *Pseudovermiculi*, was also seen; it is a worm-like organism with a nucleus in the middle, which by transformation is developed out of spherical pigmented endocorpuscular bodies. Danilewsky identifies these forms with one another, because he believes the latter to be a previous stage of the former. Such mobile worm-like bodies have not yet been observed free in the protoplasm in man; in their external form they possess a similarity to Laveran's crescentic bodies (and Danilewsky believes that they can be compared with them): they are differentiated, however, from them by the constant presence of a nucleus, by their mobility, and by their method of development.

2. *Pseudovacuolæ* (*Cystozoa*).—These are the early stages of various Hæmatozoa, and they resemble in appearance the immature forms of the malarial parasites; they form dull hyaline specks on the blood-corpuscles, and are easily mistaken for vacuoles (consequently their name). While they displace the nucleus of their host always more and more to the side, and gradually devour the hæmoglobin, they store in themselves melanin granules, which tend to swarm in the larger examples. Danilewsky found such *Cystozoa*, though few in number, *also in the white blood-corpuscles*; in this case they were naturally colourless.

In a later work Danilewsky [111] again refers to these *Leucocytozoa*, as he named the *parasites of the white blood-corpuscles*, and

[1] Danilewsky [77], in his 'Parasitologie comparée du sang,' indeed remarks pointedly that the nomenclature is only provisional.

which are especially found in the owl; and he says that these bodies are able to leave the leucocytes, whereupon they project flagella.

3. *Polymitus sanguinis avium.*—Large spherical, endocorpuscular, pigmented (or, if coming from the *Leucocytozoa*, unpigmented) bodies, possessing one flagellum or more.

This form is found in numerous birds, most frequently in the small woodpecker, the roller, and the owl; they very closely resemble the flagellated varieties of the malarial parasite (both those from the tertian spheroids and the spheroids of the crescentic series), *and it is they which Danilewsky, who has referred chiefly to the flagellated bodies of Laveran, has identified with the malarial parasites.* One must not think that Danilewsky considered the *Polymitus* and *Pseudovacuolæ* as things which had nothing to do with one another, for the opposite idea can be clearly gathered from his monograph—that the *Polymitus* represents a later stage of the *Pseudovacuolæ*.

4. *Pseudospirilla.*—Amongst these are freed flagella swimming about in the liquor sanguinis, just as they may be often seen in the malarial blood.

5. Under this heading Danilewsky describes *Trypanosoma sanguinis*, which, as an extra-corpuscular parasite, does not come into the range of our consideration.

It may also be mentioned that Danilewsky considers it probable that the young brood is infected by their diseased parents whilst feeding, because he found the parasites only in the blood of nestlings, although quite young birds have been proved non-infected. This opinion does not coincide with the generally accepted inhalations-hypothesis of human malaria.

In a yet later work Danilewsky [112] records further the interesting fact that *the birds, when the infection of their blood has reached a considerable degree, and especially when the spore-forming bodies of the* Pseudovacuolæ (*the spore-forming bodies discovered by Danilewsky*) *are present, may exhibit acute symptoms of disease which in severe cases result in the death of the bird.*

The discovery had for Danilewsky all the greater importance because through it not only the morphological and biological, but also the pathogenic similarity between the malarial parasites of man and those of the bird was proved. The birds which had fallen ill with "acute malaria" were magpies, ravens, jackdaws, and owls. The symptoms of disease were loss of appetite, weakness, sometimes convulsions, loss of weight, and rise in temperature of 1 to 1·5°. In the blood of the diseased birds very numerous endocorpuscular parasites were found which completed their cycle of development in about three or four days. At first they form exceedingly small clear specks, which lie at one pole of the oval blood-corpuscle (multiple infection is also frequent); later they show some pigment in their protoplasm, which is concentrated in the centre at the height of their development, but which does not ultimately cause the parasite to occupy more than a quarter to a third of the blood-corpuscle, for then the latter breaks up into fifteen to twenty small spores.

These parasites, then, much resemble the quotidian parasites of man (the pernicious tertian parasites of Marchiafava and Bignami). The only differences are that the parasites of birds develop more slowly (in three to four days); that they form more numerous spores; and that, lastly, their immature forms possess no amœboid movement, as is the case in those of man. For this last reason Danilewsky called them *Cystosporon malariæ-avium*, not *Hæmamœba. It is further remarkable that neither these nor the other parasites in the blood of birds are killed by quinine.*

Danilewsky [113] in his last publication differentiates an acute and a chronic malaria of birds: the first is caused by the *Cystosporon malariæ*, the second by the *Polymitus avium* and by the *Pseudovermiculi;* but the description of the diseases shows, and Danilewsky himself partly acknowledges, that the differentiation is not complete and not always possible. His attempt to distinguish between an acute and a chronic malaria in men is likely to meet with general opposition, for the commencement of every well-marked malarial infection is always acute; subsequently either a complete cure may follow, or relapses may occur, or finally a cachexia may remain which is the product of malarial anæmia and the tissue changes caused by the previous infection. None of the conditions can be called "chronic malaria." The division also of the *Polymitus* (flagellated forms) from the spore-forming bodies does not apply to men, for we know that in them the flagellated bodies occur in the tertian parasite just as frequently as they do in the quotidian parasite (spherical bodies from the crescents).

The identification of the "*Pseudovermiculi*" with the crescentic bodies is not so indisputable as Danilewsky appears to hold. Apart from the difference already mentioned between these two forms, it must also be considered that the pigment of the "*Pseudovermiculi*" does not become concentrated in the centre as in the crescents, but that it always remains at the polar regions; further, that "*Pseudovermiculi*" do not change like the crescents into flagellated spherical bodies, but that they either retain their shape or that they show a contraction which is completely unknown in the crescents; lastly, the "*Pseudovermiculi*" in birds are much rarer than all the other *Cystozoa*, whereas the crescents in malaria in man form a frequent, and in certain fevers a constant, appearance. All this taken together shows that there are between these two forms so many differences that in the meantime their identity is extremely doubtful.

In my opinion the *Polymitus avium* may be most nearly compared with the flagellated bodies of the tertian parasite, for they are both evolved from spherical bodies.

The pathologico-anatomical results of bird malaria consist, according to Danilewsky, in the enlargement of the spleen and in the pigmentation of the spleen and the liver. In "acute" malaria these appearances are said to be less in degree than they are in chronic forms.

Danilewsky's reports were followed immediately by the publications of other investigators who had occupied themselves with the study of the hæmoparasites of animals. Grassi and Feletti, Celli and Sanfelice, and Kruse have been very active in this direction, and we have to thank them for many valuable additions to our knowledge. Grassi and Feletti [114], in Sicily, found in the blood of sparrows (*Passer hispaniolensis*) and doves similar hæmatozoa to those which Danilewsky had discovered in other birds. The number of the infected birds is said to be considerable even in February, and in April and May hæmoparasites were found in the blood of all birds investigated.

Grassi and Feletti divided them into *Hæmamœba* and *Laverania* like the malarial parasites in man, and said that both genera are present in most birds, and that in some examples the crescents (*Laverania*) only were seen, but that *Hæmamœbæ* are never found alone. Like Danilewsky, these two authors say that the *Hæmamœbæ* are situated at the poles of the blood-corpuscles, and that with their growth they push aside the nucleus; whereas the *Laverania* settle themselves *by the side* of the nucleus and grow around it, so that they form at first a crescent, later on frequently a completely closed wreath. The spore-formation of the *Hæmamœbæ*, which Grassi and Feletti first recognised in sparrows, occurs after more than half of the red blood-corpuscles are replaced by them, and after the pigment has become concentrated they produce fifteen to thirty or more gymnospores. For this species of *Hæmamœbæ* from birds they employ the name of *Hæmamœba relicta*. According to them the infection of the young birds does not occur by means of the parents, as Danilewsky believes, but through the air. Later Grassi discovered in the blood of a young hawk (*Cerchneis tinnuncula*) small *Hæmamœbæ* which were *absolutely unpigmented*, and which spore without forming pigment. He calls this species *Hæmamæba subimmaculata*.

Danilewsky's *Pseudovermiculi* have not been found by Grassi and Feletti; they do not consider them, as he does, as organisms which can be compared offhand with the malarial parasites (*Laverania*), but as bodies resembling *Drepanidia*. *On the other hand, they accept, as we have seen, Danilewsky's opinion in so far that they consider the peripherally-placed, elongated, endocorpuscular parasites of birds as analogous to the crescentic bodies of man.*

It is on this point that these authors have been attacked by Celli and Sanfelice [78], and that they also partly differ from Kruse. Although Kruse's work appeared earlier, and Celli and Sanfelice agreed with his views in many respects, we will consider their work on human malaria because of their greater experience. They confirm Kruse's [115] information regarding the cycle of development of the hæmoparasites in the frog, and hold with him (in contradistinction to Grassi) that the small parasite undergoes spore-formation inside the blood-corpuscle, or that it slowly grows and leaves the blood-corpuscle as a *Drepanidium*. With reference to the parasite of the *Testudo europæa*, Danilewsky's results are confirmed by them, but they were not able to find again the spore-forming bodies which had been seen by him in the red marrow of bone.

Celli and Sanfelice chiefly studied the following birds:—*Columba livia*, *Athene noctua*, and *Alauda arvensis*. They divided the parasites found in them into three kinds, according to the rapidity of their development, as follows:

1. *Parasites with slow development.*—This is the only form which they were able to demonstrate in the *Columba livia*; its development required a duration of at least eight days—as had already been ascertained by Grassi and Feletti. The endocorpuscular forms of this species are pigmented and without amœboid movement (as with rare exceptions are all hæmoparasites of birds); they lie at the broad side of the nucleus of the blood-corpuscle, and gradually grow around it, so that the extremities of the parasite can at length meet, whereby the nucleus is encircled by the wreath-like parasite. Spore-formation has not been observed, but free, oval, and roundish bodies, usually without visible nuclei. Celli and Sanfelice compared these three forms to the *Drepanidia* of the frog and tortoise, and as the latter have shown a less complete structure and much less move-

ment than the former, they speak of a modified free phase ("si è deteriorata la fase libera").

Now, as it will be remembered, the previously-described endocorpuscular, elongated, fully-developed forms were held by Danilewsky, as well as by Grassi and Feletti, as analogous to the crescentic bodies; Celli and Sanfelice placed them parallel with the quartan parasites. I avoid giving the reasons which influenced these authors upon this question, and only remark that none of them are absolutely convincing, and that the solution of this question must in the meantime be considered as in abeyance.

2. *Forms of parasites with accelerated development.*—These are found in the *Alauda arvensis*, also in the *Passer hispaniolensis*, and correspond to the already described *Hæmamœba relicta* (Grassi and Feletti); they are compared by Celli and Sanfelice with the tertian parasite (Golgi).

3. *Parasites with rapid development* (such as *Hæmamœba subpræcox*, Grassi and Feletti), observed in the *Alauda arvensis*, *Athene noctua*, and *Passer hispaniolensis;* they form small endocorpuscular bodies which become rapidly pigmented and, at a time when they only occupy a small fraction of the blood-corpuscle, break up into some ten to fifteen spores. It is the same form whose development Danilewsky has described (see above), and which he has named *Cytosporon malariæ-avium.* Celli and Sanfelice also found here pigmented elongated bodies, often becoming free and then round, *which they compare with the crescents in man.* The whole of the third form (with rapid development) is compared by both authors with the quotidian parasite of man.

Kruse [115, 116] was the first to observe the formation of spores in the frog's hæmoparasites. Further, he found in the blood of the hooded crow (*Corvus cornix*) endocorpuscular parasites showing in their immature condition very slight amœboid movements; they either grew into "little worms," and sometimes then left the blood-corpuscles, but only when outside of the vessels (in specimens), or the elongated still endocorpuscular body became spherical, escaped from its capsule, and formed flagella (*Polymitus*, Danilewsky). Spore-formation was not observed, but sometimes a wavy contour was seen on the wreath-shaped developed forms around the nucleus, which, however, could hardly have anything to do with reproduction; similar forms have been observed by Celli and Sanfelice and by Grassi and Feletti without their ever noticing any kind of structure in the small heaps.

Attempts at inoculation have also been made upon animals by injecting the blood from infected animals into healthy ones in whose blood no alteration existed. Grassi and Feletti's experiments in this direction have been without result,—that is to say, they were never fortunate enough to infect the healthy animals; but Celli and Feletti several times obtained a positive result. They succeeded three times in six experiments in inoculating from pigeon to pigeon. The incubation lasted two to four days. The inoculation from lark to lark took in three out of twelve cases. All inoculation experiments from one species to another, as well as from animals of one class to animals of another, were negative.

The inoculation of animal hæmoparasites therefore only succeeds, if at all, when made from one animal to another of the same species and variety.

Grassi and Feletti doubt the positive results of Celli and Sanfelice, saying that so large a number of birds are infected (the infection being often missed in superficial investigation) that one can only be sufficiently guarded from errors of observation after keeping the animal to be experimented upon under observation for a long time, and ascertaining it to be free from parasites. We do not know whether Celli and Sanfelice observed these precautions or not, but the extensive experience of Celli makes us expect that his experiments have been carried out with the strictest precautions. Besides, the analogous experiments in men render the possibility of inoculations also from animal to animal likely.

Celli and Sanfelice likewise experimented on pigeons therapeutically with *quinine;* like Danilewsky, they observed that the parasites of birds are *not killed by this drug.* The alteration which certain of the parasites suffer (rounding of the elongated form, a clearer prominence of the nuclei in them) are so small as to be hardly appreciable.

It is undoubtedly a very remarkable fact, and one which deserves further investigation, that a remedy which affects the parasites in man so successfully hardly alters the hæmoparasites in birds.

From the short summary of results which have been given here on the investigations of animal blood, it may be gathered that little has been gained with regard to the investigation of malaria. The authorities apparently diverge so much in their opinions on single points, that even now it is not decided which phases and forms of the different hæmoparasites are to be brought into correlation with one another, what the method of development of the numerous forms is, how the infection of animals takes place, whether the animal hæmoparasites are pathogenic under all circumstances, or if they are to be considered as "necessary parasites."

In this place it seems necessary to say a few words concerning nomenclature. As has been already seen, no unanimity exists in the naming of the hæmoparasites. Such a number of different suggestions lie before us for their description, that one is much perplexed when it is necessary to fix upon any one of them.

We will summarise here the various suggestions.

I. *Human Parasites.*

1. *Oscillaria malariæ* (Laveran), rejected by the author himself.
2. *Hæmatozoon malariæ* (Laveran).
3. *Hæmatophyllum malariæ* (Metschnikoff).
4. *Plasmodium malariæ* (Marchiafava and Celli).
5. *Hæmatomonas malariæ* (Osler).
6. (*a*) *Hæmamœba* { *malariæ* (quartana). / *vivax* (tertiana). / *præcox* (pigmented quotidiana). / *immaculata* (unpigmented quotidiana).
   (*b*) *Laverania malariæ* (crescent) (Grassi and Feletti).

II. *Animal Parasites.*

1. *Bloodworms* (Gaule).
2. *Cystozoa* (Gaule).
3. *Drepanidium* (Ray Lankester).
4. *Pseudovacuolæ*
5. *Pseudovermiculi*
6. *Polymitus avium*
7. *Pseudospirillæ*
8. *Cystosporon malariæ-avium*
9. *Hæmogregarina*

   (4–9) } Danilewsky.
10. *Hæmoproteus* (Kruse).
11. *Hæmamœba* { *relicta* / *subpræcox* / *subimmaculata*
    Laveranum ranarum
    Laverania Danilewskii (in birds).

    (11) } Grassi and Feletti.

Of all these names only a single one, and that the least applicable, has taken root. It is the name *Plasmodium*, which was given by Marchiafava and Celli to the small unpigmented amœboid immature forms of summer fever. It is also not at all what Marchiafava intended for a spore-forming body or a crescent, for instance, to be called a *plasmodium*; indeed, this name has also been very unsuitably chosen for the small amœboid bodies for which it was first used. This has been repeatedly shown, even by the authors themselves.

Zoologists designate by the name of *Plasmodium* bodies which are formed by the conjunction of numerous *Amœbæa*, each of which maintains its nucleus. A *Plasmodium* is in reality, in a scientific sense, a multinuclear protoplasmic mass, and is utterly inapplicable to the malarial parasite, which, as is well known, possesses with hardly an exception a single nucleus. The name is also unpractical, for we have not to deal with one, but with numerous kinds varying from one another, each of which requires a designation in order that it may be readily recognised. With regard to the other designations, it is doubtless true that several of them have been rationally and practically chosen, and were certainly worth definitely retaining. I refrain, however, from choosing one of them because I am of opinion that it is the business of specialists to definitely choose a name which would completely agree with the zoological attributes.

Until they do this we will, with Laveran, and without prejudice, speak of *Hæmatozoa*, and use it as a general and provisional name for the malarial parasite. It can be used quite well as a detailed description, as will be seen later on. We desist, indeed, from bringing under consideration the blood-parasites of animals which resemble the malarial parasite, for this is of little importance to our purpose, which is chiefly the study of malarial fever in man.

CHAPTER VI.

CLASSIFICATION OF THE MALARIAL PARASITES.

Special characteristics of the different species : the quartan parasite, the common tertian parasite, the pigmented quotidian parasite, the unpigmented quotidian parasite, the malignant tertian parasite—Degeneration forms—Mixed infection.

In the last chapter we have already touched upon the question of the classification of the malarial parasite. We have seen there that Golgi divides the parasites into those of the quartan, tertian, and irregular (or long-intervalled) types; further that Grassi and Feletti differentiate five species. These five species are divided by them into two genera, *Hæmamœba* and *Laverania.* This division of the crescent from the amœboid bodies with direct spore-formation was opposed by the Roman investigators, whilst Grassi and Feletti [86] in their last detailed publication maintain their opinion and state their reasons.

As previously explained, Marchiafava and Celli found that in the blood of severe Roman summer and autumn fevers there were to be seen small unpigmented or slightly pigmented parasites. In a certain percentage of cases they also observed crescentic bodies. Marchiafava and Celli at first found these latter forms very rarely ; when, however, in consequence of the investigations of Canalis, they gave more attention to these bodies, they saw them much more frequently. Further, they first observed and described the spore-formation of the small amœboid bodies ; this occurs almost exclusively in the internal organs, so that it is most rare to find spore-forming bodies in blood taken from the finger. The unpigmented bodies are never seen in it.

Canalis [39] showed that the small parasites of this pernicious fever either spore direct or form crescents which can likewise later fall into spores. He designated this combination *as development in two cycles.*

Marchiafava and Celli also, as well as their pupils, regard the crescents—without recognising their power of spore-formation—as a form of development of the small amœboid bodies of pernicious fever previously mentioned.

Grassi and Feletti, differing from others, *imagine a complete variation in species between* (1) *the direct spore-forming and* (2) *the crescent-forming amœboid parasites.* They maintain that there are *two species* of small amœboid parasites which cannot be differentiated in their immature condition: the one falls direct into spores (like the quartan and tertian parasites) and causes the true severe pernicious fever; the other forms itself into crescents (which later likewise fall into spores), and is the cause of the mild relapsing fever with long intervals. That the spore-forming small forms with the crescents are found in the blood is explained by Grassi and Feletti as *a mixed infection with both species.* They classify the former spore-forming small bodies in the genus *Hæmamœba* (in which they also class the parasites of the quartan and tertian fevers under the name of *H. malariæ* and *H. vivax*), and they divide them, according to whether they form pigment or remain unpigmented up to spore-formation, into two species, *H. præcox* and *H. immaculata;* the others, crescent-forming parasites, they classify in the genus *Laverania,* to which (of the malarial parasites of man) only one species belongs—the *L. malariæ.* They explain their divergence from all other authorities in making this division as follows:

1. In six cases of severe pernicious fever they found the *H. præcox* and *Laverania* five times, and in one case they only found *H. præcox;* whereas the former must have been a mixed infection, the latter was a single infection.

2. In the three cases of summer fever with amœboid bodies of undetermined character and crescents, they punctured the spleen at the commencement of the attacks several times (the number is not given); they found *no* spore-forming bodies in the splenic blood, as should have been the case according to Marchiafava and Celli, but only discovered numerous crescents.

3. These cases without spore-forming bodies (without *H. præcox* and *H. immaculata*) were never pernicious, but invariably mild.

I cannot accept this classification in so far as it refers to a division of *Laverania* and *Hæmamœbæ,* because I agree with the

Roman school and Canalis that the same small amœboid bodies can either form spores or crescents; my reasons are as follows:

1. The crescents are found in such a large majority of the cases with the small amœboid parasites that it appears to me to be improbable that they can all be mixed infections. I observed crescents thirty-seven times in forty-three cases of this kind, and as these bodies are often exceedingly rare, a negative result must not necessarily be decisive.

2. The crescents indeed appear sometimes even in the first days of the illness (I have myself seen isolated ones appear on the third day). In the great majority of the cases, however, they first appear later, and are often only to be demonstrated much later; as this refers to hospital patients, in whom a second infection is excluded, the crescents can only have originated from certain bodies which were already present.

3. I have observed very severe summer fever with exceptionally few amœboid bodies and relatively numerous crescents, as also mild fevers with numerous amœboid bodies and few crescents.

4. *If the number of crescents is constantly in striking disproportion to the number of the amœboid bodies, it is on that account very improbable that they represent a necessary stage of development.*

5. The fact that in three cases Grassi and Feletti found no spore-formation is not conclusive, for sometimes we find also in tertian fevers, even in severe attacks, no spore-forming bodies; further, those three cases were treated with quinine, therefore altered to some extent, which may have hindered the undisturbed development of the parasites.

Grassi and Feletti also appear to deviate from the usual method in the recognition of the spore-forming bodies; take, for instance, the first three "spore-forming varieties" which they in their last article [86] under Fig. 6 have drawn as germinating bodies of the crescent. It is not perfectly certain in the first place that these drawings really represent spore-forming bodies, but there is no ground for supposing that they proceed from the crescents; quite the opposite, they give me the impression that they are, if anything, segmentation bodies produced from amœboid parasites.

On the basis of the facts just brought forward I do not agree with the classification of the malarial parasites into two genera, but I believe in the four species which Grassi and Feletti class in the genus *Hæmamœba*, and I divide these four species into two groups according to whether or not they form crescents—which in my opinion are syzygies.

To the four certainly known species the parasites of the Tertiana æstiva (Marchiafava and Bignami) are still to be added, and must be placed in the group of those which form syzygies.

Our classification is then as follows :

I. The malarial parasite with spore-formation without the formation of syzygies (*i. e.* without crescents).

(*a*) The quartan parasite.

(*b*) The tertian parasite.

II. The malarial parasite with spore-formation and with the formation of syzygies (that is, with crescents).

(*a*) The pigmented quotidian parasite.

(*b*) The unpigmented quotidian parasite.

(*c*) The malignant tertian parasite.

We now proceed to describe the distinguishing features of these five species.

I. The Malarial Parasite with Spore-formation without Syzygies.

The parasites belonging to this group are the chief producers of *true typical ague.* Even if this fever causes paroxysms of considerable severity, they do not present a pernicious character; they yield rapidly and completely to a rationally administered course of quinine, and when, after convalescence, a fresh infection is avoided no relapse occurs.

It must be remembered that the quartan and tertian parasites do not only produce typical ague, but that when several irregular generations are present they can produce also irregular fever; in comparing these with the rarely occurring typical cases of irregular fever, an examination of the blood will not only give the prognosis but also indicate how the quinine should be administered.

The process of development of the two species of parasites belonging to these groups has been demonstrated by Golgi, and except in minor details we need not deviate from his description.

(A) *The Quartan Parasite.*

The quartan parasite completes its cycle of development (from the spore to the formation of spores) in three times twenty-four hours.

In its immature condition it is an unpigmented body, which appears as a small clear speck upon the blood-corpuscle infected by it (see Plate II, fig. 1); it possesses a lazy amœboid movement, which is usually first seen when the warm plate is used.

The parasite remains in this stage from twelve to twenty-four hours, gaining meanwhile only slightly in size. The storing up of pigment now follows in the external layer of the parasite; it consists of fairly coarse, very dark rods and grains, and shows no movement. With the increasing formation of pigment the parasite loses the small power of moving which it had at first possessed, and it is met with therefore as a completely quiescent spherical body, already filling from one third to one half of the blood-corpuscle (see Plate II, fig. 2).

The parasite slowly grows larger and reaches in normal development the size of the red blood-corpuscle, so that when this stage of development is reached nothing more whatever is seen of the blood-corpuscle; in this condition the parasite is to be regarded as a *free* body.

It now prepares itself for spore-formation thus:—the pigment granules collect in the middle of the body and form there a compact mass, and at the periphery of the protoplasm a radial delineation becomes visible, which later on is also seen in the central part; these radiating lines, becoming gradually clearer, divide the parasite into a variable number of segments; as a rule the number does not exceed ten. (Plate II, figs. 4, 5.)

At length the grooving becomes so decided that the segments just described get separated from each other as small oval bodies ("daisy form," Golgi; Plate II, figs. 6, 7, 8); then a circumscribed bright spot makes its appearance in each of these bodies and represents the nucleolus, the appearance of which lends to the segment the character of an independent organism. There are now the completely developed spores, which hang together so loosely that slight pressure on the cover-slip is enough to make them break away from each other; also without such pressure the spores suddenly become scattered, probably in consequence of their growth and the bursting of the thin membrane enclosing them. With this the cycle of the parasite's development is accomplished. The pigment débris remaining over soon leaves the leucocytes as dead matter.

The segmentation of the parasites takes place before and during the paroxysm of fever; as a rule the first mature spore-formed bodies are seen about three hours before the onset of the cold stage, at which time, however, as Golgi [34] has shown, the temperature may be already considerably raised.

The spore-forming bodies may deviate more or less in their form and size from the normal. It may happen, for instance, that spore-formation occurs when the parasite has not yet reached the size of the red blood-corpuscle; then the number of spores tends to be less than usual (four to six). The spore-formation which Canalis [39] depicts (see Plate II, fig. 10) is interesting; it is fan-shaped, and is produced by the pigment having become excentrically concentrated: further, the nucleolus may be missed in fresh spores of the quartan parasite. (See Plate II, fig. 9.)

The red blood-corpuscles which are infected by the quartan parasites do not alter their size; in this they differ considerably from the blood-corpuscles infected with the tertian parasite. It is also worthy of note that they lose the colouring matter slowly, so that round about the mature parasite a thin, but still quite normally coloured edge, which represents the residue of the blood-corpuscles, can be often appreciated (see Plate II, fig. 4).

The several divisions of a fever cycle of the quartan type present the following parasitic appearances:

Twelve hours after the attack: small unpigmented parasites lying on the red blood-corpuscles, having either a sluggish amœboid movement or none at all.

Twenty-four hours after the attack: some of the bodies possess scanty pigment granules at the periphery, others are still without pigment; their size is about a sixth to a fifth of that of the red blood-corpuscle.

Forty-eight hours after the attack (twenty-four *before* the following attack): the parasites occupy the half or two thirds of the red blood-corpuscle; they are markedly pigmented; their form is usually round; there is no amœboid movement, the pigment is also quiescent.

Sixty hours after the attack (twelve hours *before* the next attack): the parasites fill the red blood-corpuscles so far that only a small edge, still clearly recognised by its colour, remains.

Sixty-six hours after the attack (six hours *before* the next attack): nothing more of the edge of the blood-corpuscle is to be seen on many parasites; the pigment is arranged in radii, in some bodies already loosely concentrated. Signs of commencing spore-formation can be made out in isolated parasites.

Sixty-nine hours after the attack (three hours before the next attack): isolated matured spore-forming bodies; many other parasites with concentrated pigment and the signs of commencing spore-formation.

It remains to be mentioned that in large free spherical bodies, which probably remain sterile, an active swarming of the pigment is sometimes seen; the projection of flagella is seldom observed in the quartan parasites.

In the quartan parasites the cycle of development occurs more regularly than in the remaining species of parasite, both as to duration and progress in isolated individuals. Here, too, one has the most frequent opportunity of finding spore-forming bodies in the circulating blood. The parallel progress forwards of a parasite belonging to a generation or a series makes it in this case relatively easy, when several generations are present, to recognise them and to judge of their age.

It has already been remarked in a former chapter that the quartan parasites, arranged in regular twenty-four hours of two or three generations, can form the two types of fever:—1 2 0, 1 2 0, 1 2 0, &c.; or 1 2 3, 1 2 3, 1 2 3, &c. The first is named double quartan, the second triple quartan—a form of false quotidian fever. Irregular types of fever occur not seldom (especially if sufficient quinine is not taken) through storing up of the generations, in the sense that their evolution does not occur in twenty-four hours, but in shorter or longer intervals.

The detailed relations of the structure of the quartan parasite have been studied by Grassi and Feletti [47]; as they resemble very nearly those of the tertian parasite, I refer to the following section for the necessary description.

(B) *The Tertian Parasite.*

The duration of the development of the tertian parasite covers forty-eight hours. As quite a young parasite it forms a small body having a diameter of 1 to 2 μ, which appears as a rather clear speck upon the red blood-corpuscle; in this stage the parasite is still unpigmented, or only exceedingly fine pigment dust is found in it. On the other hand, an active amœboid movement is noticeable. This can be easily established at the temperature of the room, and it continues clearly under the microscope for a long time (about an hour) after the blood is taken. It consists not only of a slight change in form, but from the periphery of the body projections (pseudopoda) go forth in different directions; they are soon again withdrawn in order to give place to another formation. In this condition (the first phase of Golgi) the parasite remains gradually growing for about twenty-four hours after its origin. It continuously collects to itself more pigment in the form of fine granules and rods, which are especially to be seen in the peripheral layers of the protoplasm, and which are mostly engaged in active swarming movement; the more the parasite contains of this pigment—the more developed it therefore is—the less becomes its amœboid movement; nevertheless it remains still so far amœboid that we see in a simple tertian fever, on the days of apyrexia, pigmented bodies, often strangely twigged by pseudopoda, which still actively continue to change their form, although at about this time they already occupy more than the half of the blood-corpuscle (see Plate II, figs. 11—18).

The red blood-corpuscle itself has in the meantime likewise undergone changes, *having lost in colour* (looking pale when compared with the non-infected blood-corpuscles), and further *having become enlarged*, often rather considerably. *Therefore the blood-corpuscles infested with the tertian parasites are very frequently distended and pale.*

After a duration of life of about forty-eight hours there follows —always, however, in only a fractional number of the parasites— *the spore-formation.* This commences as follows:—the body, which has now nearly or completely reached the size of a normal red blood-corpuscle, and still lies in the distended, already almost perfectly decolorised host, loses every motion; even the pigment stops swarming. The segmentation itself occurs, according to Golgi [37], in three different ways.

The usual method of spore-formation, which has been seen by all other authorities and which I have often been able to confirm, is as follows:—whilst the pigment concentrates itself in the middle of the body and there cakes together into a thick mass, the protoplasm of the parasite breaks down into some fifteen to twenty round, strongly refractile little balls (spores), which usually form an irregular heap, reminding one in appearance rather of a bunch of grapes or a mulberry. More rarely they lie near one another in two perfectly regular concentric rows, whereby the "sunflower" of Golgi is produced. It must not be forgotten that we view these bodies, which, in consequence of falling into spores, have a loose connection, between two glasses; and it is not impossible that by the mechanical influence, which cannot be wholly avoided in the preparation, the original regular form may be interfered with (see Plate II, figs. 20, 21).

The spores of the tertian parasite are round and smaller than the quartan parasite; they show in the fresh condition, as a rule, no details of structure. Here and there I have, notwithstanding, noticed on them a brilliant granule—the nucleolus (see Plate II, figs 22, 23).

Golgi's second method of spore-formation, which has hitherto not been confirmed by any other observer, takes place thus :—the concentrated pigment in the middle of the body, together with a small part of the protoplasm which is surrounded by a membrane, remains behind as a residual body, and only the periphery of the parasite falls into spores. After this, Golgi leaves it undecided whether the protoplasm surrounding the pigment is not subsequently segmented. In this case the second method of spore-formation would appear to be only a preparatory one to the first (see Plate III, fig. c).

In the third method of spore-formation the concentration of the pigment occurs near the periphery, a vacuole originates in the protoplasm and in this one or two bodies appear as segmentation products. Golgi himself did not know how to estimate the importance of this form with certainty; other authors, as Antolisei [117], recognise it as a form of degeneration.

Again, another method of spore-formation must be noted which not infrequently occurs and is mentioned by Celli and Guarnieri. It consists in the segmentation occurring without the pigment being concentrated at all and whilst it still forms irregular meshes lying scattered in the body. Lastly, it may happen that the pigment is concentrated in two heaps instead of in one (see Plate I, fig. A.).

According to this, then, the chief characteristic of the act of spore-formation of the tertian parasites is the formation of numerous (fifteen to twenty) *small round spores.*

The pigment is also here, as indeed always, a lifeless product; after the spores have parted from one another it becomes immediately seized on by the leucocytes in the circulating blood and in them it is again seen.

Just as in the quartan form, the act of spore-formation in the tertian form corresponds to the febrile paroxysm; here also like in the quartan, as Golgi has shown, a gradual rise in temperature begins about three hours before the commencement of the rigors and, answering to this, there are already to be found at this time isolated spore-forming bodies in the blood; they are, however, found in the greatest number during the rigors or at the beginning of the subjective heat.

Prominence must be given to the fact that in the tertian variety the spore-forming bodies are not seldom looked for in vain in the peripheral blood; it is to be supposed that in such cases only a few individuals reach the spore-forming stage and that these few remain chiefly retained in the internal organs, for which we have an analogy in the quartan parasite.

Again, now and then it happens that isolated spore-forming bodies may be found at a time far removed from an attack; it is even possible for still a second feeble generation to be present in the blood which spores at another time but is too sparsely represented to produce an attack.[1]

It must also be called to mind that in other ways the spore-forming bodies of the tertian parasite do not all show the complete typical picture which Golgi has drawn of them, but that now and then they present different appearances from the normal, and these one must be able to recognise in order to avoid erroneous conclusions.

For instance, it happens not infrequently that bodies which at first only fill a small part of the red blood-corpuscles already spore (see also the anticipating tertian); they do not then form such a large number of spores as do the fully mature parasites, but a markedly less number (see Plate II, figs. 22, 23); in this these spore-forming bodies resemble closely those of the pigmented quotidian parasite (see Plate II, fig. 35), from which they are only to be differentiated by a considerable amount of pigment and by the larger size of the individual spores. In such cases the other elements found in the blood will be conclusive.

The microscopical results obtained from a *simple tertian* fever can be expressed in the following tabular form:

One to twelve hours after the attack: small unpigmented actively amœboid-moving forms attached to the red blood-corpuscles or in part already entered into them.

Twelve to twenty-four hours after the attack: rather larger forms filling about a third of the blood-corpuscles, carrying the finest pigment dust and still possessing active amœboid movement. The infested blood-corpuscles pale and large.

Twenty-four to thirty-six hours after the attack (twenty-four to twelve hours before the following attack): the bodies fill from two thirds to four fifths of the pale enlarged blood-corpuscles; they are often of a very irregular shape, and this they change only

[1] With reference to the quartan variety, Golgi [34] makes the statement that in several cases he has seen spore-forming bodies unconnected with an attack; the temperature showed itself to be *raised*, but the patient had no knowledge of it. Such observations indeed appear to be very rare. I have never met with one, and in the literature we only find a single reference to the subject—a statement by Celli and Guarnieri [46].

very slowly, but o... coarse pigment gran... parasite itself is tremu...

Thirty-six to forty-... before and up to the nex... almost the same diamete... pigment still moves, in ... mencing and completed sp...

As an illustration of the ... and the progress of the feve... fever is given:

K—, æt. 20, had a first att... attacks on August 23rd and 25... 11 o'clock in the morning; the ... typical—cold, hot, and sweating s...

August 25th, 5 p.m.—Tempera... cold stage commenced at 11 a.m.

Under the microscope the bloo... large bodies which filled the hal... colorised blood-corpuscles; they fil... pletely. 2. Some completely form... bunches of grapes; numerous bod... tion. 3. Isolated quite small, unpigme... youngest form from which the spore... duced at the commencement of the atta... are about six hours old).

26th, 10 a.m.—Temperature 36·0° C. ...

Under the microscope are seen.— ... amœboid bodies which occupy a fifth ... corpuscles. 2. Isolated large forms with ... movement (sterile forms of the previous ...

5 p.m.—Temp. 36·3° C. (97·3° F.).

Microscopical appearances of blood: ... often markedly branched, endocorpuscu... from a quarter to a half of the blood-corpus... dropsical forms.

27th, 9 a.m.—Temperature 37·2° C. ...

Microscopical appearances: 1. Very ... which either occupy the half or the who... puscles. Many of the infested blood-corpusc... decolorised. 2. In some of the large bodies the ... cent (commencing spore-formation).

have been produced already
... No. 3).

...ly attacks of fever since
...ave a typical character—
... very anæmic; herpes
...er-breadths below the

... (98·2° F.).
...amœboid, actively
...ge parasites occupy-
...cles with actively

...vere rigors.

in less number
...poring; also
...l half-deve-
...boid move-
...ously. 3.
...generation
...ies, both

Profuse

in the
...scles
...nber
...nly

...res

11 a.m.—Temperature 39·5° C. (103·1° F.); rigors, &c.

From the above it is easy to construct a scheme for the double tertian in which the attacks occur at regular or irregular hours of the day.

To illustrate this complicated relation, the history of two patients suffering from double tertian, together with the microscopical results, are now given.

F. W—, æt. 19, worker in glass, has suffered from attacks of fever for fourteen days; at first the attacks occurred every second day, subsequently daily. Yesterday (August 11th) the attack commenced at 11 a.m.; to-day (August 12th), at 3 p.m. At 5 p.m. temperature was 39·2° C. (102·5° F.). Spleen distinctly felt, pain in limbs.

Microscopical appearances: 1. Very numerous pigmented bodies which completely fill up the blood-corpuscles. 2. Very numerous pigmented parasites in active amœboid movement which half fill the red blood-corpuscles. 3. Very numerous free pigmented balls, disintegrated forms seen in the blood-corpuscles (fever forms; see below). 4. Spore-forming bodies not found.

August 13th, 11.15 a.m.—Rigors commence. Temperature 38·2° C. (100·7° F.).

Microscopical appearances: 1. Enormous numbers of spore-forming bodies, partly regularly, partly irregularly arranged. Number of the spores about fourteen; in many spores the nucleolus is visible. 2. Fairly numerous amœboid, very slightly pigmented bodies which occupy about a third of the red blood-corpuscle. 3. Several large forms with flagella (one with five flagella).

5 p.m.—Temperature 37·5° C. (99·5° F.). Profuse perspiration.

Microscopical appearances: 1. Isolated large forms, partly with moving pigment, partly as if coagulated. 2. Numerous actively moving, slightly pigmented forms which occupy one third to two thirds of the red blood-corpuscles. 3. Numerous, very small, unpigmented, active amœboid bodies; some have only the finest points of pigment. 4. No more spore-forming bodies are to be seen.

It is at once evident that in this case we have a double tertian (that is to say, false quotidian) with *two generations* of parasites present. In the observation last noted, three generations appear to be found, but it is easily seen that the isolated large forms mentioned under No. 1 are only to be considered as the residue of that generation which had caused the paroxysm of fever that had occurred six hours previously. The immature forms from which the spores of this generation have been produced already appear as very small amœboid bodies (No. 3).

J. M—, æt. 20, has suffered from daily attacks of fever since August 1st. They occur at midday and have a typical character—cold, hot, and sweating stages. Patient not very amæmic; herpes labialis; the spleen extends for two finger-breadths below the ribs.

August 8th, 11 a.m.—Temperature 36·8° C. (98·2° F.).

Microscopical appearances: 1. Small amœboid, actively moving, but already pigmented bodies. 2. Large parasites occupying the third or the whole of the blood-corpuscles with actively swarming pigment.

2 p.m.—Temperature 38·2° C. (100·7° F.). Severe rigors.

3.15 p.m.—Temperature 40·5° C. (104·9° F.).

Microscopical appearances: 1. The large bodies in less number than at 11 a.m.; part of them appear to be sporing; also mature spore-forming bodies are present. 2. Small half-developed bodies in large numbers, possessing active amœboid movement; at the same time the pigment swarms vigorously. 3. Some small still unpigmented bodies (the youngest generation from to-day's attack). 4. Numerous disintegrated bodies, both free and more rarely endocorpuscular (fever forms).

6.30 p.m.—Temperature 40·1° C. (104·1° F.). Profuse perspiration.

Microscopical appearances: 1. Both young generations in the same condition; some of the recently infested blood-corpuscles are already swollen. 2. The large forms already less in number than two hours ago; some small spore-forming bodies with only five spores.

9 a.m.—Temperature 36·5° C. (97·7° F.). Patient still perspires profusely.

Microscopical appearances: 1. Large endocorpuscular forms; the pigment only moves slightly. 2. Small, already fully pigmented, actively moving parasites, occupying about a fifth or a sixth of the blood-corpuscles.

Patient received at 9 a.m. 0·6 grm. of bisulphate of quinine (9¼ grains).

12.45 p.m.—Temperature 37·0° C. (98·6° F.)

Microscopical appearances: 1. Large forms rather increased in number, with quiescent or moving pigment. The blood-corpuscles are either completely or three quarters filled by them. 2. The small amœboid forms less numerous than three hours ago; their amœboid movement is in part very feeble, in general considerably feebler than formerly (due to the action of the quinine). 3. Fairly numerous dissevered little balls, also endoglobular forms not infrequent (due to the action of the quinine).

Towards 3 p.m. violent rigors, which lasted till 3.30 p.m.

3.45 p.m.—Temperature 40·6° C. (105° F.)

Microscopical appearances: 1. Several developed spore-forming bodies with thirteen to fourteen spores; several indistinct spores (quinine spores). 2. A remarkable number of the amœboid immature forms are disintegrated (action of quinine and fever).

August 10th, 9 a.m.—Temperature 36·5° C. (97·7° F.). (At 7 a.m. patient took 0·6 gramme of quinine (9¼ grains)).

Microscopical appearances: 1. Several mature forms with fairly active pigment movement. 2. Younger forms exceptionally sparse.

12 p.m.—No attack of fever.

As we see, in estimating the microscopical appearances of the blood, not only must Golgi's scheme be kept in view, but other factors come under consideration which really determine the appearance of the blood.

Among these, first in importance is the circumstance *that we never have to do with absolutely one generation of parasites in the blood;* were this the case, if indeed every one of the parasites which we count as belonging to one generation were just the same age to the minute, if all formed spores and as individuals disappeared at the same moment, then the appearance of the blood would perfectly correspond to the scheme. In reality, however, parasites of the same generation are separated from each other in age by one or often by six to eight hours. To separate the generations from each other would therefore not be possible, because for this the necessary limits (Grenzen) would be wanting; the separation is, however, not needed, for we only want to place together in one group or as one generation all those parasites which cause one paroxysm of fever, whether they are of exactly the same age or whether differing by several hours.

The fact that the individual parasites of one "generation" do not form spores at the same moment, but one after another at very short intervals, obviously results in the clinical phenomenon that the paroxysm of fever also not only lasts for a few moments but for several hours, often for half a day. If the innumerable spore-forming bodies, like a volley of countless guns, *were to burst in one given moment* and strew their contents in the circulating blood, then most probably a paroxysm would result much shorter but therefore so much the more violent and disastrous in character, but as a matter of fact the spread of the spores takes place like a kind of file-firing and maintains the paroxysm throughout several hours.

This difference in the age of the parasites of one generation results naturally in a difference, though perhaps not very important, in their size, form, and other qualities at a given moment, and it would be a mistake to be misled by these unimportant differences.

One must further remember *that a large number of parasites do not reach maturity, therefore do not spore;* we do not know with certainty the reason for this, but it is a fact that has sufficient analogies in the animal world to prevent us from being particularly astonished at it. The most probable thing is that the units which remain sterile succumb in the "struggle for existence" or, to be more explicit, that they give way to those forces which the power of resistance of the human organism brings to bear in the struggle against the dangerous invaders; this will be more fully considered in the section upon spontaneous cure. These non-sporing individuals reach the size of their more successful comrades, and not seldom some are also seen which have become much larger and in which the play of the swarming pigment granules is an extraordinarily lively one. *These distended forms have already been held by Laveran to be dropsical degenerating bodies*, and it seems that this is really the case. They are still found in the blood several hours after the end of the attack, and are even to be seen on the days free from fever in pure tertian. It is clear that one cannot regard these sterile surviving spherical bodies as proofs against Golgi's law.

Another series of bodies also complicating the picture presented by the blood is found in the "*fever forms;*" these are the *débris of parasites* which are frequently found *free in the liquor sanguinis, often indeed even in the red blood-corpuscles.* They are mostly round, and several often hang together; it is not easily possible to mistake them for spore-forming bodies, because they are irregularly pigmented and differ in size (see Plate III, figs. 33, 34).

We have now to consider one more interesting form which has been noted also in the double tertian, namely, the flagellated body. These bodies are seen very frequently in tertian fevers, especially at the time of the onset of the fever or shortly before it, which, as already observed, is the reason why flagella are only produced by fully developed forms. *They are to be seen on the slide soon after the blood is drawn*; sometimes only one or two minutes elapse before their appearance, so that one is tempted to believe that they were already present in the circulating blood. This, however, is certainly not the case, for in quickly dried and subsequently coloured preparations they are never met with. The movement of the flagella is at first a very energetic one, and according to their environment it remains so for a shorter or longer time; then the energy of the movement diminishes in some or all of the flagella and they come to a standstill, but they may possibly again commence energetic lashing movements. Lastly, the complete extinction of movement follows and the flagella are then seen rolled together at the periphery of the now completely quiescent bodies.

The escape of the apparently sterile large forms of the tertian parasite from the red blood-corpuscles is a process which can likewise be observed not infrequently, but it occurs with such rapidity and in such an unexpected manner that its details cannot be appreciated.

In Plate II, figs. 25 and 26, there are two drawings of the two stages following rapidly upon one another; no visible movement was shown by the body at its excapsulation, but it appears as if it became distended and thereby shot out of the blood-corpuscle.

It must be further mentioned that this distension and decolorisation of the red blood-corpuscles infested by the tertian parasite may indeed be often, but certainly not always, observed. On Plate I these various processes are depicted. Bastianelli and Bignami [118] sometimes observed in tertian fevers copper-coloured shrivelled blood-corpuscles (Globuli rossi ottonati) like those often seen in great numbers amongst the quotidian parasites. I have never been able to see these copper-coloured bodies in tertian fever, although I had the opportunity of investigating a large number of cases; in any case they appear to be exceptional. Neither can I confirm another statement made in the same work regarding the spore-forming bodies of the *Tertiana antiponens*.

Both these authorities report that in the anticipating tertian fevers *early spore-formation* with five to ten spores (as has already been described) is frequently seen.

If we wish to refer this variety of tertian fever, which occurs not infrequently, to Golgi's law, we must accept the fact that the tertian parasite can, under certain exceptionally favorable circumstances, attain maturity a few hours earlier than it usually does, or that possibly it originally enters the infested organism with more vitality and increases there more rapidly than in forty-eight hours. In the cases of anticipating tertian fever which I have investigated, I found no difference from the ordinary tertian so far as concerns the number of spores and the size of the spore-forming bodies, but I certainly do not wish to depreciate Bastianelli and Bignami's observations; I believe rather that they are worthy of attention and require further investigation.

Of observations on the much rarer *Tertiana postponens* there are, so far as I know, no reports attainable.

The detailed relations of structure in the development of the tertian parasite are depicted in the drawings upon Plate III, fig. A.

The young parasite, which has just forced its way into the blood-corpuscle, shows a large vesicular-formed nucleus not containing chromatin. It possesses upon one side a thin layer of stained non-pigmented protoplasm, whereas at the other pole is situated the very darkly tinted round or angular nucleolus, which in this stage is always attached to the nuclear membrane, and often projects over it. With the growth of the parasite the three parts just mentioned are developed in approximately equal proportions. The cytoplasm commences to form gradually two layers, differentiated from one another, one external and containing much coarse pigment, and one internal and lying next the nucleus, either unpigmented or only slightly so. It also takes on a stain rather fainter than the external layer. These two layers I believe can be recognised as ecto- and endoplasm; the endoplasm especially often shows in later development one or more vacuoles.

The nucleus, at first free from chromatin, commences to show, especially in the neighbourhood of the nucleolus, delicate-coloured cross-bars or fine points, but they present no regularity. The nucleolus goes on growing and usually remains attached to the nuclear membrane; more rarely it parts from this so as to nourish itself near the centre of the nucleus; in this case one sometimes sees it connected with the nuclear membrane by chromatin threads.

With the increase in size of the nucleolus it decreases in colour and very dark punctate sharply-defined spaces now appear in it, which are only to be seen with the highest powers; what is the meaning of these three to seven symmetrically grouped points I do not venture to decide (see Plate II, figs. 8, 15, 16). During the appearance of these points one or more vacuoles often appear in the centre of the nucleolus, giving it a web-like appearance.

The further fate of th
I have not been able t
scribed by Grassi and Fel
parasites. I am most inclin
and dissolves with the cytop
thing appears to me certain, an
disappears. With this the pa
which is to be considered as *prep*
is characterised by the nucleus b
together with the disappearance o
taking up of chromatin in the nucl
the parasite gains an appearance differe
stages. Instead of an unstained or
almost evenly stained blue-violet body ap
distinguishable from the cytoplasm because
The sharp appearance of the nuclear me
appears, and when this has happened one c
a nucleus. Although not sharply defined, a
unpigmented part still remain for a certain tim
distinguish between these different parts, not
cally but also biologically, I name them as the
and "protoplasmic part" (see Plate II, figs. 21
body proceeding to spore-formation. In the nu
first stage of the process of spore-formation bec
when ill-defined dark-coloured balls appear in it (Plate
these are the nucleoli of the new spores. The nuclei t
in this stage not yet formed, for the separation of t
surrounding the nucleoli into a peripheral stained (p
part and a central unstained part occurs later on.
occurrence of this separation the spore-formation is
(Plate II, figs. 24, 25).

Two epochs can be distinguished in the forty-eigh
course of the life of the tertian parasite, the first vegeta
the second productive; the disappearance of the nucleolus
the point at which the second epoch puts an end to the firs.

As was mentioned in a previous section, Romanowsky
believes that the parasites divide by a species of karyokine-
A drawing given in one of his publications serves as a ba-
for this, but it cannot be considered as sufficient. Two nucle
may not infrequently be present in the most varying forms
of the malarial parasite, as is the case in the Sporozoa, with-

[1] The description of the detailed structure is taken from my publication [49].

ve not been obtained as has been the case in the
ows ian forms, but such experiments would give
proc ilts than in the mild types, because mixed
Grass igmented and unpigmented quotidian parasites
nuclear in which case the fact that the pigmented
they, like nt in the peripheral blood, whilst they are
with this al organs, usually causes confusion.

In the fir quotidian parasite describes its cycle of
the attack of y-four hours (see Plate II, fig. c); it begins
having been p the other species, as a small unpigmented
tained the del slipped from the spore-forming body, lives
parasites (disint liquor sanguinis, and then attaches itself
as far-reaching a . By means of the method which I have
of the parasites. I é and oblique illumination with a concave
the disappearance clearly, especially in these small parasites,
fact before reprodu in regard to the small forms, was right
Coccidia. After the only pressed upon the blood-corpuscles,
out it, become encyste
the nucleus usually g the quotidian parasite have active
duction. As long as th ich they first call the attention of the
methods of investiga he most part (so long as they do not
dered by zoologists as a quiescent state) they are optically so
do I not feel called upon blood-corpuscles to which they are
process in the malarial ooked by the inexperienced. Their

Finally, it must once colour slightly paler than that of
tinued or subcontinued vement of some of the bodies is
parasites when several erable time, an hour or even more,
present in the blood. emperature of the room, whereas

More frequently mixed ent soon after the abstraction of
forms originate this type in the circulating blood). *In a*
of perfectly characteristic ringlets
tres, and attract the observer's

II. MALARIAL PARASITES often at one point a small
very appropriately be compared

To this group belong infrequently contains one or
chiafava and Celli. They red substance which it has
the parasites of the first group
spores directly, these both these rings are formed:
and form crescents (syzygies, mogeneous-looking body
multiply by transverse a long time, one notices
crescents spore-formation, round in the middle, all
tation as a "second cycle"). ubtless produced by the

The parasites of this group he substance of the red

they produce those fevers which are of a stubbornly relapsing nature, leaving behind an anæmia which is difficult to cure, and has a tendency to pernicious symptoms.

The attacks are often not of a regular character like the paroxysms of mild ague; the rigors especially are frequently wanting. The patients give almost throughout the impression of being severely ill; they complain chiefly of depression, pain in the limbs, headache, and loss of appetite.

In mild cases a clear type is recognisable; it can be either quotidian or tertian, never quartan, but the type is usually blurred and difficult to analyse, in which case one has to do with an infection by several generations, which, with this rapidly evolving parasite, cause continued, remittent, &c., fevers.

Spore-formation occurs, as Marchiafava and Celli have shown, almost entirely in the internal organs, but the reason for this is up to the present perfectly unknown.

The relapses occur from eight to fourteen days after the previous paroxysmal cycle. Golgi [91] prefers to consider this subsequent fever not as a relapse, but as a type with a long interval, and rightly, because in this case we have not to do with a fresh infection, but with a rekindling of the fever which proceeds from the evolution of the crescentic bodies, the details of which are at present unknown to us. It is probable that this evolution proceeds with a regularity such as that which we have recognised in the other parasitic cycle.

(A) *The Pigmented Quotidian Parasite.*

It has already been several times mentioned that we have to credit Marchiafava and Celli with valuable information concerning the relation of the small parasite of the pernicious fever. The division of it into pigmented and unpigmented forms is indeed not the idea of the Roman investigators, for they have up to the present always maintained that it depends only upon the duration of the life of the small parasite whether it has time to form pigment or not, and that between them there is no difference in species, but only a difference in the vegetative period. Notwithstanding this, I feel bound to accept the division into two species proposed by Grassi and Feletti, chiefly because Grassi succeeded in finding in birds a parasite invariably unpigmented, and because, further, the slightly pigmented parasites have also been recognised in certain birds as a well-characterised species. Similar convincing experiments by means of inoculation upon man have not been obtained as has been the case in the quartan and tertian forms, but such experiments would give less decisive results than in the mild types, because mixed infections of the pigmented and unpigmented quotidian parasites are very frequent, in which case the fact that the pigmented forms are not present in the peripheral blood, whilst they are present in the internal organs, usually causes confusion.

The pigmented quotidian parasite describes its cycle of development in twenty-four hours (see Plate II, fig. c); it begins its existence, like all the other species, as a small unpigmented body which, after it has slipped from the spore-forming body, lives for a short time in the liquor sanguinis, and then attaches itself to a red blood-corpuscle. By means of the method which I have described (an open Abbé and oblique illumination with a concave mirror) one can see very clearly, especially in these small parasites, that Laveran, at any rate in regard to the small forms, was right in asserting that they are only pressed upon the blood-corpuscles, and not enclosed in them.

These small bodies of the quotidian parasite have active amœboid movement, by which they first call the attention of the observers to them. For the most part (so long as they do not change into the ring-form quiescent state) they are optically so like the substance of the red blood-corpuscles to which they are attached as to be easily overlooked by the inexperienced. Their contour is very delicate, their colour slightly paler than that of the blood-corpuscle. The movement of some of the bodies is actively maintained for a considerable time, an hour or even more, under the microscope at the temperature of the room, whereas the greater part become quiescent soon after the abstraction of the blood (probably also already in the circulating blood). *In a state of rest the bodies are formed of perfectly characteristic ringlets of whitish colour with reddish centres,* and attract the observer's notice at once. The ring has often at one point a small depression, in which case it can very appropriately be compared to a signet ring. The hoop not infrequently contains one or more granules of a hæmoglobin-coloured substance which it has drawn out of the blood-corpuscle.

One often sees the way in which these rings are formed: if one can fix an amœboid, moving, homogeneous-looking body under the microscope and watch it for a long time, one notices that, after it has become quiescent and round in the middle, all at once a darker spot appears, which is doubtless produced by the protoplasm becoming thinner there, and the substance of the red blood-corpuscle beginning to shine through; the thinning of the parasite in the centre may produce an opening, thus completing the ring.

If such a ring is observed with an open Abbé and oblique illumination with a concave mirror, it is definitely seen to produce in the upper surface of the blood-corpuscle a deep and sharp depression, and in the centre the substance of the blood-corpuscle projects through the hoop just as a finger through a ring. The parasite may return from the ring form into the amœboid form again; the appearance recurs sometimes repeatedly under the observer's eye[1] (see Plate II, figs. 45—47).

The immature amœboid parasite now collects exceedingly fine pigment dust, which is often only reddish; this is seen quite at the periphery of the body, where it usually shows little movement. When the parasite has replaced about a third of the red blood-corpuscle, the pigment collects in the middle or at the edge, and then the amœboid movements of the parasite cease. The pigment, after concentration, coalesces into a dark quiescent mass, and there follows, still within the infested blood-corpuscle, the breaking down of the parasite into a small number of the smallest spores (see Pl. II, fig. 35; Pl. IV, fig. 67).

As Marchiafava and Celli were able to prove in the mild cases of summer fever of the intermittent quotidian type, the concentration of the pigment and the spore-formation coincide with the febrile paroxysm. The same authors discovered the spore-forming bodies of this parasite, and called attention to the important circumstance *that the spore-formation did not occur in the peripheral blood, but in that of the internal organs*, so that during the attack, even in severe infection, few, if any, segmentation bodies are seen in blood from the finger, whereas they are present in great numbers in the splenic blood.

Owing to the infection, the red blood-corpuscles often shrink, becoming thereby copper-coloured. Marchiafava and Celli believe that the parasites enclosed in the "copper-coloured bodies" are degenerated. To this I cannot agree, on account of the staining of the structure, for one finds in these parasites the nucleolus deeply tinted (Pl. IV, figs. 13, 14). Further, the infested, and

[1] Marchiafava and Celli, who first described these ringlets, thought them to be bodies with vacuoles; then imagined them to be biconcave bodies, the red blood-corpuscle shining through the thin centre; later they thought that the centre took on blood-colouring matter, and therefore had a red colour. How both these authors can reconcile this procedure with the endocorpuscular life of the "plasmodium," which they so strongly maintain, they have not clearly shown.

in part shrivelled blood-corpuscles may also completely lose their colouring matter, in which case they form exceedingly delicate folded phantom bodies, in the interior of which the parasite lies. The "copper-coloured bodies" may be easily mistaken by the inexperienced for the "morning-star form;" it should be noted that the parasite is always to be seen on the copper-coloured bodies, and that it has usually the form of a bright ringlet, and gives to the bodies an unmistakable appearance.

After the illness has continued for several days, together with the bodies described above, others appear which belong to the crescentic series. These bodies are (1) the typical crescentic body; (2) the fusiform body blunted at the ends (cigar-shaped); (3) spherical bodies.

A detailed description of the morphology of these bodies, as well as a statement of the divergent opinions which are held with reference to their origin and importance, has been given in Chapter II.

To illustrate the correspondence between the clinical symptoms and microscopical appearances in cases belonging to this category, the following case is given as a sample.

K. S— has suffered for a week from attacks of fever daily; the symptoms are only those of heat, and occur at about 4 p.m. The patient is very weak, he cannot walk, and had to be carried to hospital; exceedingly pale typhoid appearance. The teeth dry, the papillæ at the tip of the tongue swollen, the dorsum of the tongue coated with thick grey fur. The spleen distinctly palpable. Pulse 110, dicrotic; tension normal. Daily two or three thin fluid stools.

August 4th, 1892, 5 p.m.—Temperature 38° C. (100·4° F.).

Microscopical appearances: 1. A few small amœboid bodies, all unpigmented. 2. Very many melaniferous leucocytes.

5th, 9 a.m.—Temperature 37° C. (98·6° F.).

Microscopical appearances: 1. A very few medium-sized bodies occupying a fourth to a third of the blood-corpuscle, and having a little heap of pigment. 2. Several copper-coloured bodies. No melaniferous leucocytes.

4 p.m.—Temperature 38·2° C. (100·7° F.).

Microscopical appearances: Very few small pigmented bodies. 2. A crescent with concentrated pigment.

6 p.m.—Patient received 0·66 grm. of quinine (10⅛ grains).

August 6th, 7 a.m.—Patient received 0·66 grm. (10⅛ grains) of quinine.

10 a.m.—Temperature 36·5° C. (97·7° F.). Patient very weak. Tongue dry, brown.

Microscopical appearances: 1. Isolated crescents. 2. Fairly numerous melaniferous leucocytes.

4 p.m.—Temperature 35·4° C. (95·7° F.). Patient's general condition as this morning.

From this time there was no recurrence of fever, and the threatening symptoms present at first soon gradually disappeared.

In this case the striking disproportion must be noticed between the small number of parasites, the comparatively small rise in temperature, and the severity of the other symptoms.

The crescents appeared on the eighth day of the disease.

The fever produced by the quotidian parasite is characterised by the severity of the symptoms, and this holds good for both the unpigmented as well as for the pigmented parasites. Typhoid appearance, excessive pallor, diarrhœa, severe pains in joints, and tenderness of the bones are very frequently found in these cases. They are characterised further by the cachexia which follows the fever, and by the frequency of relapse.

As already mentioned, the crescents appear in the blood with the greatest regularity soon after the commencement of the illness, as also the bodies associated with them, and they remain in the blood during the intervals, sometimes in company with isolated amœboid bodies. *When these bodies are seen in a patient's blood, it can be with certainty decided that they have originated shortly before the attack of fever. As long as the microscopical appearances consist solely of crescents and their spherical bodies there is as a rule no fever present.* Indeed, the Roman school holds the opinion strongly that these bodies are not able to produce fever, but that on each occasion when a paroxysm of fever follows, it must be ascribed to endocorpuscular amœboid bodies appearing in the blood together with the crescents. Marchiafava and Celli have seen cases in which, although there were very many crescents in the blood, the patients had no rise in temperature; similar observations have been made by other investigators, and my own experience agrees with them in the vast majority of cases, but I must mention that I have notwithstanding met with several cases having a moderate paroxysm of fever in which I have sought in vain for amœboid bodies in addition to the crescents. It might indeed be conceived that they were not in the peripheral blood, but only in the vessels of the internal organs, and indeed I hold this idea to be very probable. From a clinical standpoint these cases must not be passed over, and in the accounts of patients which follow I shall introduce several belonging to this category. But, as a rule, at the time when the crescentic bodies are alone present fever is entirely absent; the patients are in a more or less cachectic condition; the diminished proportion of hæmoglobin in the blood, as well as the diminished number of blood-corpuscles, increases slowly or not at all—sometimes indeed decreases still further, although there is no rise in temperature.

After two to three weeks periods of fever may again occur, which are accompanied by an invasion of young amœboid bodies. That these fevers are in fact not relapses, but, as Golgi believes, cycles with long intervals, is proved to us by the fact that the paroxysms occur in hospital or in other places free from malaria just as frequently as in malarial districts. Now the next question is, in which bodies in the organism have we to seek the source of the infection which has for the time been latent?

The most obvious explanation is to attribute to the crescents the cause of the relapses, and as a matter of fact this view has much probability.

To raise this probability to certainty it would be necessary to prove that spores develop either from the crescents or from the spherical bodies of their series, and during their further development produce amœboid bodies.

It has previously been mentioned that Canalis believed he had seen spore-formation in various spherical bodies. Unfortunately he has not given any certain proof of this by staining the nucleus, and therefore his views may well be doubted.

Also Celli and Guarnieri's former view that the well-known "buds" on the spherical bodies were germinating bodies is shipwrecked, owing to their non-nuclear character. Recently Grassi and Feletti state that they have found spore-forming spherical bodies (of the crescent series) in the splenic blood; the drawings which they give of these bodies, however, are not conclusive of the correctness of their opinion, so that up to the present we cannot hold that the spore-formation of the crescentic bodies is certainly proved.

On the other hand, I obtained the conviction from my own preparations that the segmentation of the crescents, first announced by Grassi and Feletti, undoubtedly occurs (see Plate III, fig. 52), and it is probable that this segmentation, in which the several limbs have a finely granulated appearance, stands in connection with reproduction.

One also frequently finds crescents of which a part is wanting, as in Plate III, fig. 40; probably these are also segmented bodies.

Golgi [91] once expressed the opinion that spores are formed at the edge of the crescents, which are scattered by the bursting of the latter; this idea would agree with segmentation. As against these attempts to learn the further development of the crescents, Bignami, Bastianelli, Celli, and Marchiafava continue to maintain an opposite view, believing the crescents to be degeneration forms which are perfectly incapable of further development, and which, after previously becoming vacuolated, disintegrate. There can be no doubt that there are degenerated crescents (see Plate IV, figs. 55, 56) in which drop-like formations are to be seen, and which one might consider to be spores if they did not change their form under the observer's eye, but from this one cannot draw the far-reaching conclusion which the above-mentioned observers wish to deduce. In the third chapter I have stated my views with regard to the body in question being syzygies, and refer the reader to that chapter.

The statements regarding the numerical relation of the crescents in the intervals free from fever, and the occurrence of the relapses do not quite agree; whereas some have observed a decrease, others say that they have demonstrated an increase or no change at all. In this connection I have noticed no remarkable or at any rate no legitimate differences, for it has happened that on one day only isolated bodies of this description were found; on the next day they were very numerous, nor have I been able to confirm the statement made by several authors that the crescents more frequently change into flagellated bodies at the time of the relapse than during the interval.

In stained preparations the young quotidian parasite appears like the immature forms of the tertian and quartan parasites. It possesses, as do they, nucleus, nucleolus, and protoplasm. In the spore-forming bodies also the new spores show complete details of structure. Before the spore-formation the nucleus and the nucleolus seem to disappear in them as in the tertian variety.

The malarial infections which occur from the pigmented quotidian parasites often show a pernicious character. In consequence of the greater adhesiveness of the parasites, the small vessels may become blocked if a sufficient number are present. Should this happen, as it may do, especially in the capillaries of the brain, then a malarial *perniciosa comatosa* occurs, which frequently ends fatally. In Plate IV, fig. 67, a drawing of a brain capillary is given, which is filled by infested blood-corpuscles. The parasites belonged to the species which we have just discussed, and they were in all the stages previous to spore-formation. This is recognised by the concentration of the pigment. I have to thank Professor Celli for this preparation, which was made from a patient who died from a comatose pernicious fever.

(B) *The Unpigmented Quotidian Parasite.*

The presence of a malarial parasite which forms no pigment, and which also forms solely unpigmented spores, has been demonstrated by Marchiafava and Celli. This appearance forms one of the most beautiful discoveries in the field of malarial ætiology made by these indefatigable and successful investigators.

With the exception of the want of pigment, this parasite resembles the pigmented quotidian parasite so completely that we can omit a separate description. It shows in the immature condition the same amœboid movement as does the other, and completes its cycle in a similar period of time, or possibly rather sooner, owing to which circumstance Marchiafava and Celli explain its want of pigment.

The spore-formation only takes place in the internal organs, and the infection must, indeed, be very severe if the spore-forming bodies are able to reach the peripheral blood. Marchiafava and Celli [71] report a case of comatose pernicious fever in which the peripheral blood contained an immense number of spore-forming bodies.

On Plate IV, fig. 66, a drawing is given of a cerebral capillary with the spore-forming bodies of the unpigmented parasite. Fig. 65 represents a transverse section of a cerebral capillary; there it is clearly seen that the infected blood-corpuscles lie along the wall of the vessel, and in this way diminish its lumen. For this preparation I have also to thank Professor Celli.

Just as with the pigmented quotidian parasites, crescents develop in these cases; and here also pigment elements come under consideration, for the crescents are, without exception, pigmented. *If, however, the patient catches the infection before the crescents have developed, one has then to deal with a completely unpigmented malaria. Indeed, Marchiafava and Celli have observed such cases.*

It is necessary to know that Antolisei and Angelini (p. 320) have often found in the spleen, the brain, and the bone marrow small pigmented bodies in cases where only unpigmented parasites were seen in blood from the finger. One cannot, therefore, from a consideration of the finger blood alone, exclude with absolute certainty the presence of pigmented bodies, for it is always possible for them to remain in the internal organs. With this reservation—for I made no puncturing of the spleen—I give here the history of a case which illustrates this subject.

D. J—, æt. 19, woodcutter, is said to have suffered from fever for a week; rigors have not occurred. Severe headache; pain in the limbs; has been constipated for a week.

August 12th, 1892, 10 a.m.—Temperature 39·5° C. (103·1° F.). Patient very ill in bed, and groans. Tongue dry and cracked. Spleen just palpable.

Microscopical appearances: Numerous small, amœboid, unpigmented bodies.

4 p.m.—Temperature 40·2° C. (104·4° F.).

Microscopical appearances: 1. Very numerous unpigmented bodies in slight movement, double infection of blood-corpuscles frequent. 2. In isolated leucocytes coarse pigment granules.

7 p.m.—Temperature 39° C. (102·2° F.); 0·33 grm. ($5\frac{1}{12}$ grains) of quinine administered.

13th, 5 a.m.—0·33 grm. ($5\frac{1}{12}$ grains) of quinine.

9 a.m.—Temperature 37·6° C. (99·6° F.).

Microscopical appearances: 1. Numerous amœboid, moving, unpigmented bodies. 2. Extremely numerous copper-coloured bodies, the parasites of which have an amœboid movement. No pigment to be seen in any of the bodies, only here and there a hæmoglobin granule.

10 a.m.—0·66 grm. ($10\frac{1}{8}$ grains) of quinine.

4 p.m.—Temperature 39·2° C. (102·5° F.).

Microscopical appearances: 1. Very numerous amœboid bodies. 2. Equally numerous copper-coloured bodies. 3. A spheroid of the crescent series.

7 p.m.—Temperature 40·5° C. (104·9° F.); 0·33 gramme ($5\frac{1}{12}$ grains) of quinine.

14th, 5 a.m.—0·33 gramme ($5\frac{1}{12}$ grains) of quinine.

9.30 a.m.—Temperature 37·2° C. (98·9° F.).

Microscopical appearances: 1. Less numerous amœboid perfectly unpigmented bodies, some with hæmoglobin enclosures. 2. Isolated crescents.

7 p.m.—Temperature 39° C. (102·2° F.); 0·66 gramme ($10\frac{1}{8}$ grains) of quinine.

15th.—Patient groans with weariness and pain in the limbs; he looks weak.

9 a.m.—Temperature 37° C. (98·6° F.); 0·66 gramme (10$\frac{1}{8}$ grains) of quinine.

Microscopical appearances: 1. Isolated unpigmented bodies. 2. Isolated crescents.

7 p.m.—Temperature 38·3° C. (100·9° F.); 0·66 gramme (10$\frac{1}{8}$ grains) of quinine.

16th, 10 a.m.—Temperature 35·8° C. (96·4° F.). Profuse perspiration.

Microscopical appearances: 1. Very few small bodies. 2. Isolated crescents.

After this the patient had no more fever.

D. J—. *Pure Quotidian* (*Unpigmented Quotidian Parasite*).

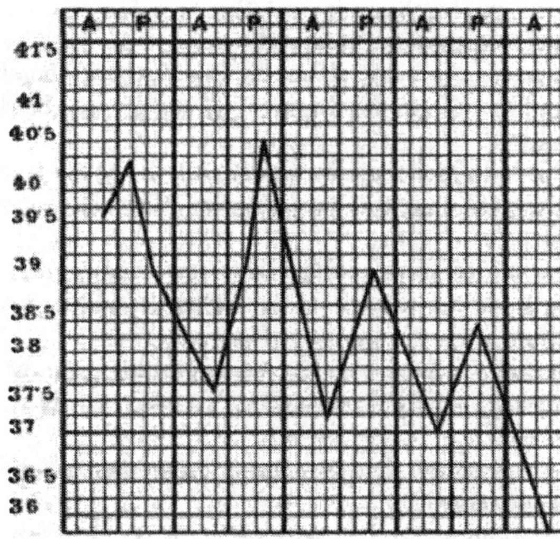

The type of fever was pure quotidian, which, to judge from the history of the patient and the beginning of the temperature curve, was preceded by a continued fever.

The pigment already observed in the leucocytes during the first days must have had its origin in crescents, for in the innumerable amœboid bodies not a granule of pigment was to be seen; spore-forming bodies were also quite absent.

The fevers caused by the unpigmented quotidian parasite, as also those of the pigmented quotidian parasite, occur most frequently in summer and autumn; I have observed most cases in the months of August and September. The single paroxysms seen in this variety also present more seldom the typical course which we are accustomed to see in the tertian and quartan varieties, and the patients as a rule complain less of heat and cold than of headache, pain in the limbs, diarrhœa, vomiting, and weakness. They very frequently appear to be very ill; the weakened condition of the organism generally continues after the period of fever, convalescence follows very slowly, and is, as already mentioned, often interrupted by relapses of fever.

Some remarks will be made later on in regard to the amount of hæmoglobin and the number of the red blood-corpuscles.

(c) *The Malignant Tertian Parasite.*

This variety of parasite has recently been separated from the other forms by Marchiafava and Bignami [99, page 100]. In its morphological relation it stands very near to the pigmented quotidian parasite, from which, as the authors themselves admit, in many stages of its development it can hardly be differentiated with certainty.

The chief differences between it and the other types which are so nearly related to it are, according to Marchiafava and Bignami, the following:

1. Its cycle of development lasts for forty-eight hours.

2. The pigment sometimes shows oscillating movements, which does not happen with the quotidian parasite.

3. The parasite reaches a considerable size; at the time of spore-forming it fills from a half to two thirds of the blood-corpuscle.

4. The advanced deeply pigmented stages still have an active amœboid movement.

5. The unpigmented stage lasts for more than twenty-four hours.

The following differences exist between it and the ordinary tertian parasite:

1. The malignant tertian parasite is in all its corresponding stages smaller than the ordinary tertian parasite.

2. It often assumes the ring form, which that of Golgi never does.

3. The pigment is more sparse, and but rarely has any movement.

4. The infested red blood-corpuscles are inclined to shrivel, whereas in the ordinary tertian form they become distended.

5. The spores of the pernicious tertian are smaller, and on an

average not so numerous (eight to fifteen) as those of the ordinary tertian.

6. The pernicious parasite forms crescents, which never happens with the others.

After noting these deviations from the other forms already dealt with, it is not necessary to give a detailed description of the pernicious tertian parasite, and we will now consider the clinical description of the pernicious tertian as sketched by Marchiafava and Bignami.

The most interesting part of it is the fever curve; we see, namely, that the apyrexial intervals are very short, and often only last several hours. The rise in temperature occurs in typical cases with great regularity at intervals of two days, and indeed suddenly, as is always the case in the fever paroxysms; the fever remains for a time, and then falls with a *pseudo-crisis,* again to rise and form a *pre-critical elevation,* which often exceeds the previous maximum; then follows sudden defervescence. *The complete attack lasts as a rule longer than twenty-four hours. It may reach a duration of from thirty to forty hours.*

The temperature curve often shows variations from this typical chart; for instance, the pseudo-crisis can be more marked, the temperature falling to 37° C. (98·6° F.), whereby the attack loses its unique character, or lasts longer than forty hours, so that, instead of apyrexia, only a remission occurs: further slight rises in temperature may occur during the apyrexia. A duplication of the paroxysm may also occur (tertian *maligna duplex*).

Under the microscope are seen, before the attack, pigmented parasites almost half filling the blood-corpuscles; at the commencement of the attack the parasites may be completely absent from the blood, and it is only after the paroxysm has lasted some (about six) hours that the forms of a new generation appear, which, as has already been mentioned, remain through twenty-four or even forty-eight hours unpigmented, so that they can be seen eight or ten hours before the attack still unaltered, or so rapidly pigmented that already at the end of the attack pigmented bodies are to be seen.

The origin of the peculiarly formed temperature curve is explained by authors in this way, that the spore-formation of the bodies present occurs not all at once, but in batches.

The spore-formation here also occurs, as in the other two species, chiefly in the internal organs; the formation of the crescents shows equally no deviation.

Typical Temperature Chart of the Malignant Tertian Fever, after Marchiafava and Bignami.

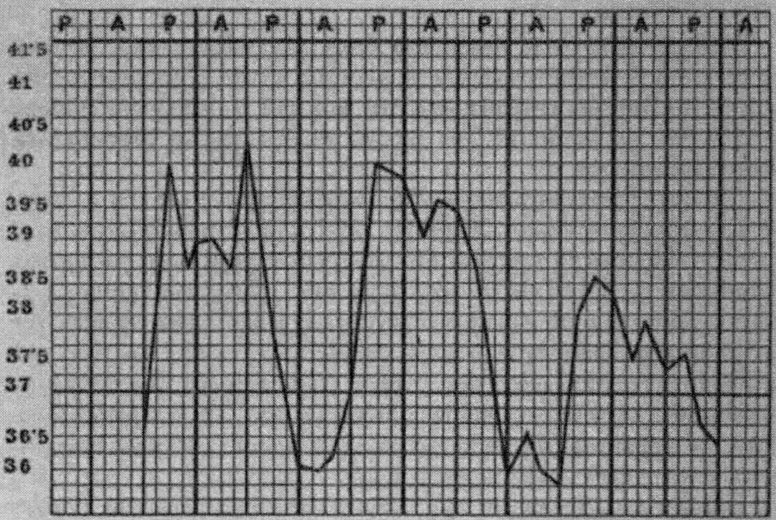

It is noteworthy that both these authors have found that the relapses in these cases usually possess the same type (often more clearly defined) as the initial fever.

Grassi and Feletti [86] do not acknowledge that this new variety of pernicious tertian fever parasite is sufficiently characterised, and they believe that in Marchiafava and Bignami's cases an ordinary tertian parasite is mixed with the pigmented quotidian parasite (*Hæmamœba præcox* and *H. vivax*).

I cannot, however, put aside Marchiafava and Bignami's opinions, as is done by Grassi and Feletti, for I have met with a considerable number of patients who definitely gave me a history of tertian fever, but whose blood showed only small bodies which could certainly not be mistaken for the ordinary tertian parasites. It did, however, turn out when observed in hospital that several of these patients had quotidian fever, *but the presence of the tertian type was demonstrated in many of them.*

Previous to Marchiafava and Bignami publishing their preliminary reports, this fact had aroused my interest in the summer of 1891, and only the wish to first study the conditions more in detail prevented me from then publishing a communication concerning the malignant tertian fever. In the summer of 1892

I was able, with further cases, to confirm the definite existence of this fever.

Of the cases met with I publish two at this place.

K. W—, æt. 42, has suffered for six days daily from severe long-continuing rigors, followed by heat and sweating; the attacks commence about 2 a.m., but sometimes not till about 8 a.m.; patient complains of severe headache, pain in the limbs, loss of appetite, and diarrhœa. The colour of his skin is slightly jaundiced, the sensorium clouded, tongue dry, spleen distinctly palpable and painful.

August 22nd, 1891, 11 a.m.—Temperature 41·5° C. (106·7° F.). At four this morning patient was attacked by rigors.

Microscopical appearances: Very numerous amœboid bodies, some of them the very smallest, others rather larger, all unpigmented.

4 p.m.—Temperature 39·8° C (103·6° F.).

Microscopical appearances: 1. Numerous very small and rather larger amœboid bodies without pigment; multiple infection of a blood-corpuscle. 2. Very many copper-coloured bodies, whose parasites contain fine pigment. 3. A melaniferous leucocyte.

7 p.m.—Temperature 38° C. (100·4° F.).

During the night profuse perspiration.

23rd, 9 a.m.—Temperature 36·4° C. (97·5° F.).

Microscopical appearances: 1. Very numerous small forms, which occupy about a fourth of a red blood-corpuscle. They move very little, and many of them contain pigment, which is throughout peripherally situated. 2. Very numerous copper-coloured bodies, most of them containing pigmented ring-shaped parasites.

About 2.15 p.m., rigors.

3.30 p.m.—Temperature 40° C. (104° F.).

Microscopical appearances: 1. Numerous quiescent endocorpuscular bodies of the size of a fourth of a blood-corpuscle, containing more pigment, which in some is still scattered and moving, in some peripherally concentrated and quiescent. 2. Several spore-forming bodies in markedly diminished blood-corpuscles. 3. Many copper-coloured bodies. 4. Numerous shrivelled and decolorised infested blood-corpuscles (diaphanous form). 5. Many very immature, still unpigmented, actively moving parasites attached to the blood-corpuscles (young generation).

5.30 p.m.—Temperature 40·7° C. (105·3° F.).

7 p.m.—Temperature 40° C. (104° F.).

24th, 9 a.m.—Temperature 38° C. (100·4° F.). (At 5.30 a.m. 0·66 gramme of quinine given—10⅛ grains.)

Microscopical appearances: 1. Numerous amœboid bodies, very small and middle-sized; all unpigmented. 2. A melaniferous leucocyte.

11 a.m.—Temperature 39·2° C. (102·5° F.).

4 p.m.—Temperature 41·6° C. (106·8° F.).

Microscopical appearances: 1. Numerous amœboid forms, middle-sized; a few pigmented amongst them. 2. Many copper-coloured bodies.

7 p.m.—Temperature 40·2° C. (104·3° F.) ·66 grm. (10⅛ grains) quinine given. Profuse night sweat.

25th, 5 a.m.—·66 gramme (10⅛ grains) quinine given.

10 a.m.—Temperature 36·5° C. (97·7° F.).

Microscopical appearances: 1. Numerous small, peripherally placed parasites, mostly immobile, all unpigmented. 2. A melaniferous leucocyte. 3. One syzygy (composed of two middle-sized bodies).

4 p.m.—Temperature 37·1° C. (98·7° F.).

Microscopical appearances: The same as this morning, all parasites unpigmented.

7 p.m.—Temperature 37·3° C. (99·1° F.).

26th, 9 a.m.—Temperature 37·5° C. (99·5° F.).

Microscopical appearances: 1. A few small unpigmented bodies. 2. Many laden melaniferous leucocytes. 3. Several crescents and spherical bodies of the crescent series.

The patient remained thereafter free of fever, and was dismissed from hospital before a relapse.

The fever chart, which, indeed, only contained one fully developed attack, notwithstanding shows clearly the tertian type, because between the two short periods of apyrexia there is an interval of exactly forty-eight hours; also the attack of fever itself shows that curve which is described by Marchiafava and Bignami as typical. The pseudo-critical fall in temperature and pre-critical elevation is perfectly well marked.

Before the attacks quiescent pigmented bodies were seen, which have for the most part filled the red blood-corpuscles; these are not enlarged, but rather shrivelled; during the attack, and especially after it, the young unpigmented generation filled the microscopic field.

It is further interesting that after the administration of the quinine the parasites did not reach the pigmented stage, and that they were no longer in a condition to digest any hæmoglobin, but became necrotic and perished.

K. W—. *Summer Tertian Fever* (*Malignant Tertian Parasite*).

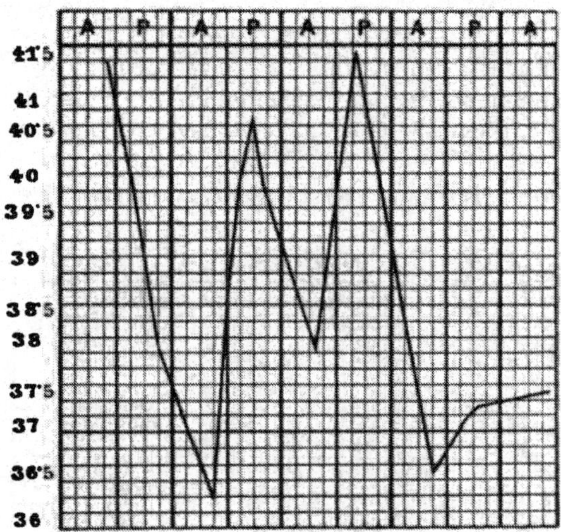

The crescents were first seen on the tenth day of the illness, after the day when fresh conjugations had been observed.

A—, æt. 27, has suffered for six days irregularly from coldness and heat; complains of severe headache and pains in the limbs.

August 19th, 1892, 4 p.m.—Temperature 36° C. (96·8° F.). The spleen distinctly palpable.

Microscopical appearances: A few isolated small forms with the finest pigment.

20th, 9 a.m.—Temperature 38° C. (100·4° F.).

Microscopical appearances: Isolated small forms, some of them with pigment masses inside.

4 p.m.—Temperature 41° C. (105·8° F.).

Microscopical appearances: 1. Very numerous amœboid unpigmented bodies. 2. Isolated ones with a small pigment mass. Multiple infection frequent. 3. A crescent which easily changes its form, and has a slight double contour; the pigment in it scattered and the grouping changing.

21st, 9 a.m.—Temperature 36·2° C. (97·1° F.).

Microscopical appearances: 1. Rather numerous unpigmented amœboid forms. 2. Separated bodies which about fill the half of the blood-corpuscle, with pigment granules which oscillate actively within a narrow space.

5 p.m.—Temperature 36·3° C. (97·3° F.).

22nd, 10 a.m.—Temperature 38·5° C. (101·3° F.).

Microscopical appearances: Very few small forms without pigment.

4 p.m.—Temperature 39·6° C. (103·3° F.).

7 p.m.—Temperature 40·2° C. (104·3° F.).

23rd.—No attack, nor on the remaining days.

A—. *Summer Tertian Fever* (*Malignant Tertian Parasites*).

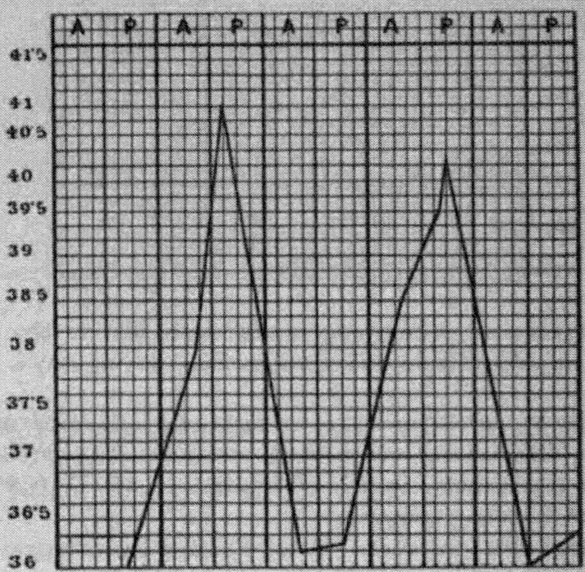

Here the curve also shows the tertian type, although of the character of the ordinary tertian without prolongation of the attacks, and with a full day's interval of apyrexia.

The existence of a tertian fever without Golgi's forms, but showing only small crescent-forming parasites, is therefore a definitely proved fact.

Another question is whether the parasites found in these fevers are to be considered as different in kind from the pigmented quotidian parasites or not.

A decided answer cannot at present be given to this question, and we will wait for the result of further investigations in this direction. In stained preparations it is seen that the details of structure of the pernicious tertian parasites correspond with those of the other kinds.

The drawings (Plate IV, figs. 1 to 12) lead one to suppose that here also the loss of the nucleus and nucleolus precedes spore-formation.

In connection with the crescent-forming parasite species, three histories of patients are given which show that fever may also occur when apparently only crescent bodies are present.

M— has suffered for fourteen days from attacks of tertian fever, which occur at about 2 p.m. with a slight rigor, soon after followed by extreme heat. The last attack occurred the day before yesterday.

August 18th, 1892, 11 a.m.—Temperature 37·2° C. (98·9° F.).

Microscopical appearances: Exceedingly few small amœboid bodies.

2 p.m.—Patient shivering slightly.

5 p.m.—Temperature 39·6° C. (103·2° F.).

19th, 10 a.m.—Temperature 36·2° C. (97·1° F.).

Microscopical appearances: One amœboid body discovered after a long search.

5 p.m.—Temperature 37·2° C. (98·9° F.).

20th, 9 a.m.—Temperature 37·4° C. (99·3° F.).

Microscopical appearances the same as before.

6 p.m.—Temperature 38° C. (100·4° F.).

21st, 9 a.m.—Temperature 36·6° C. (97·9° F.).

Microscopical appearances: A few crescents.

5 p.m.—Temperature 37·1° C. (98·7° F.).

8 p.m.—Temperature 37·7° C. (99·8° F.).

22nd, 10 a.m.—Temperature 37·1° C. (98·7° F.).

Microscopical appearances: 1. Several crescents with scattered pigment. 2. Several melaniferous leucocytes. No small amœboid bodies.

5 p.m.—Temperature 38° C. (100·4° F.).

Microscopical appearances: Several crescents, no amœboid bodies.

7 p.m.—Temperature 39·9° C. (103·8° F.).

23rd, 10 a.m.—Temperature 36·3° C. (97·3° F.).

6 p.m.—Temperature 37° C. (98·6° F.).

Microscopical appearances as before.

24th, 10 a.m.—Temperature 37·7° C. (99·8° F.).

4 p.m.—Temperature 37·8° C. (100° F.).

Microscopical appearances: Several spherical bodies of the crescent series.

7 p.m.—Temperature 40·3° C. (104·5° F.).

25th, 10 a.m.—Temperature 36·5° C. (97·7° F.).

Microscopical appearances: Several crescents and spherical bodies.

M—. *Irregular Fever* (*Crescentic Bodies*).

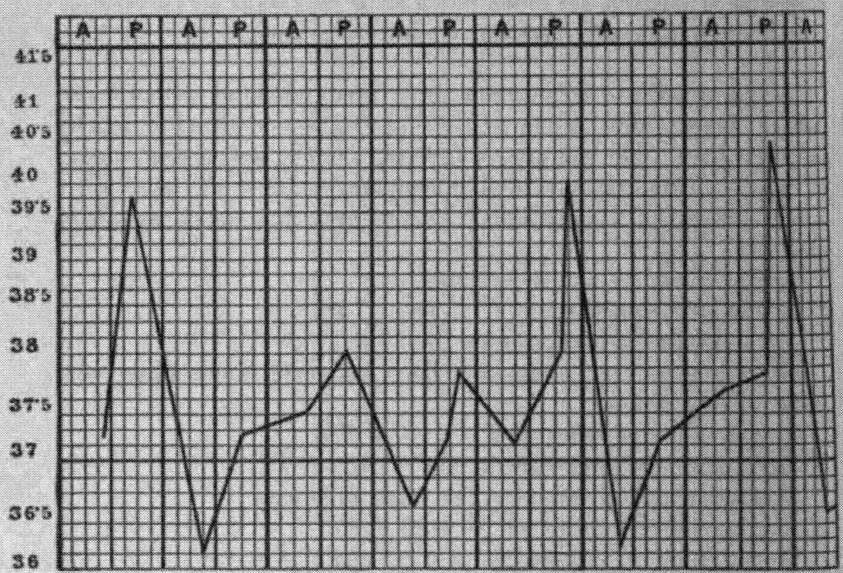

In this case there were only on the first two days exceedingly few amœboid bodies to be seen, whilst later only crescents were found; the fever had a tertian type predominating.

G. C—, canal worker, is said to have suffered for three weeks from fever, which at first was of the tertian type, but later on quotidian in type. The attacks consist sometimes of chill, sometimes of heat. There are profuse night sweats. Patient feels very weary; his whole body pains him, especially his head and legs. He is fairly pale. Spleen distinctly palpable.

October 7th, 1891, 4 p.m.—Temperature 38·7° C. (101·6° F.).

Microscopical appearances: 1. Very numerous crescents and their spherical bodies. 2. Several melaniferous leucocytes.

8th, 9 a.m.—Temperature 38·2° C. (100·7° F.).

Microscopical appearances: The same as yesterday, only rather fewer parasites. No small bodies. Hæmoglobin 70 per cent. Number of blood-corpuscles 3,217,000.

4 p.m.—Temperature 38·3° C. (100·9° F.).

10th, 9 a.m.—Temperature 36·2° C. (97·1° F.).

4 p.m.—Temperature 36·5° C. (97·7° F.).

Microscopical appearances: Numerous crescents and their spherical bodies, the latter frequently flagellated, &c.

In this case no amœboid bodies were seen, but only numerous crescents and their spherical bodies. Of the latter a remarkable number were flagellated.

K— has for a fortnight suffered from heat every evening without previous shivering. Severe headache; profuse perspirations; patient is rather anæmic; spleen on percussion found to be enlarged, but not readily palpable.

October 8th, 1891, 4 p.m.—Temperature 37·5° C. (99·5° F.).

Microscopical appearances: Innumerable crescents and their spherical bodies. No small bodies.

9th, 10 a.m.—Temperature 38·5° C. (101·3° F.).

Microscopical appearances: Very numerous crescents and their spherical bodies, the latter often flagellated.

3 p.m.—Temperature 38·3° C. (100·9° F.). Hæmoglobin 60 per cent. Number of blood-corpuscles 2,988,000.

Microscopical appearances as before; exceptionally numerous flagellated spherical bodies.

In the evening 0·66 gramme quinine (10⅛ grains) administered to patient.

10th, 9 a.m.—Temperature 35·8° C. (96·4° F.).

5 p.m.—Temperature 37° C. (98·6° F.).

Microscopical appearances as before; still many flagellated bodies.

11th, 9 a.m.—Temperature 36° C. (96·8° F.).

Microscopical appearances the same as before.

5 p.m.—Temperature 36·2° C. (97·1° F.).

12th.—The patient remained free from fever, but there are still crescents in diminished number and their spherical bodies to be seen in his blood.

In this case also the amœboid bodies were completely wanting. On the other hand, the flagellated spherical bodies of the crescents, as also the crescents themselves, were present in large numbers. It is noteworthy that though these elements still remain in his blood the fever so soon stopped.

Lastly I give a case of masked malarial fever.

A. E—, æt. 51, is said to have suffered fourteen days from typical tertian fever. The attack occurred every afternoon, the last yesterday. Pale cachectic-looking man with a distinctly palpable spleen.

September 25th, 1891, 10 a.m.—Temperature 36·2° C. (97·1° F.).

Microscopical appearances: Numerous crescents and their spherical bodies.

4 p.m.—Temperature 36·5° C. (97·7° F.).

26th, 9 a.m.—Temperature 36·3° C. (97·3° F.).

At 2 p.m. in the afternoon the patient was attacked with severe brow ague on the right side. At the same time he felt shivery and weak in his limbs.

3 p.m.—Temperature 36·7° C. (98° F.). Patient felt hot and perspired.

Microscopical appearances: Several crescents.

28th.—Patient had no fever yesterday, and appears to have felt quite well.

9 a.m.—Temperature 36·5° C. (97·7° F.).

Microscopical appearances unchanged. Hæmoglobin 60 per cent. Number of blood-corpuscles 3,281,000.

2 p.m.—Attack of brow ague in the same way as on the day before yesterday.

3 p.m.—Temperature 36·5° C. (97·7° F.).

In like manner every second afternoon there followed an attack of brow ague. The supra-orbital nerve was very sensitive to touch during this time. A fever temperature could never be ascertained. The administration of quinine remained without success, showing the well-known resistance of the crescentic bodies to this drug.

Mixed Infections.—In the previous sections it has been already repeatedly pointed out that the organism can be the host not only of *one species of parasite* in various generations, but of several species at the same time.

The combinations of the five species at present known appear to take place in all kinds of ways; most frequently the pigmented and unpigmented quotidian parasites combine together; frequently also a mixed infection between tertian and quartan parasites occurs, or between the tertian parasite and one of the quotidian parasites.

The relationship can be very complicated at times; Golgi [37] found, for instance, in the blood of a man suffering from remittent fever, three generations of the quartan parasite and two of the tertian; and the elevation of the temperature agreed completely with the microscopical appearances of the blood.

The type of fever in mixed infections is determined by the

type of the component parts, and it is comprehensible that continued, subcontinued, or even irregular fevers may frequently occur.

It is further to be noted that mixed infections may occur in which only one variety of parasite is accountable for the type of fever, whereas the presence of the second variety is only ascertained by its being found in the blood. This is the case, for instance, when anyone who has crescentic bodies in his blood, which, as we have seen, as a rule produce no fever for two or three weeks (until a relapse), receives in addition an infection with the common tertian parasite; the progress of the fever in such a case would be simply that of the tertian type, notwithstanding that, at the same time, a mixed infection is present. The following two cases are examples of mixed infection.

W. G—, æt. 43, is said to have suffered from attacks of fever during the last three weeks. At first the attacks occurred daily, later the type was irregular, and at present an attack occurs every two or three days. The paroxysms show the classical symptoms. The last attack occurred yesterday evening.

October 4th, 1891.—The patient is an anæmic and cachectic-looking weakly man. The spleen projects three fingers' breadth below the ribs.

9 a.m.—Temperature 37·7° C. (99·8° F.).

Microscopical appearances:

1. Numerous unpigmented small parasites, signet-ring shaped; amongst them also rather large, round, and amœboid parasites.
2. Several crescents.
3. Numerous copper-coloured bodies.

} Unpigmented quotidian parasite.

4. Several large pigmented forms almost completely filling the blood-corpuscles; the pigment in them is slightly moving; the infested blood-corpuscles are often hypertrophied and decolorised (mature tertian forms).

5 p.m.—Temperature 38·5° C. (101·3° F.). No previous shivering.

5th, 9 a.m.—Temperature 37·5° C. (99·5° F.). Patient feels very weak, and complains of a continual pressure in the splenic region.

Microscopical appearances: 1. Several crescents. 2. Several melaniferous leucocytes. Hæmoglobin 42 per cent. Number of red blood-corpuscles 2,217,000.

…ient has received, since yesterday mor… …uinine (15 grains) daily in three doses.

4 p.m.—Temperature 38·4° C. (101·1° F.).

6th.—Profuse night sweat.

10 a.m.—Temperature 36° C. (96·8° F.).

Microscopical appearances: 1. A few crescents. … …ucocytes with coarse pigment clots.

4 p.m.—Temperature 36·4° C. (97·4° F.).

16th.—The patient has remained free from fever sinc… …ote. Hæmoglobin 65 per cent. Number of blood-corp… …,087,000.

The infection was therefore that of an ordinary tertian … generation, which gave way to the treatment with quinine … the same time unpigmented quotidian parasites were present; these also disappeared under the quinine, and only left behind the crescentic bodies. The type of fever was quotidian; nevertheless on two days there was no absolute apyrexia, for the morning temperatures of 37·5° C. (99·5° F.) and 37·7° C. (99·8° F.) were rather fever temperatures in such a cachectic man.

F—. *Quotidian Fever (Mixed Infection of Two Generations of Tertian Parasites and the Pigmented Quotidian Parasite).*

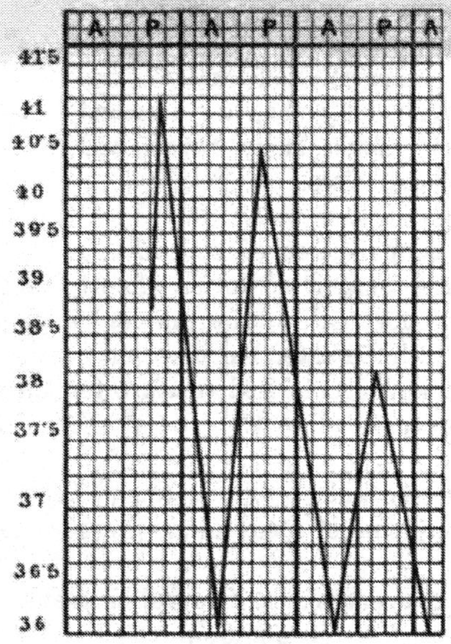

F—, æt. 29.
attack of fever
feeling, several h
ingly severe head
September 24th,
spleen projects tw
5·30 p.m.—Temp
Microscopical appea
amœboid bodies with
signet-ring shape.
endocorpuscular bodies
bodies, with many spor
blood-corpuscles.
7 p.m.—Temperature
25th, 11 a.m.—Tempera
night profuse perspiration
Microscopical appearance
forming bodies; neverthe
loped bodies.
4 p.m.—Temperature 40
patient received 0·66 gramm
26th, 9 a.m.—Temperature
(10½ grains) quinine given
Microscopical appearances:
mented forms.
4 p.m.—Temperature 38·2 C
Microscopical appearances negati
30th.—Since the 26th the patien
but he perspires considerably and
Microscopical appearances:
spherical bodies. Hæmoglobin
corpuscles 3,066,000.
October 6th.—Patient has remain
Microscopical appearances negativ
The infection consisted here of tw
tertian parasite and of the pigmented
fever had the quotidian character.

APTER VII.

ARIAL PARASITES — THE DIAGNOSTIC
ROSCOPICAL RESULTS — NEGATIVE

unnecessary, after having given
rms and phases of the malarial
to their diagnostic value.
justified by the fact that even
that substances in the blood
es which were not really so,
s that the parasites which
xperienced observer, however

only be mistaken for such
.
rpuscles, the white blood-
ducts of coagulation.
d-corpuscle has hardly
. just as little as has a
ms have not even the
But an altered crenated
copper-coloured body,
swarming fragments of
tly seen (and which
of beads, or oblong
lla. The greatest
of the red blood-
erienced, who may
f the parasite.
copper-coloured
the latter these
h oval, slightly
renated forms
of Morris?

TABLE III.—*Tabular Chart of the Characteristic Signs of the Various Parasites.*

	Duration of development.	Movement.	Pigmentation.	Maximum size.	Form of spore-formation.	Number of spores.	Crescentic bodies.	Alterations in the infested blood-corpuscles.
1. Quotidian parasite	72 hours	Small movement in the immature forms	Coarse grains; little or no movement	The size of the red blood-corpuscles	Daisy form; the single spores roughish, with distinct nucleolus	6–12	None	The red blood-corpuscles are little discoloured, and do not alter their size.
2. Ordinary tertian parasite	48 hours or less (in anticipating types)	Active amœboid movement in the immature and also in the middle-aged forms	Fine granules; in immature forms, often in the larger, actively swarming	Size of the red blood-corpuscles, sometimes even larger	Sunflower or grape-like; single spores small, round; nucleolus rarely seen[1]	15–20 (often less)	None	The red blood-corpuscles are often hypertrophied, and lose colour quickly and completely.
3. Pigmented quotidian parasite	24 hours	The unpigmented immature form very actively amœboid; less active when pigment accumulates	Very fine; later coalesces in one or two lumps; does not swarm	$\frac{1}{2}$–$\frac{1}{3}$ the size of a red blood-corpuscle	Irregularly formed heap	6–8, even more	Present	The red blood-corpuscles shrink often, and are then either darker stained (copper colour), or may be completely decolourised (Schleier).
4. Unpigmented quotidian parasite	24 hours or less	Very active amœboid movement	None	$\frac{1}{5}$–$\frac{1}{2}$ the size of a red blood-corpuscle	Star-shaped, or in irregular heaps	6–8	Present	The red blood-corpuscles shrink frequently, and are darkly stained.
5. Malignant tertian parasite	48 hours	Active; the movement remains present in the pigmented bodies	Moderately fine; often shows oscillatory movement	$\frac{1}{3}$–$\frac{2}{3}$ the size of a red blood-corpuscle	Irregular heaps	10–12, rarely 15–16	Present	The red blood-corpuscles shrink frequently; they are darkly stained, or may be perfectly colourless.

[1] N.B.—In a *fresh* condition it is always seen in a stained preparation.

CHAPTER VII.

THE DIAGNOSIS OF THE MALARIAL PARASITES — THE DIAGNOSTIC VALUE OF POSITIVE MICROSCOPICAL RESULTS — NEGATIVE RESULTS.

IT will probably appear to be unnecessary, after having given detailed descriptions of all the forms and phases of the malarial parasite, if I now once more refer to their diagnostic value.

That I do not omit doing this is justified by the fact that even until recently it often happened that substances in the blood were regarded as malarial parasites which were not really so, whilst it certainly repeatedly occurs that the parasites which *are* present are overlooked by the inexperienced observer, however good his intentions may be.

The malarial parasites can naturally only be mistaken for such bodies as are contained in human blood.

These bodies are the red blood-corpuscles, the white blood-corpuscles, the blood-plates, and the products of coagulation.

It is probable that a normal red blood-corpuscle has hardly ever been considered a malarial parasite, just as little as has a phantom blood-corpuscle,[1] for these forms have not even the remotest resemblance to the parasites. But an altered crenated blood-corpuscle might be mistaken for a copper-coloured body, or a mistake might be made between the swarming fragments of the red blood-corpuscles which are frequently seen (and which appear in the form of little balls, threads of beads, or oblong threads with snail-like motion) and the free flagella. The greatest danger, however, occurs with the "vacuoles" of the red blood-corpuscles, which may impose upon the inexperienced, who may take them to be unpigmented immature forms of the parasite.

The crenated forms are differentiated from the copper-coloured bodies in that they do not contain parasites; in the latter these are always seen as ringlets, or as bright, roundish oval, slightly pigmented or unpigmented specks; further, the crenated forms

[1] (Blutkörperchenshatten.) Invisible blood-corpuscle of Morris?

..ess pointed cogs, whereas the copper-coloured bodies ... ..eased, folded appearance (see Pl. II, fig. 49).

The swarming fragments of the red blood-corpuscles ... ..re or less the colour of hæmoglobin, whilst the swarmi.. ..gella are perfectly colourless, and sometimes have in them ... more exceedingly fine pigment granules. The swarming little ..lls and threads of beads do not, on account of their coarser ..pearance, resemble the flagella.

The "vacuoles" of the blood-corpuscles are in many respects ..ery similar to the unpigmented parasites. As is known, these ..cuoles result from mechanical injury which has occurred to the ..eparation, and the more carefully the drop of blood has been ..read out, &c., the less frequently do they occur. Vacuoles also ..ur if, for instance, a drop of oil from the lens finds its way into ..e specimen, or if the preparation is several hours old.

These vacuoles are really not what their name expresses; they ..re not small empty spaces in the blood-corpuscles, but contractions ..f the hæmoglobin substance, possibly zooids (Brücke), so that at ..he places where this contraction has occurred only the delicate ..ourless stroma (Oikoid?) which appears upon the blood-corpuscle as a bright point or ringlet, &c., according to the extent of the contraction, is to be seen. That it is indeed a contraction of the hæmoglobin substance, and in consequence of this a sinking in of the blood-corpuscle at the point in question, can be easily demonstrated in the method I have frequently before recommended, namely, of examining the object with an open Abbé and with oblique illumination from a convex mirror; with this illumination the "vacuoles" appear as furrows on the smooth upper surface of the blood-corpuscle.

The vacuoles have, further, the peculiarity of being able to change their form in a way which calls to mind the amœboid movement of the parasite.

In Plate II, figs. 67—70, a vacuole is shown in its changes of shape; these occur more actively on a warm stage. The shape and size of the vacuoles vary considerably from the finest point up to large spaces occupying two thirds of the blood-corpuscle. It also happens not infrequently that in one blood-corpuscle many small vacuoles can be seen (see Pl. II, fig. 71).

The most important difference between vacuoles and parasites is that the former possess no structure, while the latter, as living organisms, invariably do.

In fresh preparations the vacuoles are differentiated from the parasites in having a well-marked sharp contour, whilst the amœboid bodies, before they become quiescent, have an exceedingly delicate margin, which almost fades into the substance of the blood-corpuscle. The vacuoles have, further, a brilliancy which is not possessed by the parasites. The details of the differences are difficult to express shortly in words, but by a little experience it is possible in the majority of cases to decide with certainty one way or the other.

It must still be noted that the predominating ring form greatly suggests the parasite; further, that if one sees a considerable number of speckled red blood-corpuscles, whilst such are not present in another part of the preparation, it is vacuoles which are present and which have been produced by some local influence upon the preparation (pressure, oil, &c.).

The vacuoles can naturally never be mistaken for pigmented parasites, for they possess no pigment. With respect to the white blood-corpuscles, there are frequently pigment-carrying leucocytes seen in malarial blood which can be mistaken for parasites. With reference to this it should be noted that in the white corpuscles there are always one or more large compact nuclei visible, which is never the case in parasites. In fresh preparations only now and again a nucleus is seen in them, but it has always a vesicular form and a darker round disc. The nucleolus is seen in the vesicle.

The amœboid movements of the leucocytes cannot lead to any mistake, because the fully developed forms of the malarial parasite—and only these, on account of their size, need be regarded—never have amœboid movement.

Leucocytes which have taken up no pigment present no similarity to the parasites, because parasites of such a size are invariably pigmented, quite apart from the differences mentioned above.

The blood-plates may be mistaken for free spores when they lie singly and are perfectly round. When, as they often do, they lie together in little heaps they may be taken for spore-forming bodies.

Respecting the isolated blood-plates, it should be a rule never to diagnose a free spore in an unstained preparation. Such a diagnosis is in most cases impossible, for the free spores possess nothing characteristic. It is only the spores of the quartan fever which can be recognised as such on account of their visible nucleoli. Indeed, a free spore can just as well be mistaken for a round blood-plate as for a large coccus or for a yeast-cell, &c.

From this it is clear that for diagnostic purposes it is best to take no account of such-like bodies lying free in the liquor sanguinis.

In stained preparations the matter is quite different; in them we can differentiate a blood-plate from a spore with certainty (see Plate III, figs. 1, 2; Plate IV, fig. 70); whilst the former takes on a diffuse tinge and shows no structure, the latter, as is well known, behaves differently. It might be possible to take a blood-plate to be a piece broken off a large parasite; this would occur all the more easily because under very high powers a few granules may be seen in a blood-plate.

The blood-plates in groups are distinguished mostly from spore-forming bodies by the fact that they have no pigment, whilst, with few exceptions, no spore-formation without pigment residue occurs; and with reference to this exception, namely, the spore-forming bodies of the unpigmented quartan parasites, they are differentiated from the blood-plate conglomerations by the simple fact that they lie in red blood-corpuscles; indeed, this spore-formation, as has been said, hardly ever occurs in peripheral blood.

In stained preparations the same marks of difference obtain which we have given for the isolated blood-plates.

Lastly, with reference to the products of coagulation in the blood, clots, which however occur less frequently, must be considered. They appear as amorphous uniform bodies; they are always floating freely in the liquor sanguinis, and are not likely to be mistaken for parasites.

Together with these constituents of the blood, one must guard against such matters as epithelium, dust, and particles of rust, which foreign bodies may be present in the preparation notwithstanding all care and cleanliness.

Unless attention is paid to it, there are very frequently indefinable black particles, which may produce much doubt when pigment is searched for. It is quite certain that the malarial pigment may be present in a free state in the liquor sanguinis at the time of spore-formation, before the leucocytes appointed for the purpose have cleared away this fæcal matter of the parasites; and as a matter of fact, in preparations which have been made at the time of a fever paroxysm, these freely floating lumps of malarial pigment are frequently seen. Therefore, for diagnostic purposes, too much weight must not be laid upon such appearances, and from them alone the presence of a malarial infection must not be assumed.

It is much more significant when pigment is found in the leucocytes of *fresh preparations*; even if it be only a few granules, they form an important aid to diagnosis, especially if there is no me-

picion of a relapsing fever, for in such a condition pigment occurs in the blood.[1]

After a patient is cured, pigment remains for a short time visible in the circulating blood. It is, however, soon deposited by the leucocytes in the well-known positions. Usually in two or three days after the last paroxysm of fever (produced by tertian or quartan parasites) no more melaniferous leucocytes are present in the blood, but after fevers produced by the crescents it is different, for in such cases pigment-bearing leucocytes are met with in the blood as long as the crescents themselves.

Finally, the possibility must be considered of a poisoning with bisulphide of carbon or sulphurated carbonic oxide, which can rapidly produce pigment in the blood, as has been shown by C. Schwalbe (loc. cit.). I have repeatedly made experiments on mice, by subcutaneously injecting them with a few drops of bisulphide of carbon, and can fully confirm Schwalbe's statements. In such cases the history of the illness will clear up any doubts. But the alterations in the blood of animals so poisoned show a completely different picture from that given by the malarial parasites. I do not consider it necessary to give details, because, so far as I know, the alterations of the blood in question have not yet been observed in man.

In the blood of rabbits which have been poisoned with dinitrobenzol Huber observed an enormous formation of vacuoles in the red blood-corpuscles; the picture given in his work will serve as an interesting object of comparison with the immature malarial parasites.

Being now in a position to accurately recognise the malarial parasites, the question comes to be—what use can we obtain from this knowledge?

The answer is that the presence of even one single malarial parasite in the blood settles the diagnosis of a malarial infection.

I will not go in detail into those assertions which were made a few years ago, according to which, in the most different infectious diseases and cachexias, "similar bodies" in the blood had been found, through which the pathognomic and ætiologic importance of Laveran's malarial parasites was to be depreciated, for most authors on the subject have gradually admitted that they erroneously took things—they were almost always the "vacuoles" of the blood-corpuscles—for parasites which were not so. By means

[1] Recently the statement has been made that pigment is found in the blood in Addison's disease. I have not been able to confirm this in two cases which I have investigated with regard to it.

of the numerous investigations of blood which are at the present time pursued for diagnostic purposes, one has daily opportunity of convincing oneself that the malarial parasites exist exclusively in the blood of malarial patients.

From the microscopical appearances of the blood one can not only diagnose the presence in general of a malarial infection, but it is also possible to decide the species of the fever, the type, and often even the approximate severity of the attack. But, indeed, this accurate estimation of the results of the investigation of the blood can only be fully appreciated by those who have had considerable experience, and who are thoroughly acquainted with all the forms of the parasite.

It was Golgi who, after he had learnt to differentiate one parasite from the other, employed this knowledge to accurately settle the diagnosis with reference to type of fever, time of the attack, severity of the same, &c. Since that time his communications have always found increasing confirmation, to which I can add still further, because I have been able in many cases to clearly analyse the microscopical results according to Golgi's statements. The few contradictions which he has met with proceeded only from those investigators who, having had very little material to go upon, were not able to give an adequate opinion on the matter.

It is natural at the present time, after the gradual increase of and considerable advance in our knowledge, recently obtained through the work of Marchiafava and Bignami, that we should take into consideration the results obtained now, together with Golgi's original statements.

I pass over a detailed expression of opinion concerning the diagnosis of type, for were I to do so it would necessitate my repeating what has already been reported at length in regard to the special characteristics of the species of parasites, and this I would rather avoid. Anyone may obtain, from the description given in previous sections, the necessary information with regard to the diagnosis of the species.

I will only refer in few words to those points to which attention is chiefly necessary.

When a positive result has been obtained, one seeks in the first place to decide whether the species of parasite found belongs to the first group (which does not form crescents) or to the second group (which does), or whether, indeed, both groups are present in the blood. The experienced observer decides that in a short time, if large pigmented endocorpuscular forms are in the majority, they must be relegated to the first group; on the other hand, numerous small and slightly pigmented or non-pigmented parasites indicate the second group; if, however, crescents or spherical bodies of the crescent series are present, then it is at once decided that the second group is represented. These spherical bodies can be at once, even after very little experience, differentiated from the spherical bodies of the tertian and quartan parasites by the sharp, often double, contour, by the peculiar residue of the blood-corpuscles, by the frequent wreath-like arrangement of the pigment, and by the peripherally placed "buds."

Both the species of the first group can be differentiated by the activity of the amœboid movement, the shape and colour of the infested blood-corpuscles, and, in case such are present, by the shape of the spore-forming bodies, and the size, number, and structure of the spores. When, then, the species present in the individual case is recognised, one next seeks to ascertain whether one or more generations are present. This is the most difficult point for the beginner to decide, because he may be easily led astray by the sterile large forms which have lived through the attack, and then by the slight difference in size between the units of the same generation; so that he finally believes that he sees all stages present—therefore innumerable generations in the blood, whereas in reality probably only two, or indeed only one is present.

The idea must be held fast that we have here to do with living organisms which are not to be calculated in all their phases with mathematical accuracy, but which show variations within well-marked limits; a conclusion must be drawn from the average appearances, and exceptional extremes must not lead to a false conclusion.

To the determination of the number of generations follows the approximate estimate of the degree of development of the majority of the parasites present, for if this is known it is not difficult to estimate the time for the formation of spores, and therefore that of the paroxysm. The degree of development is fixed by the size, the amount of movement, and the pigmentation. The severity of the attack is, according to Golgi, proportionate to the number of parasites present.[1]

One proceeds in like manner in dealing with the parasites of

[1] In general I can confirm this view of Golgi's, but I must admit that individual idiosyncrasy and possibly also the virulence of the parasite may considerably influence the severity of an attack.

the second group. As may be imagined, it is more difficult to come to a conclusion in the mixed infections as they are more complicated, but in most cases the difficulties to be overcome are not insuperable.

We now turn to the negative microscopical appearances. It has happened to me, as well as to other observers (especially to Baccelli, who has occupied himself with this side of the question), that I have not been able to find any parasites, in spite of repeated diligent search, in the blood of patients who, according to all the symptoms, the progress of the disease, and the action of quinine, suffered from malaria. These cases were indeed very rare —in all three in some 130 cases—where positive results were obtained.

That negative results in general are of little importance has been repeatedly proved in other instances. With reference to the malarial parasite, it is still to be mentioned *that in perfectly fresh infections—that is to say, during the first days of the illness—the parasite is sometimes missed.* This occurs also in those cases in which experimental illness has been induced by the injection of malarial blood.

The cause of this is either that during the first days the parasites are only present in small numbers, and in consequence are difficult to find, or that they do not get into the circulating blood immediately.

In order to clear up the matter with certainty, when the first examination is negative, it is advisable to wait until one or more paroxysms have occurred, and thereafter to repeat the examination of the blood at a specially favorable time (before the paroxysm) ; in such cases also puncture of the spleen might be justifiable.

Further, it must be mentioned here that in malarial districts, where the disease plays a chief rôle in medical practice, one is very much inclined to attribute to malaria the most varying pathological conditions, the nature of which is not otherwise to be explained. I do not doubt the extraordinarily grave appearances of the malarial symptoms, for I have had opportunity enough to confirm them, but that it is too much to expect that in cases of gastritis, or gall-stone, or sepsis the malarial parasite should be demonstrated, every one will allow ; that just such cases in some of their forms resemble malaria very much, renders it comprehensible that often a false diagnosis is made. If, indeed, quinine does its duty, then the correctness of the diagnosis cannot be doubted for a second, and the negative parasite statistics are increased by one case more. How cautious one must be here, and with what care one must compare the symptoms with the microscopical results obtained from the blood, does not require further elucidation.

By the examination of the blood becoming general in malarious regions, the diagnosis of malaria will gain an immense advantage; the physician will be enabled to base an indisputable diagnosis upon positive irrefragable facts, and thereupon to base his therapeutical measures. The hesitation for days or weeks as to whether a case is typhus, or malaria, or sepsis, will now occur much less frequently than has been the case up to the present.

But it is not only for physicians in malarious regions that the knowledge of the malarial parasite is of great use; it is also nearly as important for all physicians, for there are a whole row of diseases which at times present the appearance of a typical intermittent fever, also a form of malaria which is sporadic, and which may occur at any time and everywhere. I will not go into particulars, but only call to mind how frequently obscure sepsis may for days or even weeks produce a perfectly typical fever, which can either be quotidian or tertian in type; the same occurs in miliary tuberculosis. Also in commencing typhus abdominalis, in pneumonia, in abdominal tumours, in gall-stone, and in sarcomata, typical fevers occur all too frequently.

In all these cases the exclusion of malaria by an investigation of the blood is a pressing necessity. From these short remarks it is sufficiently illustrated how rapidly the comparatively recent discovery of Laveran has won for itself a prominent and definite place in the diagnosis of internal disease.

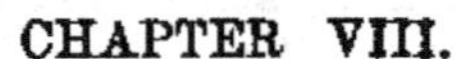

CHAPTER VIII.

ERNING THE CAUSAL RELATIONSHIP BETWEEN [illegible] PARASITES AND THE SYMPTOMS OF THE DI[illegible]

HAVING now considered the malarial parasites from [illegible] al standpoint, we will proceed to consider [illegible] ther and to what extent the symptoms of mala[illegible] ined through the presence of the microbes in [illegible] ether it is at the present time possible to erect a new [illegible] malaria based on the new discovery, and in a satisfactory [illegible] ace the former theories, or whether this is not yet [illegible] ly the case.

Two important and, as I th[illegible] two of the most important [illegible] ms of malaria may be co[illegible] l now as completely clear[illegible] by the discovery of the [illegible] rasites, and these symptoms [illegible] the *anæmia* and the *m*[illegible]

Before Laveran's discov[illegible] xplanation of the melanæmia, to which every one had instinctively turned with the greatest interest, as of chief importance, offered to clinicians and pathologists the very greatest difficulties, and much sagacity was expended in finding for it the correct solution—with what result we have seen in former chapters.

The melanæmia is to-day explained convincingly and indubitably by the fact that the parasites transform the hæmoglobin by which they are nourished by means of their metabolism into melanin. Melanin is therefore nothing but the undigested residue of nourishment which the parasites form and heap up in their bodies: the granules and rods can be conveniently termed fæcal matter, notwithstanding that they are not thrown out; for nothing seems to prove that they are stored-up "reserve nourishment."

It appears that the hæmoglobin undergoes several stages of decomposition in the body of the parasite before it finally forms the black pigment. It has already been mentioned that amongst the pigment granules all shades of colour, from that of hæmoglobin to the black of the completed pigment, may be seen;

and these differen...
chemical change.

After the spore-...
either concentrated ...
residue, which is imm...
these are the polyn...
leucocytes, whose pr...
sometimes only in the ...
more or less coarse lum...
ment is seen in a single ...

The leucocyte can on...
free in the liquor sang...
time of the attack, and co...
in consequence of this, ...
numerous melaniferous leu...
worthy that melaniferous leu...
attack of fever in the finge...
discover pigmented parasi...
amœboid bodies. This app...
ginner, is explained by the ...
bodies may be found in the ...
them is found in the periphera...

In general the melaniferous ...
in the diagnosis of malaria, be...
of having to come to a diagno...
especially the case in the inter...
fever if the crescentic bodies ...
often occurs in the mild quartan ...
the apyrexia a pigmented leuco...
than a parasite.

The *anæmia* is explained in ju...
the melanæmia, because we can ...
parasites the infested blood-corpuscle...
It is further also clear that the gre...
there are, the more blood-corpuscle...
consequent anæmia will be the more gr...

By proper methods of staining, ...
picric acid fixing, as I have advised, ...
the infested blood-corpuscles appear ...
possible that this is due to a precipita...
tion, produced by the parasites, or ...
ducts, in the hæmoglobin of the ...
I have frequently seen in the blo...

... per cent. of hæmoglobin and about

... I ascertained on the fourth day of the
...k every day of true quotidian fever
...rasites), hæmoglobin 100 per cent.,
...4,978,000; two days later (during
...urred), hæmoglobin 85 per cent.,
...012,000; after further two days (no
... hæmoglobin 60 per cent., number

... patient, although he had suffered
... of the blood proved to be normal
...gain suffering from an attack, a
...dy reduced blood-composition
...d is probably explained by the
... for an explanation of the last
...tion previously given, that the
... the dissolved poison of the

...ort that after the fever parox-
...e red blood-corpuscles rises
...lobin, and that at the time
...hlorotic appearance. This
...or *I found that for several*
proportion of hæmoglobin
...d-corpuscles began to in-

..., who had suffered for
...th quotidian parasites
... number of blood-cor-
...ring which the patient
...nt., number of blood-
...globin contained fell
...lood-corpuscles rose

...three weeks from
..., hæmoglobin 65
...; five days after,
...bin 55 per cent.,
... of hæmoglobin
... blood-corpuscles
...s from typical

cases, non-infested blood-corpuscles which were damaged, because numerous points in them were stained with methylene blue (see Plate IV, fig. 68). This method of degeneration of the red blood-corpuscle was, as is well known, described by Ehrlich. It is possible that this damage to the non-infested blood-corpuscles is due to the parasitic poison which is dissolved in the liquor sanguinis.

So we see that the red blood-corpuscle in malarial patients may be attacked in two ways, but their destruction is far more due to direct invasion by the parasites than to the dissolved poison.

In malarial patients the anæmia may reach a very considerable degree; in this connection we have to thank the French investigator Kelsch [66] for very thorough investigations. He has, indeed, taken a very successful part in the study of malaria in various directions.

Kelsch saw a diminution of the red blood-corpuscles as low as 500,000 per cubic millimetre. This diminution occurs according to him irregularly, and is greater at the commencement of the illness, therefore during the first attack, than during the later attacks. Kelsch saw in one patient the number of blood-corpuscles diminished by 2,000,000 in the course of four days.[1]

Dionisi [122] has recently likewise determined the number of blood-corpuscles in malarial patients, and he was able to prove that after single pernicious attacks a diminution of from 500,000 to 1,000,000 occurred.

Hayem and Halla [123] found a diminution in the number of blood-corpuscles of 1,182,760, or 2,800,000. In some of the malarial patients observed by me I have undertaken the estimation of the hæmoglobin and the enumeration of the blood-corpuscles, and was able to determine in each case a considerable diminution in both figures from the normal and in the following manner—that the poverty of the blood in blood-corpuscles, as in hæmoglobin, was parallel, and showed a picture of simple anæmia. I take the opportunity of stating the following figures in this connection.

In the case of a man, M—, suffering from pernicious tertian fever, I ascertained on the fourth day of the illness the amount of hæmoglobin to be 60 per cent., the number of blood-corpuscles 3,131,250; on the seventh day of his illness, hæmoglobin 45 per cent., number of blood-corpuscles 2,112,500.

Between these two days one attack occurred, and the patient

[1] It may be said once and for all that the number of blood-corpuscles always refers to the number per the cubic millimetre, the hæmoglobin percentage to results obtained from von Fleischl's hæmometer.

lost in consequence 15 per cent. of hæmoglobin and about 1,000,000 blood-corpuscles.

In a second patient, F—, I ascertained on the fourth day of the illness (patient had an attack every day of true quotidian fever caused by unpigmented parasites), hæmoglobin 100 per cent., number of blood-corpuscles 4,978,000; two days later (during which time two attacks occurred), hæmoglobin 85 per cent., number of blood-corpuscles 4,012,000; after further two days (no other attack having occurred), hæmoglobin 60 per cent., number of blood-corpuscles 3,310,000.

It was remarkable that in this patient, although he had suffered from three attacks, the condition of the blood proved to be normal at first, and that later, without again suffering from an attack, a further diminution of the already reduced blood-composition occurred. The first result obtained is probably explained by the small number of parasites found; for an explanation of the last result I fall back upon the supposition previously given, that the blood-corpuscles may be damaged by the dissolved poison of the parasites, as a possible cause.

Kelsch and Kiener [98, p. 543] report that after the fever paroxysms have ceased, the number of the red blood-corpuscles rises more rapidly than the amount of hæmoglobin, and that at the time of convalescence the blood presents a chlorotic appearance. This I have not been able to observe exactly, for *I found that for several days after the last paroxysm of fever the proportion of hæmoglobin still fell, whilst the number of the red blood-corpuscles began to increase.*

For instance, in the case of a man, P—, who had suffered for some long time from quotidian fever (with quotidian parasites without pigment), hæmoglobin 65 per cent., number of blood-corpuscles 2,544,000; three days thereafter, during which the patient was free from fever, hæmoglobin 45 per cent., number of blood-corpuscles 3,711,000. Therefore the hæmoglobin contained fell about 20 per cent., whilst the number of blood-corpuscles rose about 1,200,000.

In the case of M—, who had suffered for three weeks from irregular fever (unpigmented quotidian form), hæmoglobin 65 per cent., number of blood-corpuscles 2,717,000; five days after, the patient having been free from fever, hæmoglobin 55 per cent., number of blood-corpuscles 3,191,000. The loss of hæmoglobin was therefore 10 per cent., whereas the gain of blood-corpuscles amounted to nearly 500,000.

In the case of S—, who suffered for three weeks from typical tertian (Golgi's form), I found hæmoglobin 55 per cent., number of blood-corpuscles 2,476,000; three days after, during which there was no fever (the temperature rose once to 38·2° C. [100·7° F.]), hæmoglobin 40 per cent., number of blood-corpuscles 2,650,000. Therefore a loss of 15 per cent. of hæmoglobin, whilst the red blood-corpuscles slightly increased—about 200,000.

It cannot be said with certainty how this paradoxical condition arises; one thing is certain, that after the attacks cease new blood-corpuscles are rapidly formed. (Kelsch and Kiener, like Marchiafava and Celli, have sometimes proved the presence of nucleated red blood-corpuscles.) The loss of hæmoglobin is, as we have seen, not only not balanced, but goes on increasing for a time.

Nevertheless, I cannot consider the condition mentioned to be a constant rule, for in other cases the reproduction of the hæmoglobin has kept pace with the increase in the number of blood-corpuscles. For example, the blood of a man G—, after a three weeks' fever (mixed infection of tertian and unpigmented quotidian), showed hæmoglobin 42 per cent., number of blood-corpuscles 2,217,000; eleven days later, during which time the temperature had only once reached 38·4° C. (101·1° F.), hæmoglobin 65 per cent., number of blood-corpuscles 3,087,000; so that the hæmoglobin showed a gain of 23 per cent. and the red blood-corpuscles a gain of about 900,000.

The third principal symptom of malaria, the fever or the paroxysm of fever, with its typical or atypical formation, cannot be explained in such a satisfactory manner with our present knowledge of the malarial parasite, as is the case with the melanæmia and anæmia. Our ideas are, however, led in a very definite direction owing to the facts already lying before us, and it may be with great probability expected that after the elucidation of several moot points this direction will prove to be the right one.

Amongst the facts pointing in this direction, the very first is that found by Golgi in the correspondence between spore-formation and the attack of fever in the quartan and tertian fevers, which like correspondence Marchiafava and Celli also confirm for the true quotidian parasites.

It was, indeed, not too bold a step, and a not altogether unjustifiable application of the saying—elsewhere in physical science not well accredited—"post hoc ergo propter hoc," to bring the fever paroxysms into causal relation with the spore-forming mass of parasites.

Golgi states the matter thus, that, in consequence of the

bursting of the sporing bodies, an immense number of spores, and most probably also other substances which are formed in the parasites and are poisonous to man, get into the blood, and that these injurious bodies together cause the paroxysm.

This conception is supported by the numerous confirmations respecting the frequent correspondence of the spore-formation with the fever paroxysm. There are, however, some facts on the other side which are not yet cleared up; these are the occurrence of paroxysms without spore-formation, indeed even without parasites being found in the blood at all on the first days of fever.

It is upon the last circumstance that Baccelli [124] lays especial weight, and to illustrate it he recently reported a case of *Status perniciosus with hæmoglobinuria in which no parasites were found*, the malarial nature of which was proved by the success of its treatment with quinine. There is, however, in the history of the illness a contradiction, for on the 22nd of November, after many investigations, *a few pigmented leucocytes and amœboid parasites were found*. So that this case cannot be considered as perfectly conclusive, even if one has to allow that the severity of the illness stands in striking disproportion to the small number of parasites noted on one day.[1]

In face of such cases, in which for the time being no parasites were found, we must be particularly careful in regard to the diagnosis of malaria; we must keep in mind that against a very important number of positive results there are only an exceedingly small number of negative results, and that the latter would certainly be still further decreased if blood from the internal organs, where the parasites are most numerous and which contains the most developed forms, had been investigated. Further, it is not at present fully known *what consequences may follow the invasion by the parasites, after they themselves have again disappeared*. True, we know several of these results—the malarial cachexia with the ague cake, the chlorosis or sometimes even pernicious anæmia in consequence of the condition of the blood, the post-malarial delirium, the post-malarial hæmoglobinuria, &c., but it is not yet certain that these are the only consequences of the previous parasitic invasion, and that there are not other conditions possessing a more acute character which possibly might be added to them. The Italian investigators, as well as

[1] E. Grawitz [125] observed a case of malaria biliosa hæmoglobinurica, also without parasites in the blood; but it appears questionable whether it was not in this patient only an illness following a previous infection.

Sakharoff, say that there is a *Febris secondaria post malariam*, a fever which lasts for some days or even weeks after the parasites have ceased to be found, and which does not react to quinine. If I have not been able to observe this secondary fever, which indeed appears rarely to occur, I can at any rate point to another fact, previously mentioned, which follows the parasitic infection, namely, the decrease in the amount of hæmoglobin after the paroxysms of fever cease, as a condition which may be with certainty considered as the result of the action of the parasites which have disappeared. I mentioned, when describing the condition, that it was probably caused by the action in the blood of a poison produced by the parasites which had not been perfectly eliminated.

As we have seen, Golgi believes that a poison may be present in the spore-forming bodies, causing the paroxysm. In the present state of our knowledge of bacteriology such a view can hardly be denied, and all the less so because several facts are known which point to the paroxysms of malaria being accompanied or followed by the elimination of poisonous substances.

Roque and Lemoine [126] report that the urine voided after the fever acts as a poison to rabbits, whilst that passed before or during the fever has a markedly less poisonous action.

Further, Queirolo [127] has been able to kill rabbits by injecting them with the sweat of malarial patients.

These points respecting the production of a poison by the malarial parasites are indeed very meagre, but they show at any rate that the suggestion of a poisonous substance produced by the parasites is not altogether groundless. This poison in its action resembles the poison which is produced by septic parasites, chiefly, it appears, the Streptococci.

As a matter of fact, the clinical pictures of malaria and sepsis resemble one another, which appears to justify the idea that there is a near relationship between the agent causing the illness in both diseases.

Not only do rigors with fever, followed by sweating, form the chief clinical symptoms of both diseases, but we find in both resemblances between the accompanying symptoms; those occurring in the stomach and the intestines, as vomiting, diarrhœa, gastro-duodenal catarrh with consecutive jaundice, are just as much symptoms of sepsis as of malaria; dyspnœa also accompanies the malarial paroxysms, as those of sepsis; even ecchymosis of the skin has been repeatedly observed in malarial fevers, giving them an exceedingly similar appearance to that caused by sepsis.

These analogies between the two diseases cannot surprise us now-a-days, for in both conditions analogous processes occur in the organism, in that sepsis is produced by an infection of the mass of the blood with bacteria and their poisonous products, and malaria by an infection of the blood with protozoa and their products.

We can in the meantime regard malaria as a protozoa sepsis, and compare it with the ordinary bacteria sepsis.

Just as we refer the septic fever paroxysms (rigors, vomiting, fever, dyspnœa) to an irritation of the medullary centres, the septic jaundice and the diarrhœas to an irritation of the mucous membrane caused by the septic bacterial poison, so we must seek to explain the analogous appearances in malaria by the action of the protozoa poison upon the same central organs and mucous membranes. In this way the old theory concerning the nervous origin of the malarial paroxysm again presses to a certain extent to the front, although not in the sense understood by Trousseau [97], who described malaria as a direct neurosis, but rather in the sense of Griesinger [128], who in 1864, with wonderful acuteness, expressed himself as follows: "The cause of the periodicity of fever is therefore not found chiefly in a disposition of the nervous apparatus to rhythmical vital actions, as one formerly frequently tried to do, but it must, at least according to the present, although faulty, standpoint of our knowledge concerning the causes of heat, be attributed to something periodically taking place in the blood, which is connected with the increased formation of heat."

The "future" has abundantly justified Griesinger, for this periodic "something" taking place in the blood at the time of the paroxysm has, as we have seen, *been proved to be the spore-formation of the malarial parasites occurring at more or less regular intervals of time.*

How simply the fever type is explained by the period of evolution of the species of parasite present has been repeatedly mentioned. Also the change of type, for which formerly no reason at all could be found, is now fully explained by the addition or the death of one or more generations of parasites. But it must be mentioned that we have not sufficient knowledge concerning the reason for this change in the number of generations. It is frequently seen that a simple tertian may become a double tertian by doubling the generations, but why and how this doubling has taken place we do not know; still less can we explain why the generations are so frequently found at exactly twenty-four hours' intervals from one another.

In old authors we find it stated, and by Griesinger also, that by gradually postponing the attacks a tertian fever may change into the type of a quartan fever. It is to be seen whether such a case will be observed now that temperatures are taken so generally.

The postponing paroxysms can be easily explained by a slower development of the parasite; also the falling out of individual generations with consequent change of the type of fever—for instance the change of a double quartan into a simple quartan—does not cause any difficulty to our comprehension. The spontaneous cure of malaria is of frequent occurrence, and it is comprehensible that single generations from some cause, either in themselves or in the organism, may be isolated and die out.

This species of change of type, as well as the postponing paroxysms and also the obliteration of the cycle, may be experimentally produced by means of a corresponding administration of quinine.

Long known pathologico-historical causes are responsible for the enlargement of the spleen, which in malaria is very seldom absent. The recognition of the malarial parasite has caused fresh investigations in this direction, as those by Guarnieri and A. Bignami, whose results will be referred to subsequently when the phagocytes are considered.

Hæmoglobinuria is another symptom of malarial infection which frequently occurs.

Kelsch and Kiener [98, p. 383] have proved that in every severe case of malaria, even in every malarial cachexia, hæmoglobinuria may be observed, and they believe on these grounds that hæmoglobin is probably dissolved in the liquor sanguinis of every malarial patient. This opinion gains much in probability when we consider that all the hæmoglobin substance of the infested blood-corpuscles is not consumed by the parasites, but that usually more or less coloured débris of the blood-corpuscles is left behind (see also the process of excapsulation, Pl. II, figs. 55 and 56); it may be assumed that the hæmoglobin in this residue is dissolved, and if so, all that is necessary for the production of the hæmoglobinuria is present.[1]

Bastianelli and Bignami always found in several cases of fever with severe hæmoglobinuria the small forms of the crescent-

[1] Possibly lesions of the renal epithelium also deserve consideration, as recently again pointed out by Bignami.

forming parasites in the blood, and they state that the infested blood-corpuscles were colourless, therefore had given up their hæmoglobin. They have also observed cases in which the relapses, as well as the corresponding primary fever, were accompanied with hæmoglobinuria, from which they justifiably draw the conclusion that a certain individual tendency of the blood-corpuscles (which manifests itself in the easy surrender of the hæmoglobin under the influence of the parasites) is a concurring cause of hæmoglobinuria.

It may be admitted that these were specially severe cases, but it must not be forgotten that, as already mentioned above, Kelsch and Kiener have demonstrated the very frequent occurrence of hæmoglobinuria in malaria.

Another equally frequent symptom of the malarial infection consists of severe pains in the extremities, especially the legs; these are bone pains which may be increased by tapping the bones. These pains remind one of those in leucocythæmia, and when we take into consideration the excessive call which is made on the blood-forming marrow during the malarial infection, and think how very fluid, excessively hyperæmic, and filled with large melaniferous cells the marrow is found to be in malarial corpses, we shall clearly understand why the bones have been so tender during the illness.

In severe malarial infections the cerebral symptoms play an important *rôle*. Delirium, convulsions, paralysis, and coma may manifest themselves.

Heschl, Planer, Frerichs and others have for a long time explained these symptoms as due to thrombus caused by pigment cells and also to white thrombus; Kelsch and Kiener added to this the presence of endothelial swellings in the small cerebral vessels, with consequent diminution in their lumen.

But, as Frerichs has pointed out, all cases of malarial coma cannot be explained by the blocking of the cerebral vessels with pigment, because the autopsies in many cases of coma show no pigment or but very little.

On this point Marchiafava and Celli's results give some light; they find that blood-corpuscles infested with small amœboid parasites may impede the circulation, because they attach themselves to the walls of the vessels, especially in the cerebral vessels (see Pl. IV, fig. 66).

Bastianelli and Bignami's investigations are also worthy of mention with regard to the capillary hæmorrhages from the thrombosis of the smallest arteries of the white substance of the brain, which are frequently found after malarial coma. The extravasated blood-corpuscles showed themselves to be non-infested, whilst the walls of the vessels were lined by infested blood-corpuscles. This observation teaches that the infested blood-corpuscles, probably on account of a certain adhesiveness, attach themselves to the walls of the vessels and so impede the circulation.

It may be that besides this anatomical disturbance in the region of the cerebral vessels, the poisonous products of decomposition of the malarial parasites aid in the production of the cerebral symptoms.

In like manner the *hæmorrhages into the retina* may be explained; such hæmorrhages are not infrequent in pernicious fevers, but the numerous *hæmorrhages of the skin*, which are less often seen, are more probably caused by the action of poison.

In the cases of malaria accompanied by *choleraic diarrhœa*, Bignami found a high degree of hyperæmia of the stomach and intestinal mucous membrane, with punctiform hæmorrhages; microscopically there were found enormous accumulations of blood-corpuscles containing parasites within the blood-vessels, and extensive superficial necrosis of the mucous membrane and small-celled infiltration.

For several rare complications of malaria, such as *algid malaria, cardiac malaria, masked neuralgic malaria*, there are not up to the present sufficient results obtained, so that we cannot enter into any discussion with regard to them.

Besides those points of view just mentioned, there are still some general ones to be considered which relate to the severity of the infection, the individual tendency, and the toxicity of the virus.

Golgi established it as a rule that the severity of the attacks was parallel with the abundance of the parasites.

One has now, indeed, frequent opportunities of confirming this rule, as one usually sees very numerous parasites followed by severer attacks than is the case when the parasites are few.

This rule of Golgi's holds good in many, perhaps in most, cases, but one also finds not a few in which it does not obtain, especially in those cases where the most violent attacks are frequently seen with relatively few parasites. The contrary of this is much more rarely the case.

Bearing in mind the pathogenic nature of the parasites, we must, in such paradoxical cases, consider especially the heightened individual tendency; this might consist in a heightened irritability of the nervous system or in a chemical constitution of the blood, which would offer to the parasites a soil adapted to the production of particularly poisonous substances. Further, a difference in the strength of the toxicity of the parasites must not be forgotten.

That these factors in the infection of malaria certainly have an influence one sees most plainly in the diversity of the course of the disease under apparently similar circumstances.

It happens, for example, not infrequently that with many patients who are infected by the small quotidian parasite spontaneous cure sets in, the parasites becoming always fewer and at last quite disappearing, while other patients infected with the same quality and quantity pass through a severe illness, due to rapid increase of the parasites, and eventually, in spite of energetic therapeutic measures, succumb.

That the individual tendency plays a very important rôle in malaria we learn from the reports of doctors who practise in tropical regions, and have there the opportunity of comparing the morbidity and mortality of the natives with that of immigrant Europeans. Martin [130], who practised for seven years at Deli, in Sumatra, says that Europeans were attacked by the severest forms of fever, while the Malays, natives of Java, and especially the Tamils (of the Coromandel coast), suffered much more seldom than the Europeans, and then chiefly from the mild forms like quartan and tertian.

Schellong [131], in Finschhafen (Kaiser Wilhelmsland), reports similar observations; if he denies that the native population have almost an immunity from malaria, he nevertheless admits that they show a smaller tendency to it than the Europeans.

One must, however, take into consideration the exact conditions under which these observations were taken, and remember that in those countries the Europeans are hygienically much better off than the native population as regards nourishment, dwellings, clothing, and occupation; that the number of those who suffer among them would be much greater than is now the case if they did not enjoy these advantages, each one of which may be regarded as a partial protection against malaria.

It is thus seen that the personal tendency, as well as the number of the parasites (of the same kind understood), influences the severity of the disease in large measure.

We possess no direct proofs of the difference in the strength of the poison of the parasites, but it may be conjectured from the fact that persons who suffer from the same forms of fever at different times develop sometimes milder and at other times severer symptoms. One might, of course, suppose a temporarily heightened or decreased predisposition in these cases; but this question of toxicity can only be settled with certainty by experimental methods, indeed by means of cultivations at which we have not yet arrived, or by obtaining the hypothetical poison from the urine, sweat, &c.

CHAPTER IX.

SPONTANEOUS CURE OF MALARIAL FEVER—PHAGOCYTOSIS—INFLUENCE OF QUININE UPON THE MALARIAL PARASITES.

THAT many cases of malaria, mild cases of ague, as well as severe illnesses resulting from the small forms of parasites, may be cured spontaneously, especially when the patients are brought under favourable hygienic circumstances, has been known for a long time. We not seldom see that the illness spontaneously disappears soon after the arrival of the patient in hospital without quinine or any other means being administered. It is clear from this how carefully one must estimate the therapeutic effect of a new remedy in regard to malaria, and that certain conclusions can only be arrived at after considerable experience.

The reason for the spontaneous cure during hospital treatment (or also by treatment at home) must be ascribed first of all to rest in bed, better nourishment, and general bodily restoration, which factors strengthen the organism in its struggle against the enemy that has broken in.

Secondly, the protection against fresh infection must be considered as an important factor, although in regard to this one must remember that malaria has generally a period of incubation of from eight to fourteen days, so that the possible fresh daily infection cannot take effect at once.

In spontaneous cure the number of parasites diminishes rapidly, and after a few days at the most only a few will be found, if any. For example—

J. L—, æt. 19, is said to have had an attack daily for fourteen days; never had fever before. He is a strong lad, rather pale, skin slightly jaundiced, spleen easily palpable. He has pain in the spleen and weakness in the limbs.

October 6th, 1892, 10 a.m.—Temperature 36·5° C. (97·7° F.).

Microscopical appearances: 1. Large pigmented parasites which are nearly as large as blood-corpuscles; the pigment actively swarming. 2. Rather numerous, also deeply pigmented parasites, which half fill the blood-corpuscles. The infested blood-corpuscles are many of them distended and decolorised.

This is then the picture of a double tertian, and it agrees with the patient's statement.

3 p.m.—Temperature 37° C. (98·6° F.).

6 p.m.—Temperature 37·5° (99·5° F.). The expected attack did not occur; no sweating during the night.

7th, 10 a.m.—Temperature 36·2° C. (97·1° F.).

Microscopical appearances: The same as yesterday afternoon, but in addition many pigment-carrying leucocytes.

4 p.m.—Temperature 37·5° C. (99·5° F.).

Microscopical appearances: Very few large parasites.

6 p.m.—Temperature 38° C. (100·4° F.).

8th, 10 a.m.—Temperature 36·3° C. (97·3° F.).

Microscopical appearances: After a long search a large free parasite with active pigment movement was found.

Patient remained free from further attacks of fever. Nothing more was found in his blood.

P—, æt. 47, states that he has suffered daily for four days from a severe typical attack of fever.

September 21st, 3.30 p.m.—Temperature 40·3° C. (104·6° F.). Pulse 120. Tension below normal. Slight jaundice. Spleen extends to three finger-breadths below the ribs.

Microscopical appearances: A few unpigmented amœboid parasites.

22nd.—During the night patient perspired profusely.

9 a.m.—Temperature 35·8° C. (96·4° F.).

Microscopical appearances: Several small quiescent parasites of ring shape; no pigment.

4.30 p.m.—Rigors. Temperature 39° C. (101·2° F.).

5.30 p.m.—Temperature 40° C. (104° F.). The rigors continue.

8 p.m.—Temperature 40·2 C. (104·3° F.).

23rd, 9 a.m.—Temperature 36·7° C. (98° F.). Patient very weak; the spleen has enlarged since yesterday.

Microscopical appearances: Very few small quiescent parasites of ring shape.

6 p.m.—Free from fever.

24th.—Free from fever.

Microscopical appearances: Two pigment-carrying leucocytes. No parasites.

28th.—Patient has remained free from fever since last note.

Microscopical appearances: Crescents.

In this case there were small unpigmented quotidian parasites present, which as a rule, unless energetically treated, may easily originate a pernicious fever, whereas they spontaneously disappeared in this case without any treatment, and at the same time the attacks of fever ceased.

Respecting the means possessed by the organism to combat the malarial parasites, we are taught by Metschnikoff [32] that the macrophages of the spleen and the marrow of bones develop an energetic destructive action against the parasites. As a fact A. Bignami [50] also found in the spleen and in the marrow large single nucleated cells in which numerous parasites, and among them frequently spore-forming bodies and even whole infested blood-corpuscles, were enclosed. In the cerebral vessels the endothelium also develops some, though considerably less, phagocytic action.

Together with the macrophages possessing well-stained nuclei, Bignami also frequently found others with a non-stained nucleus which are to be considered as necrotic phagocytes. These necrotic macrophages with spore-forming bodies inside them originated Bignami's opinion, previously mentioned, that the relapses were caused by spores which had escaped from the disintegrated cells. The frequency of the presence of phagocytes in the organs just mentioned lends to Metschnikoff's theory regarding malaria considerable support, especially the fact of whole groups of spores being consumed, and it can hardly be doubted, therefore, that the phagocytes play a considerable rôle in the spontaneous cure of malaria. It is desirable that it might be proved by puncture of the spleen that the phagocytic action by the macrophages does not only occur post mortem, as we see it in the leucocytes of the blood under the microscope.

Less weight is to be laid upon the frequent observation of phagocytosis by means of the leucocytes in the blood.

In preparations which are examined for half an hour to an hour under the microscope it is often seen how a moving leucocyte may gradually enclose in its substance a free parasite, even one which is flagellated; the movement of the pigment in the parasite continues for a time in the leucocyte; it then stops, and the contour of the parasite is gradually lost until at length only a small heap of pigment represents the body which has been devoured.

This process does not appear to occur in the circulating blood, because one never finds, either in a fresh unstained preparation or in dry preparations, a leucocyte which has a clearly recognisable parasite within it. It is not alone the circulating blood which hinders the process of phagocytosis, as may be concluded from the circumstance that the leucocytes no doubt very frequently contain pigment which they have taken up, if no parasites, and this must have been absorbed in the circulation. It is indeed, however, possible that the slower circulation in the spleen and in the marrow renders phagocytosis easier in those places. Another circumstance which renders highly improbable phagocytosis of the malarial parasites by the circulating white blood-cells is, that the leucocytes in malaria are frequently found to be diminished in number.

Kelsch [132] pointed out that the number of leucocytes rapidly diminished during an attack of fever, so that the numerical relation of the white and red blood-corpuscles can become 1 in 2000. When one remembers that the absolute number of the red blood-corpuscles has likewise greatly diminished, the absolute diminution of the white blood-corpuscles appears far greater than the above proportion expresses. Kelsch also found in cases of malarial cachexia a marked diminution of the leucocytes, and only in fevers with pernicious symptoms has he always found a conciderable increase in the leucocytes as much as 1 in 48.

This difference in the relation of the leucocytes in cases of malaria of mild and of pernicious character is inexplicable, and is worth further detailed research.

Kelsch was able to prove that the leucocytes which had disappeared from the blood were stored in the spleen, because after energetic faradisation and consequent contraction of that organ, the number of leucocytes in the blood was raised; one or two hours later, with the fresh gradual distension of the spleen the former condition of things obtained.[1]

This remark is not intended to serve as an explanation of the phenomena in question, but only as a stimulus to further investigations.

Golgi, who estimates the phagocytosis by means of the white blood-corpuscles higher than my experience permits me to do, believes that a rhythm may be found in the process which runs parallel with the type of the fever. In quartan and tertian

[1] It is possible that the phagocyte theory could be imagined thus—that at the time of the malarial attack the leucocytes collect in the spleen; there, under more favourable circumstances than are found to obtain in the circulating blood, to employ their parasite-destroying activity, and that those malarial cases become pernicious in which this collecting of the leucocytes (in the spleen) does not occur (from what reason is at present unknown), and in which the blood is therefore not impoverished of leucocytes, but indeed richer in them than it is in other cases

fevers he finds that the phagocytosis commences with the attack and lasts three or four hours longer than it does. Later on, the parasites taken up by the leucocytes are digested, and it is possible to estimate approximately the time which has passed since the attack by the amount of change which the parasites in the leucocytes show.

It must be remarked, however, that Golgi himself allows that he has rarely seen leucocytes containing parasites in fresh blood.

In many hundred stained preparations I have never seen such an instance, but only been able to find pigment; neither have I succeeded in ascertaining more from the melaniferous leucocytes than that an attack of fever has occurred; it appears to me that the data are insufficient on which to base an opinion of the time of the occurrence of the attack.

I can thoroughly confirm the statement that the melaniferous leucocytes are to be found in the blood both at the time of the attack and for twelve to twenty-four hours thereafter (and even longer), and I believe that these leucocytes containing pigment only appear during and after the attack, because it is only at that time that the pigment is free in the blood, which it is their function to take up, and therefore that the absorption of pigment from the blood is not a "cyclical function" *sui generis* of the leucocytes, but to be considered simply as a consequence of the circumstance mentioned.

In blood aspirated from the spleen during an attack of fever, Golgi also frequently found many large extremely pigmented cells (macrophages); unfortunately it is not said whether living parasites or indeed recognisable parasitic bodies were to be seen enclosed.

Marchiafava and Bignami [100] likewise found in the fevers caused by the malignant tertian parasite that the melaniferous leucocytes were to be seen in the greatest numbers chiefly at the time of the attack and shortly afterwards. In multiple infection with continued or remittent fever they found these cells, in the same number, at all times, for reasons which may be easily understood.

These authors appear to put the phagocytosis of the leucocytes in the blood down to a mere cleansing of the blood from the freed pigment and the dead bodies of the parasites, whilst, on the other hand, they state that the large granulated single nucleated macrophages of the spleen, the marrow, and the endothelium of the cerebral vessels (as Metschnikoff, Guarnieri [134] and Bignami have shown, and which has been already mentioned) as a matter of [illegible] absorb whole parasites, spore-forming bodies, even copper-[illegible]red bodies or decolorised infested blood-corpuscles.

[illegible] usefulness of the activity of the macrophages is believed [illegible] influenced, however, by the circumstance mentioned by [illegible], that many of the gorged macrophages again degenerate [illegible] they have digested the spores.

[illegible] methods of resistance may come into play as well as the [illegible] in the battle against the parasites, for one frequently [illegible] fevers spontaneously cured, just as in those which have [illegible] treated with quinine, the large free parasites, *which we [illegible] to recognise as sterile forms*—those, therefore, which [illegible] at spore-formation and yet retain their species, but [illegible] probably also by phagocytosis or by disintegration. [illegible] large sterile bodies are very often met with amongst [illegible] parasites. They remain in the blood after the single febrile [illegible] after the conclusion of the so-called paroxysmal cycle [illegible] forty-eight hours.

[illegible] attack itself *acts injuriously upon a large part both [illegible] of the perfectly mature parasites*, either by the [illegible] temperature of the blood or by the pyrogenic sub-[illegible] from the sporing parasites.

[illegible] found disintegrated tertian parasites, and less [illegible] parasites during the febrile paroxysms. These [illegible] bodies (see Plate III, figs. 33 and 34) may be found [illegible]puscular or free, according to whether the injurious [illegible] has acted upon an immature or a rather more [illegible]

[illegible] show, the disintegration occurs in nume-[illegible], and there can be no manner of doubt that [illegible] vitality and the power of life and reproduction [illegible]. The endocorpuscular disintegrated parasite [illegible] if accurately observed, for amœboid bodies, [illegible] the fever, are found in especially active movement; [illegible] one sees that the isolated fragments are [illegible] so that it cannot be objected that it is a multiple [illegible] blood-corpuscle.

[illegible] *malaria depends, therefore, upon three [illegible] phagocytic action of the macrophages in the [illegible] less upon the epithelium of the cerebral [illegible] that [illegible] parasites remain [illegible] action of the fever paroxysm, [illegible] the disintegration of [illegible] immature and [illegible]ites.*

We meet with the sterility and the disintegration of the parasites in a considerably increased measure when quinine has been administered, but this subject will be dealt with immediately.

The action of quinine upon the malarial parasites has, since Laveran's discovery, been studied both by him and by several other investigators.

Laveran investigated the matter thus: From one patient he prepared at the same time two specimens of blood; the one he treated with a very weak solution of quinine, the other served as a control, and was examined under the microscope without any addition to it. Laveran found that whilst in the control specimen the parasites remained in active movement for a considerable time, in the preparation treated with quinine all the parasites lay quiescent and lifeless, whereby the direct poisonous action of the drug upon the parasites was proved.

Later experiments confirmed this appearance, but they limited its importance in so far that they showed that other indifferent substances added to the preparation also killed the parasite. Thus Marchiafava and Celli [19] found that the parasites ceased their movements if a solution of common salt or distilled water was added to the preparation. Grassi and Feletti [135] showed also that if malarial blood was shaken with distilled water for an hour and then injected into a healthy man no infection followed, because on account of this procedure the malarial parasites had died.

As the action of quinine could not be studied directly with sufficient success, I undertook to investigate the parasites in the blood of patients who were being treated with quinine, and to give to the structural details of the cinchonised parasites especial attention. About the same time, and independently of me, Romanowsky did the same with his method of staining. Baccelli, Golgi, Marchiafava, and Bignami have also methodically examined fresh blood at short intervals, with reference to the action of quinine, and in this way tried to clear up the question.

The total result of all these investigations consisted in the proof that quinine in the organism killed the parasites in the blood.

This action of quinine upon the malarial parasites is analogous to its action upon Infusoria, as shown by Binz [79] in 1867, and later on further studied by him and his pupils, and we shall see *that the alterations which the malarial parasites show when poisoned with quinine are exceedingly like the changes which Binz has described in the poisoned Infusoria.*

If we examine in the first place the quartan and the ordinary tertian parasites with reference to their reaction against quinine, we find the following appearances:

As soon as three hours after the administration of 0·5 to 1·0 gramme of quinine (8—15 grains), to cases in which the *amœboid form of the tertian parasites* is present, a considerable diminution in the amœboid movement can be demonstrated. From three to six hours later the number of the parasites is also considerably diminished, and of those which remain many are disintegrated, so that they form several little balls lying within the red blood-corpuscles, which are no longer connected together; of this one may be convinced by long-continued observation.

After the administration of quinine the mature forms of the tertian parasite show either a complete standstill of the movement of the pigment which gives the parasite a clotted, shining, homogeneous appearance as if coagulated, or a dropsical distension of the parasite occurs with a most active oscillating movement of the pigment, or lastly, the parasite breaks up into several particles just as does the immature endoglobular variety.

The last two methods of alteration, namely, the disintegration of the parasite and the dropsical distension, we have learnt to know as the appearances which also occur during the febrile attack without the action of quinine; whilst the disintegration may be doubtless considered as the death of the parasite, the distension may be perhaps rather considered as a kind of interference with development or rather with reproduction, therefore a sterilising of the parasite.[1]

It must further be borne in mind that a short time after the administration of quinine the middle-sized tertian parasites may be met with in most active, so to say, writhing movement; a somewhat similar appearance may be occasionally observed during febrile attacks; it appears, therefore, that the parasites sometimes are stimulated to increased movement before they coagulate and are brought to a standstill in consequence of the quinine. Binz has described similar appearances in the Infusoria.

The spore-formation of the tertian parasite takes places in part in a normal manner under the influence of quinine (if the quinine is given in two or three 0·5 gramme [8 grains] doses four to six hours before the attack), whilst it remains incomplete in others, to which we shall refer when describing the details of structure of the "quinine forms."

[1] According to Binz, Herbst [136] found in 1867 that quinine in a weak solution prevented the power of reproduction in Infusoria; stronger solutions caused death.

Golgi observed that under the influence of quinine the medium-sized quartan parasites show a rather fine granulation, a metallic lustre, and a tendency to shrivelling; the large forms are distended, they have an active oscillating movement of the pigment, and sometimes contain vacuoles or abortive spores.

As one sees, the complete resemblance between these two nearly related forms of parasite also holds good when under the influence of quinine.

The small crescent-forming parasites are not so well studied in fresh preparations as in stained ones with reference to their behaviour under quinine.

Baccelli [124] observed that shortly after the administration of quinine the amœboid bodies showed an increased activity, and that twenty-four hours afterwards most of the bodies had often disappeared without leaving a trace. I have found in cases of true quartan, mild in character, that even three hours after the administration of a dose of quinine, 0·5 gramme (8 grains), part of the amœboid bodies show a nucleolus badly stained or not stained at all. If the quinine is continued, it is found in these cases after further twelve hours that only isolated parasites possess a nucleolus; the remainder have either a nucleolus which will not stain or is already disintegrating, so that in the most altered forms only a few shapeless fragments are found (see Plate IV, figs. 57—62).

A commencing necrosis of the small parasites is indicated by the nuclear chromatin remaining unstained; this is followed, as it appears, very rapidly by a complete disintegration of the bodies, so that after forty-eight hours not a trace of them is to be found.

In like manner the action of quinine on the tertian parasites is to be explained. I found that a few hours after the administration of the first dose of quinine, the greater part of the small and middle-sized varieties did not possess a nucleolus that would take on the stain, whilst the clear vesicle which represented the nucleus was to be seen as formerly; the further fate of these necrosed parasites consists likewise in disintegration (see Plate III, fig. 35).

I have found, moreover, that many of the spore-forming bodies can undergo peculiar changes owing to the administration of quinine several hours before an attack (see Plate III, figs. 36 and 37).

These spore-forming bodies show, indeed, a segmentation which in fresh preparations might possibly appear as complete; in stained preparations, however, the interesting fact is brought out *that only a small portion of the segments formed consists of spores capable of life, for they only* show a well-developed structure, *whereas the larger part of the segments possess no nucleolus,* and therefore cannot be considered as having the power of life.

On the basis of these drawings I think I am justified in considering that segmentation under the influence of quinine takes place in a faulty manner, and in consequence I named these non-nucleated segments "*stillborn spores.*" It is, however, possible (according to an observation of Golgi's to be mentioned immediately) that the spores perished only after they had become capable of life. There is, however, really no difference between the two possibilities.

Romanowsky [48] has recognised a decided action of quinine upon the mature large parasites, for he found them frequently without a nucleolus and with only a diffusely stained nucleus. I have previously mentioned that I do not consider the diffuse staining of the nucleus and the disappearance of the nucleolus in the large forms as a necrosis in every case, but also as a preparation for spore-formation. Therefore I consider the immature forms without a nucleolus as distinctly more characteristic of the action of quinine than that described by Romanowsky. The faulty tinting of the nucleoli (his nucleus) in his spore-forming bodies Romanowsky describes in agreement with me.

From observation of stained preparations we see, therefore, that quinine causes a necrosis in malarial parasites of different species and different ages, and that in this way, on the one hand the specific action of quinine in malaria receives a thorough explanation, and on the other hand the pathogenic nature of the malarial parasite is supported by the susceptibility to quinine which they are proved to possess.

It must, however, still be mentioned that all the parasites do not immediately become necrosed after the administration of the first doses of quinine. We know, indeed, that after commencing treatment, no matter when the quinine is given, further attacks of fever may follow both in the quartan and tertian fevers, especially in fevers of the second group. Indeed, notwithstanding the abundant subcutaneous injection of quinine in pernicious fevers, the disease may either result in death, or relapses persistently occur for a long time.

The causes of this faulty action, or even of the absence of action of the quinine, may be very various. The method of the administration of the drug has of itself an influence upon its action. It is known to all physicians who are practically acquainted with malaria that the administration of quinine in the form of powder by the mouth retards the rapidity of its action when compared with the administration of the same doses in solution. The reason for this is easily seen. Without doubt, in order to exert definite action upon the parasites, the quinine must be dissolved in the blood in a definite amount, and unless there is this proportion, a slighter action only upon some especially susceptible parasites will be obtained, or even no action may result. The quinine must be present in the organism in such a way that the blood contains for some time as strong a proportion of quinine as possible. This result is certainly less obtained by the administration of the drug in the form of powder than when it is given in solution; the solution is more rapidly absorbed than the powder, which is only gradually dissolved in the stomach and absorbed in small portions. In this connection it must be remembered that the quinine is eliminated by the urine very rapidly. The elimination already commences ten minutes after the drug has been given, increases considerably six hours later, and is almost completed in twelve hours (Thau [135]). Later (from forty-eight to sixty hours) only traces of it can be demonstrated in the urine.

Still better than by the administration of solutions of quinine by the mouth, the desired results may be obtained by the hypodermic injection of the drug. The following solution recommended by Vitali and Galignani [136] may be most conveniently employed.

Chininum Muriat.	10·0
Aquæ Dest.	7·5
Acid. Mur. dilut.	2·5

This solution contains 0·73 gramme of the muriate of quinine in the cubic centimetre (nearly 11¼ grains in 16 minims).

Baccelli [137] has recently introduced the intra-venous injection of quinine with much success for the gravest malarial infections, in which the greatest possible concentration of the drug and the most rapid action is needed. It can be recommended for cases of *malaria comatosa*, which very frequently terminate fatally.

Baccelli employs the following solution:

Chininum Mur.	1·0
Natrium Chlorat.	0·075
Aquæ Dest.	10·0

The solution should be boiled and filtered before use; the injection should be made into a small vein in the arm. It may be injected direct through the skin, which has been previously thoroughly disinfected.

Apart from the method of administration there may be other circumstances which retard the action of quinine, as, for instance, imperfect action of the mucous membrane of the stomach or intestines or of the subcutaneous connective tissue which delays absorption, blocking of the cerebral capillaries with infested blood-corpuscles, on account of which the parasites cannot come in contact with the quinine, and possibly also a heightened power of resistance on the part of some species of the parasite.

One series of the malarial parasites is completely unsusceptible to the action of quinine, namely that of the crescentic bodies. All observers are at one in stating that these bodies remain unaltered even by the most energetic administration of quinine, and that the treatment in these cases likewise plays no prophylactic rôle is shown by relapses occurring whether or not quinine has been given during the periods of apyrexia.

This fact also militates against Bignami's view of latent spores which have escaped out of the phagocytes causing relapses. Through all the various stages of the development of the malarial parasite the spores are the most susceptible to the action of quinine. Golgi [140] has constructed the following scale of susceptibility to quinine for the various phases of development of the quartan parasite, based upon his experience of fresh specimens of blood.

I. Spores.

II. Mature forms before the commencement of the process of segmentation.

III. Endocorpuscular younger forms.

The spores are the most susceptible bodies; then follow the large bodies which have completely replaced the blood-corpuscles, and finally the endocorpuscular younger bodies whose blood-corpuscle envelope Golgi considers as a relative protection against quinine. Of the tertian parasites Golgi has found, as I have, the endocorpuscular immature forms very susceptible, and he believes that the quinine can more easily penetrate into the hypertrophied more flexible blood-corpuscles.

In quartan and tertian fevers Golgi has tried to ascertain, by observing the appearance of the parasites, at what time the administration of quinine is of the greatest use in the smallest dose, and he came to the conclusion that the most beneficial time was three to five hours before the attack. The next attack, indeed, follows with full severity, but the following attacks do not occur, often indeed without the further administration of quinine. Golgi has observed that parasites preparing for segmentation were not influenced by quinine, but that they completed that process notwithstanding the drug; on the other hand, he found that the young spores were exceedingly susceptible to quinine.

Now, if at the time mentioned (three to five hours before the attack) 1 gramme (15 grains) of quinine is administered, then the blood at the time of the attack will contain so much dissolved quinine that the spores just formed, the whole young brood so to say, are killed in *statu nascendi* and thereby the attack which should follow is rendered impossible.

It has been long known and has been recently confirmed by Golgi that when quinine is administered about six or eight hours before an attack it will be postponed and weakened; in this way a postponing type can be artificially produced. In multiple infections with quartan parasites Golgi succeeded sometimes in killing one generation after another, and thereby changing a triple quartan (quotidian) first into a double and finally into a single quartan. This experiment can be performed if a small dose of quinine, about 0·4 gramme (6 grains), is given two hours before the attack; with this small dose one succeeds in killing a large part of, or under certain circumstances all, the spores newly formed during the attack, so that one generation is removed. The large forms of another generation which may be present are not at all or only slightly injured by the small dose of quinine; they remain uninfluenced and produce the corresponding fever type. This experiment does not invariably succeed, because the differences in susceptibility of the various stages of the parasite are by no means very great, so that small doses may cause damage to all the generations and thereby prevent the gradual production of the attacks. By the administration of quinine, not at the favorable period of the spore-formation, but at an haphazard period, the type of fever is often delayed. The paroxysms which formerly occurred at regular intervals can be either separated further from one another or drawn nearer together, according to whether the therapeutic measures have curbed one or other generation of parasites in its development or left it intact.

Similar observations to those which Golgi has made with regard to tertian and quartan fevers have been made by Marchiafava and Bignami [100] with malignant tertian fever. They found that when the quinine was administered towards the end of the paroxysm the young generation of parasites either stopped developing, and after twelve to twenty-four hours (more rarely thirty-six to forty-eight hours) disappeared from the blood, or that a part of the generation developed, only in a sluggish manner, or lastly (and this one must probably be put down to a special resistance in the parasites to the alkaloid) that the entire generation went on developing and propagating undisturbed. According to these three possible courses, the following attack either did not occur, or it followed later and remained abortive, or it came at the right time and in full force. The last course was especially noticed to follow the administration of the drug in one single dose.

If the quinine be administered during the apyrexia, at the time that the pigmented parasites are already preparing to form spores, then the young generation is not seen to make its appearance at all; if the temperature is, however, rising at the time of the administration of the drug, then the young generation is seen either to make its appearance during the attack of fever and soon after disappear, or it is first seen in the blood-corpuscles several hours (up to twenty-four) after the commencement of the attack.

Corresponding to this, when the drug is administered during the apyrexia the next following attack breaks out in full force, but the later ones generally do not occur.

When there is multiple infection with these parasites—and that is indeed by far the most usual case—the various generations disappear one after the other. After the spores, the pigmented bodies are believed to be the most susceptible, while the immature already endocorpuscular parasites have more power of resistance and are to be found during one or two days, though perhaps in diminished numbers.

We see also in these fevers, presupposing that apyrexia is recognisable in them (that they therefore are caused by only one generation), *that the quinine has the greatest effect if administered several hours before the attack.*

The same may be said of the quotidian fever. It must, however, be borne in mind that the three crescent-forming species of parasites occur mostly in multiple generations, so that therapeutical measures cannot, in the case of the resulting continued or remittent fevers, be directed upon the single paroxysm. In these cases it is important to begin the administration of quinine as soon as the diagnosis is made, and to continue the same in

0·5 to 1·0 gramme (8 to 15 grains) doses, given at intervals of four to six hours; smaller doses also, as 1·0 gramme (15 grains) in three doses, taken in the morning, mid-day, and evening, give good results in these fevers when they are not too severe.

Marchiafava and Bignami report that in the Roman hospitals, in summer fevers of ordinary severity, they give at first 2 grammes of sulphate or muriate of quinine (30 grains) in two doses at an interval of from two to four hours, and then give 0·5 to 1·5 gramme (8 to 24 grains) doses every twelve hours. In the severer forms of this fever a subcutaneous injection of 1 to 2 grammes (15 to 30 grains) is given at first; in fever with pernicious symptoms one of from 2 to 3 grammes (30 to 45 grains), at the beginning every four to six hours, later 1 gramme (15 grains). These fevers are, as has already been mentioned, most successfully met with the intra-venous injections of Baccelli.

Besides the therapeutical, the prophylactic use of quinine must also be mentioned; this is employed with success in many malarial districts, and consists in the following treatment: that people should take daily a fairly large dose of from 0·3 to 0·4 gramme (5 to 6 grains), generally in brandy. In Pola this prophylactic treatment by quinine was introduced some years ago among the soldiers who were posted at very bad malarial spots (such as the Brionic Islands, certain marine fortresses, &c.), and I have heard from the naval surgeons that it has done very good service. Similar results are reported from the English and French navies.

The destructive action of quinine upon the lower animals appears, according to Binz [141], to be connected with the power of this alkaloid to arrest oxidation. It has also been ascertained by Bonwetsch, Binz, and Rossbach that quinine causes a more stable combination between the hæmoglobin and the oxygen, the latter being therefore less readily given off; quinine also weakens considerably the ozone reaction of the blood, whether the quinine be incorporated in the living animals or mixed with the blood.

Binz is therefore justified in giving expression to the opinion *that the Infusoria are destroyed by asphyxia*, the quinine robbing the protoplasm of the ability to take up oxygen.

It was mentioned above that the malarial parasites present appearances under treatment by quinine very similar to those which Binz observed in the Infusoria. In support of this statement his work [142] in 1869 may be referred to, where, amongst other things, it is remarked that if there is a small concentration of the solution of quinine, an irritation of the larger Infusoria is proved by the action of the quinine; we have above described the same thing as occurring in the malarial parasites. In a further publication Binz [141] writes: "One often sees how they (the Infusoria) are almost immediately disintegrated by quinine, or they burst, their distended nucleus springs forth, and within a few minutes every trace of the cellular form and the organism vanishes. It is an act of destructive force which the quinine exercises upon the structure of many living albuminous bodies when present in not too weak a solution." Binz saw sweet-water amœbæ rolling themselves together as if tetanised in a solution of 1 in 50,000 of neutral muriate of quinine.

On account of his observations Binz, in 1868, drew the following conclusion with regard to malaria, which at that time was generally considered to be a neurosis. "It is now undeniable that malarial diseases, many typhus fevers, the pyæmia of the surgeons and, as Semelweiss's investigations clearly show, the puerperal fever, are processes of fermentation, which are caused by the absorption of septic matter into the blood. These matters are of varying nature, as is their influence upon metamorphosis. In one important point, however, they agree with one another, in causing illness with a high temperature and rapidly penetrating disintegration of the connective-tissue substance. In some of them the ferment is reproduced and becomes easily infectious; in others this is still doubtful. That this ferment is a very low form of organism, as in other fermentative and putrefying processes, requires a final judgment."

As we know to-day, the "final judgment" has, in the case of malaria, proved Binz to be thoroughly right.

It still remains to mention a point or two concerning *the action of quinine upon the leucocytes.*

It is known that Binz [143] found that the colourless blood-corpuscles became immediately granulated and died under the influence of a solution of quinine of 1 in 2000;[1] further, that the number of the leucocytes in the circulation was diminished to one quarter by the administration of large doses of quinine.

It may not be too great an assumption to imagine that the phagocytes in the internal organs have their functions rather weakened than stimulated by quinine, and that we cannot therefore refer the cure of malaria by quinine to a stimulation of the phagocytic

[1] Engelmann found that even a solution of 1 in 20,000 slowed the amœboid movement of the leucocytes.

action of the cells, but entirely ascribe it to the specific destruction of the parasites within the circulating blood.[1]

It is finally interesting once more to call attention to the fact that the hæmoparasites of birds are not influenced by quinine; possibly this results from the difference of the soil, for we must remember that, according to Binz, the *sweet*-water amœbæ but *not* the *salt*-water amœbæ are killed by quinine; also that the *Euglenea* show themselves refractory to the alkaloid.

[1] It may be mentioned that Golgi also observed after the administration of quinine a later and weaker phagocytic action in the circulating blood.

CHAPTER X.

CULTIVATION EXPERIMENTS—CONJECTURES AS TO THE EXISTENCE OF PARASITES EXTERNAL TO THE ORGANISM—MODE OF INFECTION OF MALARIA—INCUBATION.

It has already been repeatedly indicated that all attempts at cultivating the malarial parasites, though so numerous and varied, have failed to yield any but negative results. Besides the employment for this purpose of the soils generally used in bacteriology, other materials have been used which would be *a priori* supposed to offer to the malarial parasites the most favorable conditions for development; it was believed that soils containing hæmoglobin would suit the parasites, but success did not follow this attempt, and the experiments made with blood obtained by venesection and sealed up in tubes were just as little fruitful.

The only thing gained by these experiments was the retention (alive) of some parasites—especially the large bodies of the quartan and tertian parasites—for two or three days. I was able in my warm damp oxygen chamber to keep apparently alive for two or three days the unaltered forms of the varieties above mentioned as well as of the crescentic bodies.

Once an immature spore-forming body of the tertian parasite arrived at maturity; the spores separated from one another and assumed those appearances which we are accustomed to see in the immature parasites twelve hours after rupture of the spore-forming body, but I found them all to be dead.

Just as little success attended the attempts to plant the malarial parasites in a cavity of another animal or to retain them capable of reproduction.

Rosenbach [144] saw living tertian parasites after an interval of forty-eight hours in leeches which he had applied to a patient—at least they showed pigment movement; the same result was obtained by Sacharoff when he placed leeches replete with blood upon ice.

I repeatedly fed flies with malarial blood, rich in spore-forming bodies or in crescents; the bodies in this case only remained alive for a short time, but did not increase in number.

After all these unsuccessful attempts, it appears to be more and more probable *that the malarial parasites do not exist in the external world as saprophytes, but must live as parasites either in animal or vegetable organisms.*

Laveran's supposition that possibly the gnats are the hosts of the parasites is disproved by Grassi and Calandruccio [100] on account of the negative experiments in feeding which were made by Calandruccio. These investigators have occupied themselves with a thorough investigation of the question as to the existence of the malarial parasite in the external world, and they believe that they are justified in drawing the conclusion from their investigations that certain species of amœbæ—especially the *Amœba guttula* (or *gracilis*)—may be regarded as their extra-parasitic form.

Grassi and Calandruccio start with the assumption that the malarial parasites are to be sought amongst those Rhizopoda which are found in all malarial districts. Therefore they investigated marsh water, moist soil, rice fields, macerated hemp and linen, in a word all possible malarial seats, for Rhizopoda, and found in all of them species of the genus Amœba and of those genera nearly related to them—the *Hyalodiscus* (*Dactylosphærium*)—present in great numbers. They imagined that the infection of men and animals occurred by the encysted amœbæ being inhaled in consequence of their imponderability and presence in the air currents. They were also able, although very rarely, to prove the presence of amœboid cysts in dew; further they discovered them in the nasal secretion of pigeons which they had exposed for several nights to the evaporation from marshes or from malarial earth.

They explain the impossibility of cultivating the parasites taken from the blood of men or animals back to the amœbæ of the external world by stating that the parasites of the animal organism have been, so to say, "spoilt," so that they lose their capacity to again return to an independent mode of life.

The most weighty objection which can be raised against Grassi and Calandruccio's hypothesis is this, that the amœbæ mentioned by them are more widely distributed in the world than malaria itself. The weight of this objection is recognised by both authors themselves, and they reply to it that it is the greater number of the amœbæ which causes the malarious regions to be such plague spots.

It is impossible at present to fully estimate this proposed hypothesis, and it is important in the first place to wait for the detailed publication of the results obtained by the Sicilian investigators before passing a judgment on the correctness of their argument. With all reserve, and without in the least drawing the slightest conclusion from it, I may mention that I once had the opportunity during a cultivation experiment (with tertian parasites) in the moist oxygen chamber to find in the preparation, twelve hours after the commencement of the experiment, two cysts which appeared to completely resemble the cysts of the *Monas guttula*, Ehrenberg.

That the malarial germs may be inhaled with the air there can be no possible doubt after innumerable experiences, although there are observations reported from time to time which point to the fact that it is also possible to acquire malaria through the intestinal tract, especially by means of drinking water.[1]

These observations are, however, very few as against the general experience as to the dangerous nature of the air in malarious districts; indeed, it appears that a number of these communications are not completely free from objection with reference to the correctness of the diagnosis of the cases of disease in question. In the well-known case of the ship "Argo," which was reported by Boudin and which has been quoted repeatedly since then, the circumstances are also, as Colin pointed out, not irrefutable, and it is by no means certain that those of the crew who are said to have suffered from malaria at sea, owing to the use of bad drinking-water, really suffered from malaria, and not rather from some typhoid condition, as Colin finds reason to suppose.[2]

In my opinion the same objection can be raised also against Senise [146], who three years ago reported on the outbreak of a malarial epidemic in Basilicata, where, in consequence of damage to the aqueduct, the population used impure drinking water. The cases of illness appear to have chiefly presented appearances of gastro-enteritis and liver complaints. Unfortunately, Senise neglected the investigation of the blood, and from what we know now the diagnosis of malaria must be doubted.

That, on the other hand, drinking of even very bad swamp water need not produce malaria has been repeatedly proved, as indeed by Marchiafava and Celli [19] several years ago,

[1] Büchner's [145] observation may be given as a curiosity, namely, that an ague could be given by a malarial patient to a healthy person with whom he slept in the same bed.

[2] Colin, quoted by Kelsch and Kiener [98, page 843].

who permitted six persons to drink water from the Pontine marshes for eight to sixteen days without seeing one of them attacked by malaria. Two years ago Salomone Marino [147] made similar experiments, also with negative results.

That the malarial parasites, or the blood-corpuscles infested by them, can pass through the placenta is proved by the cases in which the fœtus has been infected by the suffering mother, as shown by the reports of Dinstl, Schramm, Duchek, and Playfair; the nurse also has been observed to infect the suckling (Schramm, Baxa, and Luc), and the reverse condition has likewise been maintained (Sons [145]).

It may be mentioned here that Dochmann [148] succeeded in inoculating a healthy man with the contents of an herpetic vesicle of a patient suffering from quartan fever, and produced a fever after a few hours' incubation which was of the quartan type; in the same way he inoculated three men with quotidian fever, once with a positive, twice with a doubtful or negative result.

Nothing is up to the present known as to the contents of an herpetic vesicle containing parasites, but after Dochmann's experiments it is highly probable that the parasites must have been in the serum of the vesicle.

I have repeatedly investigated *sweat* without result.

It does not lie within the scope of this book to consider the telluric and atmospheric conditions which cause and aid in the production of malaria, but it may be pointed out at this place that the rules which have been gained by a study of those conditions, and have been thoroughly appreciated by numerous authors, in no way militate against the supposition of a living malarial virus. The most important conditions under which malaria breaks out are, as is well known, *slight porosity of the soil, moderate moisture and warmth*, and indeed most authorities on malaria state that a rainy spring and a warm but not too hot summer following, which does not completely dry the soil, results in the appearance of far more numerous and severe cases of malaria than when the opposite conditions obtain. In our climate the most severe malarial season is August and September; in tropical countries, as for instance in Algiers and Tunis, September and October (see Kelsch and Kiener, loc. cit., p. 816).

It must, indeed, be admitted that those circumstances which have been named as favouring malaria completely agree with the conditions which present the best opportunity for growth to a low organism having either a parasitic or saprophytic character.

Finally, concerning the incubation of malaria, we know that

it can be very various. The duration of incubation appears to be most frequently eight to fourteen days, as is shown not only by numerous observations in spontaneous illness, but, as we have seen, in experimentally produced cases of malaria.

Less frequently the incubation occupies a shorter period, but cases with one or two days' or even only a few hours' incubation are not altogether rare.

All these cases may probably be explained by the quantity of the parasites inhaled or injected.

Looking at the experimentally produced malaria, we must imagine that a relatively very small quantity of parasites are injected with 0·5 to 1·0 cm. of blood, and of these it is highly probable that the greater part perish, especially in subcutaneous injections, and are therefore not capable of producing fever immediately, and it is only after eight to fourteen days that they have increased sufficiently to produce a requisite number of parasites to cause a paroxysm of fever. If the whole mass of the blood of a malarial patient were at one time carried into a healthy man, then he would probably show immediately fully developed symptoms of fever; similarly I believe I may take for granted that the same thing takes place also in spontaneous malarial illness; the amount of the parasites taken up may determine the period of incubation. This, however, does not exclude the possibility of individual predisposition, according to which the multiplication of the parasite is favoured or retarded.

The cases of sudden illness after a visit to malarial regions make it appear very improbable that the parasites are taken up in a form which requires a longer interval (about fourteen days) for metamorphosis in order to exert the pathogenic action—in order, therefore, to become the malarial parasites of man.

The not infrequent cases of malaria having an incubation of several months are still completely inexplicable in the present state of our knowledge; they may be placed by the side of rabies, in which also there may be a long period of incubation; indeed there is an extreme similarity between the differences in the duration of the incubation of these two diseases.

PLATE I.

A. *A composite microscopic field from a case of simple tertian ague at the time of the attack.*

In the upper part of the field two spore-forming bodies; one of the same at the lower right-hand corner. The remainder intra-corpuscular pigmented parasites in an advanced stage of development. Most of the infested corpuscles are hypertrophied and discoloured. In the left-hand corner an eosinephile; below, a polynuclear leucocyte.

B. *A composite microscopic field from a double tertian ague at the onset of the attack.*

Besides two spore-forming bodies, several parasites in an advanced stage of development are to be seen; further several partially developed parasites (*i. e.* the second generation which would cause the attack of the next day); lastly, there are also seen two immature parasites of circular form; these originate from spores which have just become free and have already found hosts; they would attain maturity in forty-eight hours. The infested blood-corpuscles are hypertrophied and pale. To the right a leucocyte.
Stained with methylene blue and eosine.

× 1000; Zeiss's apochromatic lens, 3 mm. focus; aperture 1·40; compensation eye-piece 12.

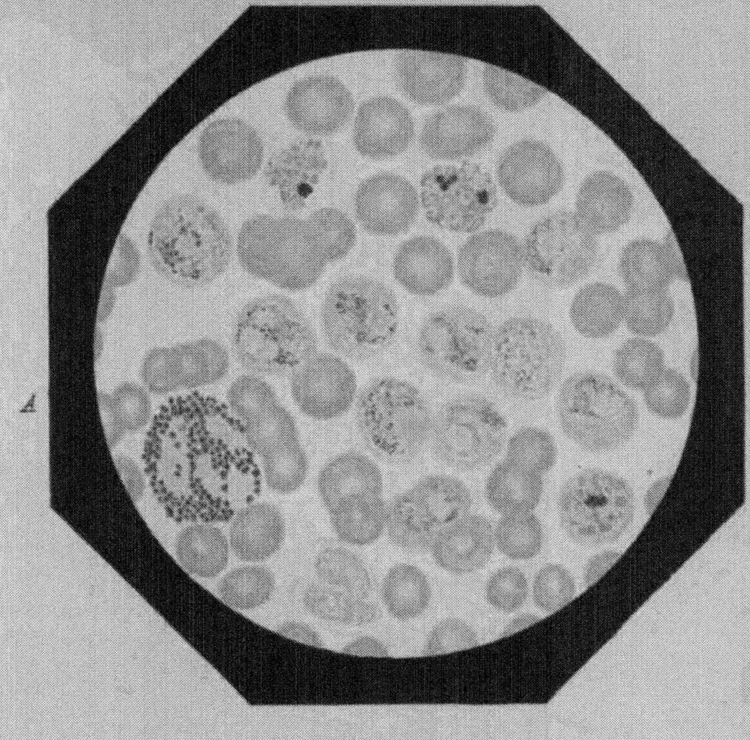
A

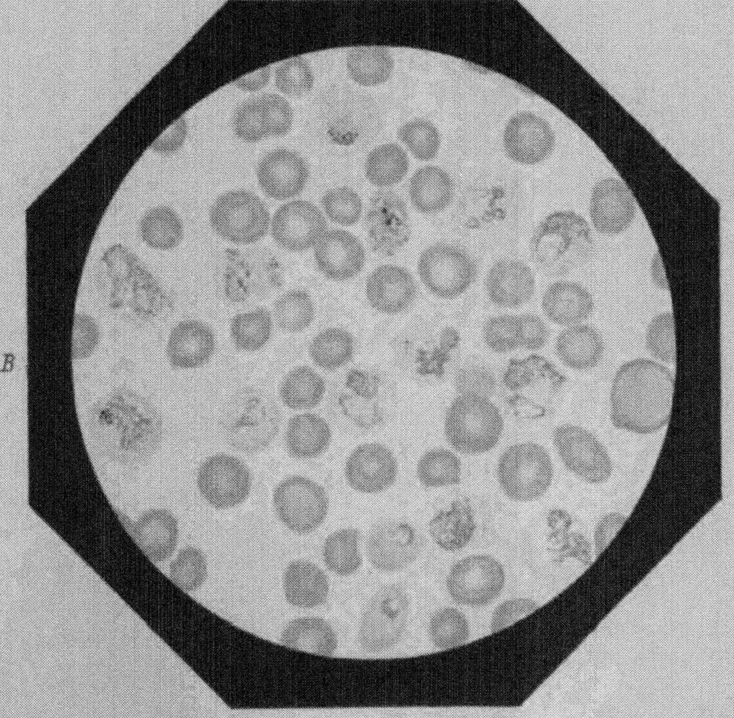
B

Th.Bannwarth,lith.et imp.Vienna.

PLATE II.

A. *The process of development of the quartan parasite.* (Figs. 1—8 after Golgi.)

FIGS.

1. Unpigmented parasite, slightly amœboid.
2. Pigmented parasite.
3. Fully developed parasite.
4. Preparatory stage to spore-formation.
5. Concentrated pigment; radiating striation as the commencement of spore-formation.

6—8. The spores developed, each with a visible nucleolus.

9. Spore-forming body, in which the spores *in vivo* have exhibited no nucleolus.

10. Fan-shaped spore-formation, after Canalis.

B. *The process of development of the tertian parasite.*

11. Unpigmented amœboid corpuscle.

12—14. Parasite with a marginal pigment granule showing actual amœboid movement.

15—18. Gradual progressive development, amœboid movement being less but still present.

19. Body quiescent before forming spores.

20, 21. Ordinary spore-forming bodies.

22, 23. Abnormal spore-forming bodies, with few spores and a visible nucleolus.

24. Large free body, very granular, with vacuolated nucleus and nucleolus.

25. Large pigmented parasite.

26. Escape of the same from the blood-corpuscle.

27. Free parasitic débris.

28. Large free parasite.

29. Flagellated parasite.

C. *The process of development of the pigmented quotidian parasite.*

30—35.

D. *The process of development of the unpigmented quotidian parasite.*

36—39. Parasites with amœboid movement.

40. Body quiescent, containing a fragment of hæmoglobin.

41, 42. Parasites situated at the periphery (of blood-corpuscles). The spore-formation of this parasite is depicted on Plate IV, fig. 68.

E. *The process of development of the malignant tertian parasite.*

43. Immature amœboid unpigmented body.

44. Peripherally situated parasite, already containing pigment.

45—47. Transformation of quiescent body (ringlet) into the amœboid condition, and *vice versâ.*

48. Spore-formation in a very much shrivelled blood-corpuscle.

F. *Forms common to the last three varieties.*

49. Copper-coloured corpuscle (*glob. rossi ottonati*).

50. A sphere of the crescent series with double contour.

51, 52. Fusiform body of the crescent series; the double contour disappeared suddenly under the microscope.

53—55. Coalescence of two small amœboid bodies observed under the microscope.

56. Syzygy.

57—61. Transformation of a crescent into a spherical body, whereby the residue of the blood-corpuscle has re-absorbed the hæmoglobin colour. During the transformation the original double contour was lost.

62—66. The escape and separation of a spherical body of the crescent series out of the capsule of a blood-corpuscle, with subsequent formation of flagella.

G. *Vacuoles changing their shape.*

67—70.

71. The punctiform vacuolisation of a blood-corpuscle.

× 1000; Zeiss's apochromatic lens, 3 mm. focus; aperture 1·40; compensation eye-piece 12.

Malarial Parasites (J. Mannaberg)

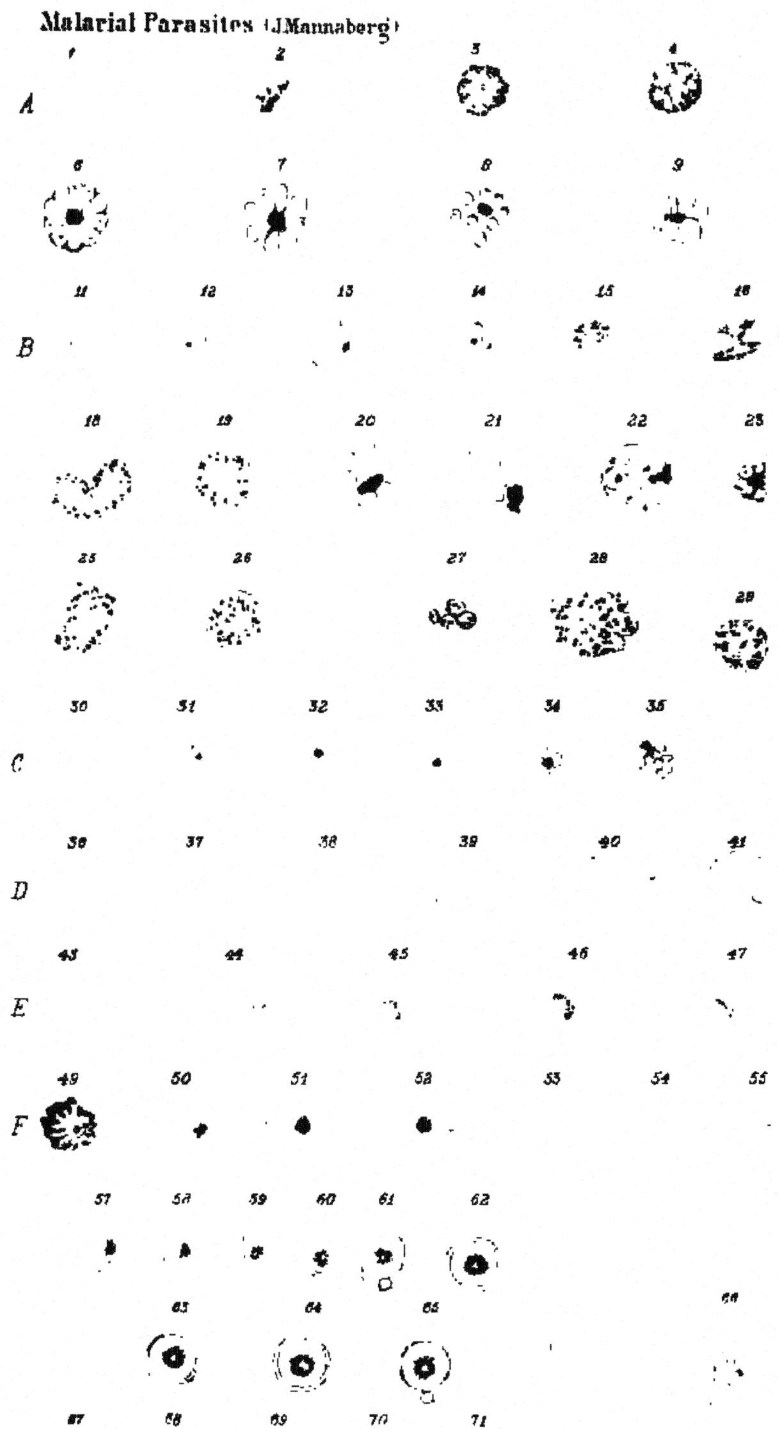

PLATE III.

A. *Illustrations of the forms of the tertian parasite.*

FIGS.

1. Free spore, consisting of protoplasmic capsule and nucleolus.
2. Free spore, consisting of protoplasm, nucleus, and nucleolus.
3. Unpigmented immature form.
4. Pigmented form partially developed: a vacuole and a nucleolus.

5—7. Partially developed forms.

8—18. The nucleolus gradually disappears (through coalescence with the protoplasm); sometimes (8, 15, 16) symmetrically arranged points are to be seen in it.

19. Chromatin band in nucleus, the nucleolus having entirely disappeared.
20. The nucleus begins to gain chromatin.
21. The nucleus containing chromatin.
22. Separation into nuclear part and protoplasmic part.
23. Preparing to form spores.
24. Spore-formation; each spore shows protoplasm, nucleus, and nucleolus.
25. Spore-formation, with development of the nucleoli before the nuclei.
26. Abnormal spore-formation with very few spores.

27—30. Various free spores, sometimes two united.

31. Irregularly shaped medium-sized parasite.
32. Excessive vacuolisation.

B. *Fever and quinine types.*

33. Disintegration of parasite within blood-corpuscle in febrile paroxysm.
34. Disintegrated febrile form.
35. Coagulated and disintegrated quinine form.

36, 37. Spore-forming bodies under the influence of quinine. Only a small number of the spores are normally formed; most are "stillborn."

C. *Golgi's scheme of the spore-formation of the tertian parasite.*

D. *Golgi's scheme of the spore-formation of the quartan parasite.*

Figs. 1—15, 27—30, 35—37, fixed with picric acid and stained with hæmatoxylin.

Figs. 28, 31—34, stained with Sahli's borax-methylene-blue (after Malachowsky).

× 1000; Zeiss's apochromatic lens, 3 mm. focus; aperture 1·40; compensation eye-piece 12.

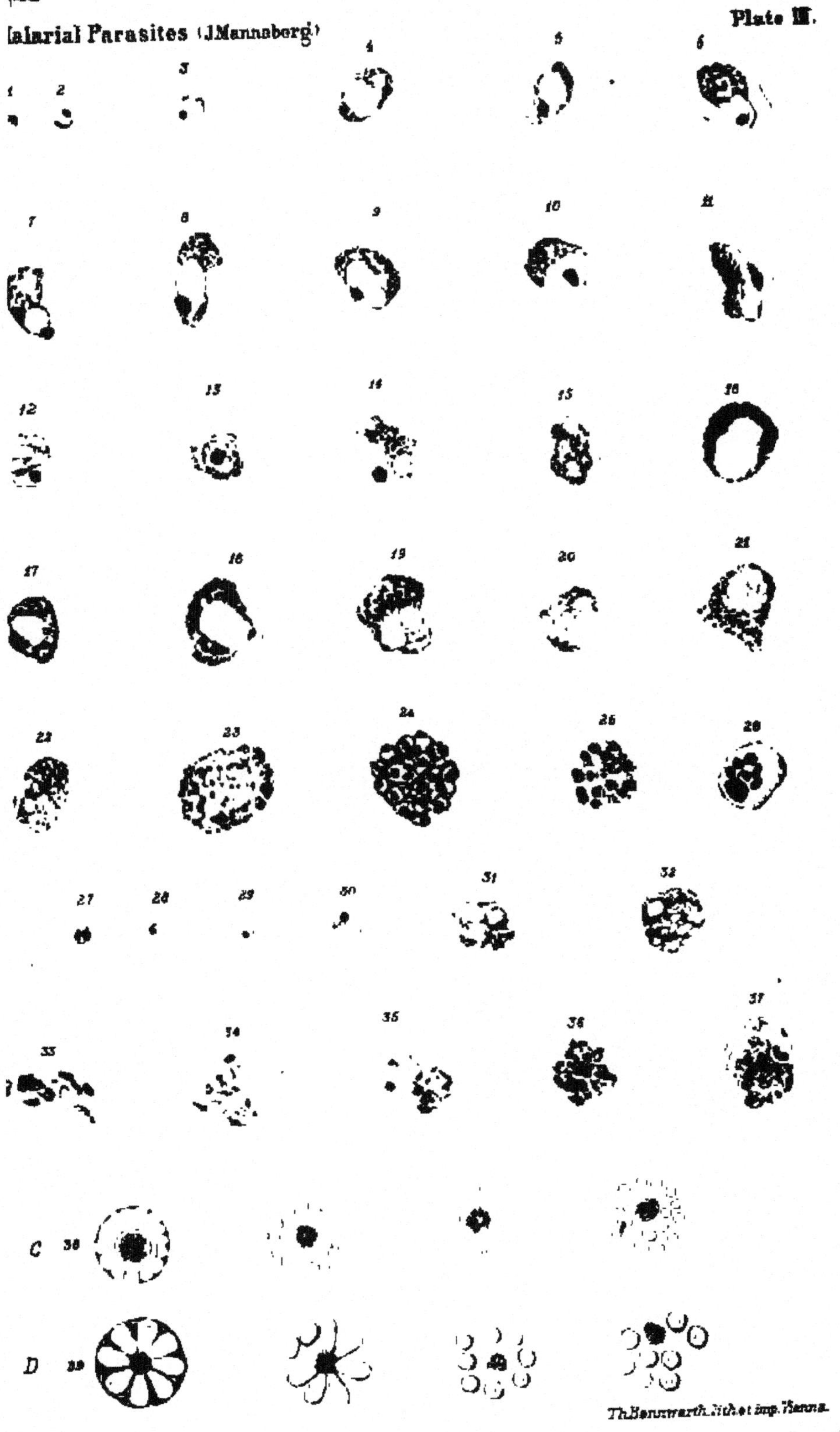
Malarial Parasites (J. Mannaberg)
Plate III.
C
D
Th. Bannwarth lith. et imp. Vienna.

PLATE IV.

FIGS.

1—12. Structural details of the malignant tertian parasite. From fig. 5 onwards the nucleolus is missing; from fig. 8 onwards the nucleus also. Fig. 12, completed spore-formation.

13, 14. Small copper-coloured bodies (the blood-corpuscles are decolorised in consequence of treatment with acetic acid). The small parasite with nucleolus is clearly seen.

15, 17. Small parasites with two nucleoli.

16. Small copper-coloured body.

18—21. Small amœboid parasites in different stages of development.

22. Small amœboid parasite with vacuole.

23. Amœboid parasite lying at the periphery.

24—26. Multiple invasion by small amœboid parasites.

27—30, 32. Sysygy composed of two parasites. In fig. 32 several pigment granules are already visible.

31. Syzygy composed of four parasites.

33, 34. Two crescents decolorised by treating with ammonia. A transverse bridge is seen in which lie two slightly stained points, and which divides the crescent into two parts.

35—39. Crescents and oval bodies in various stages of development.

35—38, 46—48. Distinct division of the pigment, with two parts often in the form of an 8.

40, 41. Very slightly pigmented crescents.

42, 50. Asymmetrical distribution of pigment.

39, 50. Stained granules in the substance of cell wall.

47. Fragment of hæmoglobin in crescent.

44, 47. Crenated remains of blood-corpuscle.

51. Division of pigment, side nicked.

52. Transverse segmentation of crescent; the protoplasm finely granulated throughout.

53. Half of crescent.

54. Truncated crescent.

55, 56. Phenomena of degeneration in a crescent consisting of circles which alter their shape.

63, 64. A spherical body of the crescentic series with a double contour and remains of blood-corpuscle (altering the focus causes the two appearances depicted).

57—62. Action of quinine upon small amœboid bodies.

65. Transverse section of a small vessel in the brain from a case of *malaria comatosa*. The blood-corpuscles at the periphery are invaded by unpigmented parasites. (Stained with hæmatoxylin, a preparation of Prof. Golgi's.)

66. Brain capillary from a case of *malaria comatosa*, filled with spore-forming bodies of the unpigmented parasites. (Preparation of Prof. Golgi's.)

67. Brain capillary and escaped blood-corpuscles; each blood-corpuscle is invaded by small pigmented parasites. (Stained methylene blue, a preparation of Prof. Golgi's.)

68. Spotted red corpuscle.

69. Melaniferous leucocyte.

70. Blood-plates.

Figs. 1—12, 17, 43—45, 51—53, 57—62, stained with borax methylene blue; figs. 16, 46—49, after Romanowsky's method; the remainder, with the exception of figs. 65, 66, and 67, with picric acid and hæmatoxylin.

× 1000; Zeiss's apochromatic lens, 3 mm. focus; aperture 1·40; compensation eye-piece 12.

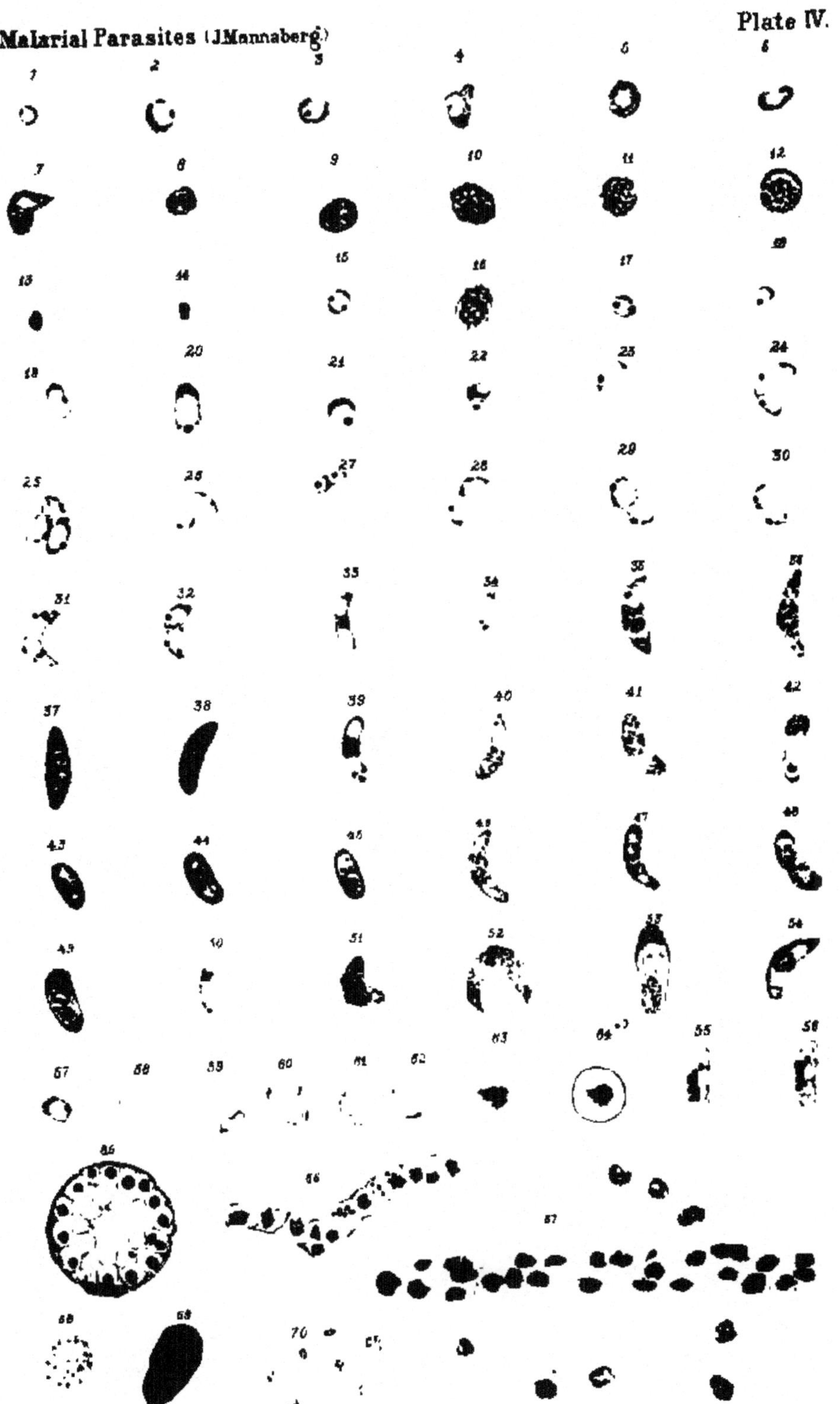

Malarial Parasites (J. Mannaberg.)

Plate IV.

Th.Bannwarth Lith.et imp. Vienna.

BIBLIOGRAPHY.

1. H. Meckel. Ueber schwarzes Pigment in der Milz und im Blute einer Geisteskranken. *Zeitschr. f. Psychiatrie*, 1847, S. 198.
2. R. Virchow. Zur pathologischen Physiologie des Blutes. *Virchow's Archiv*, Bd. ii.
3. R. Virchow. *Cellularpathologie*, 1858.
4. Heschl. *Zeitschrift der k. k. Gesellschaft der Aerzte in Wien*, 1850.
5. Heschl. *Zeitschrift für praktische Heilkunde*, 1862, S. 750.
6. Planer. Ueber das Vorkommen von Pigment in Blute. *Zeitschrift der k. k. Gesellschaft der Aerzte in Wien*, 1854.
7. A. Laveran. Note sur un nouveau parasite trouvé dans le sang de plusieurs malades atteints de fièvre palustre. *Note communiquée à l'Académie de médecine*, Séance du 23 Novembre, 1880.
8. Laveran. Deuxième note, &c. *Note communiquée à l'Académie de médecine*, Séance du 28 Décembre, 1880.
9. Laveran. Nature parasitaire des accidents de l'impaludisme, 1881, Paris, chez Baillière et fils.
10. Laveran. Communication à l'Académie des sciences sur la nature parasitaire des accidents de l'impaludisme. *Comptes rendus*, 1881.
11. E. Richard. Sur le parasite de la malaria. *Comptes rendus*, 1882, Séance du 20 Février.
12. Cuboni und Marchiafava. Neue Studien über die Natur der Malaria. *Archiv f. experimentelle Pharmakologie*, 1881.

Note.—The works numbered 1—146 have been referred to in the foregoing pages; the remaining publications, even if not directly mentioned in the text, have been taken into consideration. The works marked † have only come to the knowledge of the author after the conclusion of his work.

13. Marchiafava e Cuboni. Atti della R. Acc. dei Lincei, 1891. Ref. in *Archivio per le scienze med.*, vol. v.

14. Max Schultze. Ein heizbarer Objecttisch, &c. *Arch. f. mikroskopische Anat.*, Bd. i, S. 25.

15. Marchiafava und Celli. Die Veränderungen der rothen Blutkörperchen, &c. *Fortschritte der Medicin*, Bd. i, 1883.

16. Marchiafava e Celli. *Memorie della R. Acc. dei Lincei*, 1883.

17. Marchiafava e Celli. Les altérations des globules rouges dans l'infection par malaria, &c. *Archives italiennes de biologie*, 1884, tome v.

18. A. Laveran. Traité des fièvres palustres, 1884. *Paris, chez O. Doin.*

19. Marchiafava und Celli. *Fortschritte der Medicin*, 1885, Nr. 11 u. 24.

20. Marchiafava e Celli. Nuove ricerche sulla infezione malarica. *Archivio per le scienze mediche*, vol. ix, 1886.

21. Sternberg. The Malarial Germ of Laveran. *The Medical Record*, New York, 1886.

22. Councilman. *Fortschritte der Medicin*, 1888, Nr. 12—13.

23. Osler. *The British Medical Journal*, 1887, p. 556.

24. Maurel. Recherches microscopiques sur l'etiologie du paludisme, *Paris*, 1887, *chez Doin.*

25. James. The Micro-organisms of Malaria. *The Medical Record*, 1888, p. 269.

26. N. Sacharoff. Ref. in *Centralblatt f. Bakteriologie*, 1889, S. 452.

27. Paltauf. *Wiener klin. Wochenschrift*, 1890.

28. Plehn. Aetiologische und klinische Malariastudien, *Berlin*, 1890, *bei Hirschwald.*

29. Quincke. Ueber Blutuntersuchungen bei Malariakranken. *Mittheilungen des Vereines Schleswig-Holst.*, Aerzte, 1890.

30. v. Jaksch. *Prager med. Wochenschrift*, 1890.

31. Chenzinsky. Ref. in *Centralblatt f. Bakteriologie*, 1887, Bd. i.

32. E. Metschnikoff. Russkaia med., 1887, Nr. 12. Ref. in *Centralblatt f. Bakteriologie*, 1887, Nr. 21.

33. C. Golgi. Sur l'infection malarique. *Archives italiennes de biologie*, 1887, t. viii.

34. C. Golgi. Sull' infezione malarica. *Archivio per le scienze med.*, 1886, vol. x, Nr. 4.

C. Golgi. *Fortschritte der Medicin*, 1889, Nr. 3.

36. C. Golgi. Interno al preteso "Bacillus Malariae" di Klebs-Tommasi-Crudeli e Schiavuzzi. *Archivio per le scienze med.*, 1889, vol. xiii.

37. C. Golgi. Sul ciclo evolutivo dei parassiti malarici nella febbre terzana. *Archivio per le scienze mediche*, 1889, vol. xiii.

38. Marchiafava e Celli.—Sulle febbri malariche predominanti nell estate e autunno, &c. *Archivio per le scienze med.*, 1890, vol. xiv.

39. P. Canalis. Studi sulla infezione malarica. *Archivio per le scienze med.*, 1890, vol. xiv.

40. Tommasi-Crudeli. *Rendiconti dei Lincei*, 1886–7.

41. Maragliano. II. Congresso della Società Italiana di Medicina int. Roma, 1889. Ref. in *Rif. med.*, 1889, Nr. 254.

42. A. Mosso. Degenerazione dei corpuscoli rossi, &c. *Rif. med*, 1887, p. 260.

43. A. Mosso. Die Umwandlung der rothen Blutkörperchen, &c. *Virchow's Archiv*, 1887, Bd. cix, S. 264.

44. A. Mosso. Congress für innere Medicin in Rom, 1889. Ref. in der *Wiener klin. Wochenschrift*, 1889, Nr. 48, 49.

45. Cattaneo e Monti. Alterazioni degenerative dei corpuscoli rossi, &c. *Archivio per le scienze med.*, vol. xii, 1888.

46. Celli e Guarnieri. Sulla etiologia dell' infezione malarica. *Archivio per le scienze med.*, vol. xiii, 1889.

47. Grassi und Feletti. *Centralblatt für Bakteriologie*, 1890.

48. Romanowsky. Zur Frage der Parasitologie und Therapie der Malaria, *St. Petersburg*, 1891.

49. Mannaberg. Beiträge zur Morphologie und Biologie des Plasmodium malariae tertianae. *Centralblatt für klinische Medicin*, 1891, Nr. 27.

50. Amico Bignami. Ricerche sull' anatomia pat. delle perniciose. *Atti della R. Accad. med. di Roma*, anno xvi, vol. v, Ser. 2.

51. Gruby. Sur une nouvelle espèce d'hématozoaire. *Comptes rendus*, 1843.

52. Lankester. *Quarterly Journal of Microscopical Science*, 1871.

53. Osler. *Proceedings of the Royal Society*, xxii, p. 391. Quoted from Gaule (56).

54. Lewis. *Quarterly Journal of Microscopical Science*, 1879, p. 109. Quoted from Gaule (56).

55. Gaule. Ueber Würmchen, welche aus den Froschblutkörperchen auswandern. *Archiv für Anatomie und Physiologie*, 1880.

56. Gaule. Beziehungen der Cytozoën zu den Zellkernen. *Archiv für Anatomie und Physiologie*, 1881.

57. Gaule. Kerne, Nebenkerne und Cytozoën. *Centralblatt für med. Wissenschaften*, 1881, S. 561.

58. E. Malachowski. Zur Morphologie des Plasmodium malariae. *Centralblatt für klinische Medicin*, 1891, Nr. 31.

59. Freund. Ueber die Ursache der Blutgerinnung. *Medicinische Jahrbücher der k. k. Gesellschaft der Aerzte in Wien*, 1888, S. 259.

60. Gerhardt. Ueber Intermittens-Impfungen. *Zeitschrift für klin. Medicin*, 1884, Bd. vii.

61. Marchiafava et Celli. Nouvelles études sur l'infection malarique. *Archives Italiennes de biologie*, 1887, tome viii.

62. Antolisei e Angelini. A proposito delle forme semilunari di Laveran. *Riforma medica*, 1889, Nr. 237.

63. Frerichs. *Klinik der Leberkrankheiten*, 1858.

64. Mosler. Ueber das Vorkommen von Melanämie. *Virchow's Archiv*, 1877, Bd. lxix.

65. Arnstein. Bemerkungen über Melanämie und Melanose. *Virchow's Archiv*, 1874, Bd. lxi.

66. Kelsch. Contribution à l'anatomie path. des maladies palustres endémiques. *Archives de physiologie*, 1875, II Serie, tome ii.

67. C. Schwalbe. Die experimentelle Melanämie und Melanose. *Virchow's Archiv*, 1886, Bd. cv.

68. B. Afanassiew. Beitrag zur Pathologie der Malaria-Infection. *Virchow's Archiv*, 1881, Bd. lxxxiv.

69. E. Marchiafava. Commentario clinico di Pisa, 1879. Quoted from Celli and Marchiafava in *Festschrift zu Virchow's* 70, Geburtstag, Bd. iii.

70. O. Rosenbach. *Deutsche med. Wochenschrift*, 1890, Nr. 16.

71. E. Marchiafava ed A. Celli. Sulla infezione malarica. Memoria quarta. *Archivio per le scienze med.*, 1888, vol. xii.

72. Grassi e Feletti. Sui parassiti della malaria. *Riforma med.*, 1890, p. 62.

73. Celli und Marchiafava. Ueber die Parasiten der rothen Blutkörperchen. *Festschrift zu R. Virchow's 70, Geburtstag*, Bd. iii.

74. Danilewsky. Die Hämatozoën der Kaltblüter. *Arch. für mikr. Anatomie*, 1885, Bd. xxiv.

75. Danilewsky. Zur Frage der Identität, &c. *Centralblatt für med. Wissenschaften*, 1886, Nr. 41 u. 42.

76. Danilewsky. Ueber Polimitus malariae. *Centralblatt für Bakteriologie und Parasitenkunde*, 1891, Nr. 12.

77. Danilewsky. *La parasitologie comparée du sang*, i u. ii, Kharkoff, 1889.

78. A. Celli e F. Sanfelice. Sui parassiti del globulo rosso nel uomo e negli animali. *Annali dell' istituto d'igiene sperimentale della R. università di Roma*, 1891, vol. i (Nuova Seria).

79. Binz. Ueber die Wirkung antiseptischer Stoffe auf Infusorien von Pflanzenjauche. *Centralblatt für med. Wissenschaften*, 1867, Nr. 20.

80. Hayem. *Du sang et de ses altérations*, pag. 2, Paris, chez Masson, 1889.

81. Richard. *Revue scientifique*, 1883, p. 114.

82. E. Antolisei. (Veröffentlicht durch A. Angelini.) Considerazioni intorno alla classificazione dei parassiti della malaria. *Riforma med.*, 1890, p. 590.

83. Grassi und Feletti. Weiteres zur Malariafrage. *Centralblatt für Bakteriologie und Parasitenkunde*, 1891, Nr. 14.

84. A. Laveran. Des hématozoaires du paludisme. *Annales de l'Institut Pasteur*, 1887, t. 1.

85. A. Bignami e G. Bastianelli. Osservazioni nelle febbri malariche estivo-autunnali. *Riforma medica*, 1890, p. 1334.

86. Grassi e Feletti. Contribuzioni allo studio dei parassiti malarici. *Memoria*, S. A.

87. Mannaberg. Beiträge zur Kenntniss der Malariaparasiten. *Verhandlungen des XI. Congresses für innere Medicin zu Leipzig*, 1892, Wiesbaden, Bergmann.

88. A. Laveran. Du paludisme et de son hématozoaire. *Paris*, 1891, *chez Masson.*

89. C. Golgi. *Fortschritte der Medicin*, 1886, Nr. 17.

90. C. Golgi. Ref. in *Fortschritte der Medicin*, 1886, Nr. 21.

91. C. Golgi. Sulle febbri intermittenti malariche a lunghi intervalli. *Archivio per le scienze mediche*, 1890, vol. xiv.

92. Marchiafava e Celli. Intorno a recenti lavori sulla natura della causa della malaria. *Bullettino della Reale Accademia med. di Roma*, 1890.

93. Celli. Ueber die Malariakrankheiten. X. internationaler med. Congress in Berlin. Ref. in der *Wiener klin. Wochenschrift*, 1890, Nr. 48.

94. P. Gualdi e E. Antolisei. Una quartana sperimentale. *Riforma medica*, 1889, Nr. 264.

95. Di Mattei. Quoted from Grassi and Feletti (86).
96. Calandruccio. *Ibidem.*
97. Trousseau. *Clinique médicale*, 7 édition, tome iii.
98. Kelsch et Kiener. Traité des maladies des pays chauds, *Paris*, 1889, *chez Baillière et fils.*
99. Marchiafava e Bignami. *Rif. med.*, 1891.
100. Marchiafava e Bignami. Sulle febbri malariche estivo-autunnali, *Rom.*, 1891, *bei Loescher et Comp.*
101. G. Bein. Aetiologische und experimentelle Beiträge zur Malaria. *Charité-Annalen*, 1891.
102. E. Antolisei. L' ematozoa della quartana. *Rif. med.*, 1890. p. 68.
103. Waldenberg. *Archiv für path. Anatomie*, 1867, Bd. xl, S. 438; Quoted from R. Leuckart, Die Parasiten des Menschen, 2 Aufl., 1879, Leipzig, Winter, S. 233.
104. R. Pfeiffer. Beiträge zur Protozoënforschung. *Berlin bei Hirschwald*, i, 1892.
105. Claparède, Lieberkühn, Gabriel. Quoted from Bütschli (106), S. 538.
106. O. Bütschli. *In H. G. Bronn's Classen und Ordungen des Thierreiches*, Bd. i, Protozoa, 1889, Leipzig, bei Winter.
107. Gualdi e Antolisei. Due casi di febbre malarica sperimentale. *Rif. med.*, 1889, Nr. 225.
108. E. Antolisei e A. Angelini. Due altri casi di febbre malarica sperimentale. *Rif. med.*, 1889, Nr. 226.
109. P. Gualdi ed E. Antolisei. Inoculazione delle forme semilunari di Laveran. *Rif. med.*, 1889, Nr. 274.
110. Danilewsky. Développement des parasites malariques dans les leucocytes des oiseaux (Leucocytozoaires). *Annales de l'institut Pasteur*, 1890, p. 427.
111. Danilewsky. Sur les microbes de l'infection malarique aiguë et chronique chez les oiseaux et chez l'homme. *Annales de l'institut Pasteur*, 1890, p. 753.
112. Danilewsky. Contribution à l'étude de la microbiose malarique. *Annales de l'institut Pasteur*, 1891, p. 758.
113. Grassi und Feletti. Malariaparasiten in den Vögeln. *Centralblatt für Bakteriologie und Parasitenkunde*, 1891, Nr. 12—14.
114. W. Kruse. Ueber Blutparasiten. *Virchow's Archiv*, Bd. cxx.
115. W. Kruse. Ueber Blutparasiten. *Virchow's Archiv*, Bd. cxxi.
116. E. Antolisei. Sull' ematozoo della terzana. *Rif. med.*, 1890, p. 152.

117. Bastianelli e Bignami. Sull' infezione malarica primaverile. *Rif. med.*, 1890, p. 860.

118. E. Antolisei e A. Angelini. Nota sul ciclo biologico dell' ematozoo falciforme. *Rif. med.*, 1890, p. 320.

119. A. Huber. Zur Giftwirkung des Dinitrobenzols. *Virchow's Archiv*, Bd. cxxvi.

120. Dionisi. Variazioni numeriche dei globuli rossi, &c. *III. Congresso della soc. di med. int.*, 1890. *Rif. med.*, 1890, Nr. 258.

121. Hayem und Halla. Quoted from E. Reinert. *Die Zählung der Blutkörperchen*, Leipzig, 1891, bei Vogel.

122. Baccelli. Ueber das Wesen der Malaria. *Deutsche med. Wochenschrift*, 1892, Nr. 32.

123. E. Grawitz. Ueber Bluntuntersuchungen bei ostafrikanischen Malaria-erkrankungen. *Berliner klin. Wochenschrift*, 1892, Nr. 7.

124. Roque et Lemoine. Recherches sur la toxicité urinaire dans l'impaludisme. Ref. in *Centralblatt f. Bakteriologie*, 1891, Nr. 10.

125. Queirolo. II. Congresso della soc. ital. di medicina int., Roma, 1889. Ref. in *Rif. med.*, 1889, Nr. 254.

126. Griesinger. Infectionskrankheiten in *Virchow's Handbuch der speciellen Pathologie und Therapie*, 1864.

127. Bastianelli e Bignami. Osservazioni sulle febbri malariche estivo-autunnali. *III. Congresso della Soc. ital. di med. int.*, Roma, 1890. Ref. in *Rif. med.*, 1890, Nr. 251.

128. Martin. Die Malaria der Tropenländer, *Berlin*, 1889, *bei Springer*.

129. Schellong. Die Malariakrankheiten, *Berlin*, 1890, *bei Springer*.

130. Kelsch. Nouvelle contribution à l'anatomie path. des maladies palustres endémiques. *Archives de physiologie*, 1876, II Série, tome iii.

131. C. Golgi. Le phagocytisme dans l'infection malarique. *Archives italiennes de biologie*, 1889, t. xi.

132. Guarnieri. *Atti della R. Accademia med. di Roma*, 1887.

133. Grassi und Feletti. Weiteres zur Malariafrage. *Centralblatt für Bakteriologie und Parasitenkunde*, 1891, Nr. 16.

134. Herbst. Beiträge zur Kenntniss der antiseptischen Eigenschaften des Chinin. *Inaug. Diss.*, *Bonn*, 1867.

135. Thau. Quoted from Nothnagel und Rossbach. *Handbuch der Arzneimittellehre*, Berlin, 1887, 6 Aufl., S. 653.

136. VITALI und GALIGNANI. Quoted from BINZ. *Vorlesungen über Pharmakologie*, Berlin, 1891, Hirschwald, S. 576.

137. BACCELLI. Le iniezioni intravenose dei sali di chinina nell' infezione malarica. *Rif. med.*, 1890, p. 14.

138. C. GOLGI. Ueber die Wirkung des Chinins auf die Malariaparasiten und die diesen entsprechenden Fieberanfälle. *Deutsche med. Wochenschrift*, 1892, Nr. 29—32.

139. BINZ. Artikel Chinin in *Eulenburg's Real-Encyklopädie*.

140. BINZ. Pharmakologische Studien über Chinin. *Virchow's Archiv*, 1869, Bd. 46.

141. PINZ. Ueber die Einwirkung des Chinin auf Protoplasmabewegung. *Schultze's Archiv für mikr. Anat.*, iii.

142. O. ROSENBACH. *Berliner klin. Wochenschrift*, 1891, Nr. 34.

143. BÜCHNER, DINSTL, SCHRAMM, DUCHEK, PLAYFAIR, BAXA, LUC, SONS. Quoted from Thomas. Ergebnisse aus Wechselfieberbeobachtungen. *Archiv für Heilkunde*, 1866, vii Jahrg.

144. SENISE. *II. Congresso della società ital. di med. int. Roma*, 1889. Ref. in *Rif. med.*, 1889, Nr. 254.

145. SALOMONE MARINO. Dell' acqua dei luoghi malarici. *Congresso med. Roma*, 1890. Ref. in *Rif. med.*, 1890, Nr. 251.

146. A. DOCHMANN. Zur Lehre von der Intermittens. *St. Petersburger med. Zeitschrift*, 1880, Nr. 20; Ref. in *Virchow-Hirsch Jahresbericht*, 1880, ii, S. 11.

147. O. BARBACCI. Ueber die Aetiologie der Malaria-Infection, &c. Zusammenfassendes Referat. *Centralblatt f. allg. Path. und path. Anat.*, 1892, Nr. 2.

148. BASTIANELLI e BIGNAMI. Note cliniche sull' infezione malarica. Soc. Lancisiana, 12th April, 1890; Ref. in *Rif. med.*, 1890, p. 574.

149. C. BINZ. Ueber Chinin und die Malaria-Amöbe. *Berliner klin. Wochenschrift*, 1891, Nr. 43, S. A.

150. BOSSONI. *II. Congresso della società italiana di medicina interna in Roma*, 1889. Ref. in *Rif. med.*, 1889, Nr. 254.

151. P. CANALIS. Sopra il ciclo evolutivo delle forme semilunari, &c. Nota preventiva. *Rif. med.*, 1889, Nr. 41.

152. P. CANALIS. Studien über die Malaria-Infection. *Fortschritte der Medicin*, 1890, Nr. 8—9, Schultze's Archiv.

153. P. CANALIS. Sulle febbri malariche predominanti nell' estate e nell' autunno in Roma. Risposta ai professori Celli e Marchiafava. *Archivio per le scienze mediche*, 1890, vol. xiv.

154. P. CANALIS. Intorno a recenti lavori sui parassiti della

malaria. *Lettera al presidente della R. Accad. med. di Roma*, 1890, S. A.

155. A Celli. Ulteriore contributo alla morfologia dei plasmodi della malaria. Nota preventiva. *Rif. med.*, 1889, Nr. 189.

156. Celli e Guarnieri. Sulla intima struttura del Plasmodium malariae. Nota preventiva. *Rif. med.*, 1888, Nr. 208.

157. Dieselben. Sulla intima struttura, &c. Seconda nota preventiva. *Rif. med.*, 1888, Nr. 236.

158. Celli e Marchiafava. Sulle febbri malariche predominanti, &c. *Atti della R. Accad. med. di Roma*, anno xvi, vol. v, Seria ii.

159. Celli und Marchiafava. Ueber die Malariafieber Roms, &c. *Berliner klin. Wochenschrift*, 1890, Nr. 44.

160. G. Dock. Die Blutparasiten der tropischen Malariafieber (Galveston, Texas). *Fortschr. der Medicin*, 1891, Bd. ix, Nr. 5.

161. Dolega. *Verhandlungen des IX Congresses für innere Medicin zu Wien*, 1890.

162. Dolega. Blutbefund bei Malaria. *Fortschr. der Medicin*, 1890, Nr. 20.

163. Doulet. Ètude clinique sur l'étiologie du paludisme, 1891, *Paris, chez Baillière et fils.*

164. Feletti e Grassi. Sui parassiti della malaria. *Rif. med.*, 1890, p. 62.

165. Feletti e Grassi. Sui parassiti della malaria. *Rif. med.*, 1890, p. 296.

166. Gerhardt. Ueber Lungenentzündung mit mehrfach unterbrochenem Fieberverlauf. *Festschrift zu R. Virchow's* 70, *Geburtstag*, Bd. iii.

167. C. Golgi. Demonstrationen der Entwicklung der Malariaparasiten durch Photographien. *Zeitschrift für Hygiene*, 1891, Bd. x.

168. B. Grassi. I protozoi parassitici dell' uomo. *Congresso med. di Pavia.* Ref. in *Rif. med.*, 1887, Nr. 228.

169. P. Guttmann und P. Ehrlich. Ueber die Wirkung des Methylenblau bei Malaria. *Berliner klin. Wochenschrift*, 1891, Nr. 39.

170. Heinemann. Ueber Malariakrankheiten in Vera-Cruz. *Virchow's Archiv*, Bd. cii.

171. H. Hertz. Malaria-infectionen. *V. Ziemssen's Handbuch der spec. Pathologie und Therapie*, 1886, Leipzig, bei Vogel.

172. A. HIRSCH. Handbuch der historisch-geographischen Pathologie, 2 *Aufl.*, *Stuttgart*, 1881.

173. N. IWANOVSKI. Ueber die pathologisch-anatomischen Erscheinungen bei einer in Charkow endimischen Krankheit. *Festschrift zu R. Virchow's* 70, *Geburtstag*, Bd. iii.

174. JILEK. Ueber die Ursachen der Malaria in Pola, *Wien*, 1868.

175. E. KLEBS. Ueber die Kerne und Scheinkerne der rothen Blutkörperchen der Säugethiere. *Virchow's Archiv*, 1867, Bd. xxxviii.

176. KLEBS und TOMMASI-CRUDELI. Einige Sätze über die Ursachen der Wechselfieber, &c. *Archiv f. exp. Pathologie u. Pharmakologie*, 1879.

177. KLEBS und TOMMASI-CRUDELI. Studien über die Ursache des Wechselfiebers, &c. *Ibidem.*

178. R. KOCH. *Mittheilungen ans dem Reichsgesundheitsamt*, 1881, Bd. i.

179. A. M. KOROLKO. Ueber Malaria (Russian). *Petersburg*, 1892.

180. A. M. KOROLKO. Autoreferat in den *Fortschr. f. Medicin*, 1892, Bd. x, Nr. 21.

181. † A. LABBÉ. Sur les hématozoaires de la grenouille. *Comptes rendus*, 1891, 12th Octobre.

182. † A. LABBÉ. Sur les hématozoaires des vertébrés à sang froid. *Comptes rendus*, 1892, Schultze's Archiv.

183. A. LAVERAN. Troisième note relative à la nature parasitaire des accidents de l'impaludisme. *Note communiquée à l'Académie de médecine*, 1881, Séance du 25th Octobre.

184. A. LAVERAN. Des parasites du sang dans l'impaludisme. *Comptes rendus*, 1882, 23rd Octobre.

185. A. LAVERAN. Les hématozoaires de l'impaludisme. *Annales de l'institut Pasteur*, 1887, tome i.

186. † A. LAVERAN. Parasites des fièvres palustres. *Comptes rendus de la société de biologie*, 1892, Nr. 34.

187. † A. LAVERAN. De la nature des corps en croissant du sang palustre. *Ibidem*, Nr. 36.

188. E. MARAGLIANO e P. CASTELLINO. Sulla necrobiosi lenta dei globuli rossi, &c. *Rivista clinica*, 1891, 4 fasc.

189. MARCHAND. Kurze Bemerkungen zur Aetiologie der Malaria. *Virchow's Archiv*, 1882, Bd. lxxxviii.

190. F. MARCHIAFAVA. *I. Congresso della società italiana di med. int. di Roma*, 1888. Ref. in *Rif. med.*, 1888, Nr. 292.

191. E. MARCHIAFAVA. *II. Congresso della società italiana di med. int. di Roma*, 1889. Ref. in *Rif. med.*, 1889, Nr. 254.

192. MARCHIAFAVA e CELLI. Sui rapporti fra le alterazioni del sangue, &c. *Bullettino della R. Accad. med. di Roma*, anno xiii, fasc. 7.

193. E. MARCHIAFAVA ed A. CELLI. Sulle febbri malariche predominanti nell' estate e nell' autunno in Roma. Nota preventiva. *Rif. med.*, 1889, Nr. 214.

194. MARCHIAFAVA und BIGNAMI. Ueber die Varietäten der Malariaparasiten und über das Wesen der Malaria-Infection. *Deutsche med. Wochenschrift*, 1892, Nr. 51 u. 52.

195. MAUREL. Contribution à l'étiologie du paludisme. *Archives de médecine navale*, 1887.

196. MITROPHANOW. Beiträge zur Kenntniss der Hämatozoën. *Centralblatt f. Biologie*, 1883–4, Bd. iii.

197. PEPPER. De la malaria, 1891, *Paris, chez Masson.*

198. L. PFEIFFER. Das Vorkommen der Marchiafava'schen Plasmodien im Blute von Vaccinirten und von Scharlachkranken. *Zeitschrift f. Hygiene*, 1887, Bd. ii.

199. L. PFEIFFER. Beiträge zur Kenntniss der pathogenen Gregarinen. *Zeitschrift f. Hygiene*, 1890, Bd. viii.

200. L. PFEIFFER. Die Protozoën als Krankheitserreger, 1891, 2 *Aufl., Jena, bei Fischer.*

201. F. PLEHN. *Berliner klin. Wochenschrift*, 1890, Nr. 13.

202. F. PLEHN. Beitrag zu der Lehre von der Malaria-Infection. *Zeitschrift f. Hygiene*, 1890, Bd. viii.

203. F. PLEHN. *Virchow's Archiv*, 1892, Bd. cxxix.

204. ROMANOWSKY. Ueber die specifische Wirkung des Chinins bei Malaria, Wratsch, 1891, Nr. 18. Ref. in *Centralblatt f. Bakt.*, Bd. xi, Nr. 6 u. 7.

205. ROSIN. *Deutsche med. Wochenschrift*, 1890, Nr. 16.

206. N. A. SACHAROFF. Ueber Malariabeobachtungen an der transkaukasischen Eisenbahn (russisch), *Tiflis*, 1889.

207. N. A. SACHAROFF. Recherches sur le parasite des fièvres palustres irrégulières. *Annales de l'institut Pasteur*, 1891, t. v.

208. W. SCHEWIAKOFF. Ueber die karyokinetische Kerntheilung bei Euglypha alveolata. *Morph. Jahrbücher*, 1888, Bd. xiii.

209. SCHIAVUZZI. Untersuchungen über die Malaria. *Beiträge zur Biologie der Pflanzen von Ferd. Cohn*, 1890, Bd. v, 2 Heft.

210. SCHUETZ. *Archiv f. Heilkunde*, 1868, S. 69.

211. v. SCHLEN. Studien über Malaria. *Fortschr. der Medicin*, 1884, Nr. 18.

212. SPENER. Ueber die Krankheitserreger der Malaria. Zusammenfassender Bericht, *Leipzig, bei Besold.*

213. STADELMANN. Toluylendiamin und seine Wirkung auf die Thierkörper. *Archiv f. exp. Pathologie u. Pharmakologie,* 1881, Bd. xiv.

214. S. STRICKER. Skizzen aus der Lehranstalt für experimentelle Pathologie, 1892, *Wien, bei Hölder.*

215. WERNER. Beobachtungen über Malaria, 1887, *Berlin, bei Hirschwald.*

216. WITTICH. Spirillen im Blute von Hamstern. *Centralblatt f. med. Wissenschaft,* 1881.

PRINTED BY ADLARD AND SON,
BARTHOLOMEW CLOSE, E.C., AND 20, HANOVER SQUARE, W.

CPSIA information can be obtained
at www.ICGtesting.com
Printed in the USA
LVOW03s1021300816
502467LV00014B/218/P